Advanced Topics of Embryonic Stem Cells

Advanced Topics of Embryonic Stem Cells

Edited by **Jack Collins**

FOSTER
ACADEMICS

New Jersey

Published by Foster Academics,
61 Van Reypen Street,
Jersey City, NJ 07306, USA
www.fosteracademics.com

Advanced Topics of Embryonic Stem Cells
Edited by Jack Collins

International Standard Book Number: 978-1-63242-030-5 (Hardback)

Printed in the United States of America.

Contents

Preface

This book illustrates the advancements made in embryonic cells. The eventual medical employments of embryonic stem cells require methods and protocols to turn these unspecialized cells into fully functioning cell types found in a wide variety of tissues and organs. This book presents an overview of contemporary research on differentiation of embryonic stem cells to a wide variety of cell types, including neural, cardiac cells. Also, induced pluripotent stem cells and other pluripotent stem cell sources have been described. The book will prove to be a valuable resource for engineers, scientists, and clinicians as well as students in a wide range of disciplines.

The researches compiled throughout the book are authentic and of high quality, combining several disciplines and from very diverse regions from around the world. Drawing on the contributions of many researchers from diverse countries, the book's objective is to provide the readers with the latest achievements in the area of research. This book will surely be a source of knowledge to all interested and researching the field.

In the end, I would like to express my deep sense of gratitude to all the authors for meeting the set deadlines in completing and submitting their research chapters. I would also like to thank the publisher for the support offered to us throughout the course of the book. Finally, I extend my sincere thanks to my family for being a constant source of inspiration and encouragement.

Editor

Part 1

Endothelial Differentiation

Endothelial Differentiation of Embryonic Stem Cells

Peter Oettgen

Division of Cardiology,
Division of Molecular and Vascular Medicine,
Department of Medicine, and the Center for Vascular Biology Research,
Beth Israel Deaconess Medical Center, Harvard Medical School, Boston, MA,
USA

1. Introduction

Embryonic stem (ES) cells are a rich source of multiple different cell types of diverse lineages. Significant advances have recently been made in our understanding of the molecular mechanisms by which ES cells differentiate into endothelial cells. The differentiation of ES cells into endothelial cells can be enhanced by certain growth factors, environmental cues, cell-cell interactions, and extracellular matrix. A wide variety of signal transduction pathways and transcription factors have been shown to participate in this process. The use of ES cells for endothelial differentiation are not only of interest with respect to the molecular mechanisms but also for identifying sources of endothelial cells that can be used for a number of therapeutic purposes. The purpose of this chapter is to review recent advances in the molecular mechanisms underlying ES differentiation into endothelial cells and how endothelial cells derived from ES cells are being used therapeutically.

2. Culture conditions

ES cells are derived from the inner cell mass of a growing blastocyst [1]. As such, they have the capacity to differentiate into all the cell types of an organism [2]. To maintain their undifferentiated state ES cells are generally grown in the presence of feeder cells or leukemia inhibitory factor (LIF). In the absence of inhibitory factors ES cells can spontaneously differentiate into cells with characteristics of one of three germ layers; mesoderm, endoderm, or ectoderm. A variety of approaches have been used to differentiate human and mouse ES cells that include: (1) aggregating ES cells into three-dimensional cell masses called embryoid bodies (EBs); (2) by co-culturing the ES cells with other cell types; and (3) by culturing the ES cells on specific matrix surfaces together with defined media.

Murine ES cells have been used for several years to study differentiation along multiple lineages. Culturing ES cells into EBs has been the most frequently used model to study EC differentiation. The appearance of structures consisting of immature hematopoietic cells surrounded by endothelial cells and the formation of vascular-like channels suggests that the EBs produce factors necessary not only for endothelial differentiation but also for vasculogenesis. These structures closely resemble the so-called blood islands of the yolk sac. One of the major advantages of this culture method is the highly reproducible timing of molecular events that occurs during the process of differentiation. The induction of both hematopoietic and endothelial markers at precise time points during the differentiation has greatly facilitated investigation of factors that promote or inhibit EC differentiation or hematopoiesis. Their close association has also led to commonly held belief that the hematopoietic and endothelial lineages stem from a common precursor known as the hemangioblast. The markers of hematopoiesis and endothelial differentiation also permit the isolation of specific populations of cells at different stages of differentiation. An example of one of the earliest markers of the endothelial lineage is VE-cadherin, and of the hematopoietic lineage is CD41. One of the potential disadvantages of this model is that only a fraction of the cells, on the order of 5-10%, ultimately become endothelial cells.

Human ES cells have also been used to generate EBs as a model of EC differentiation or hematopoiesis. endothelial cells can be isolated and propagated from human EBs at vary time points during differentiation. The EBs can also be used as a model of angiogenesis in addition to EC differentiation and vasculogenesis. 11-day old EBs are cultured within three dimensional type 1 collagen matrix gels that is supplemented with angiogenic growth factors including VEGF and FGF2 [3]. The sprouting of new vessels can be observed radiating out from the EBs into the surrounding matrix.

A second mouse model of ES cell differentiation is a two dimensional system that takes advantage of the calvaria stromal cell line OP9. ES cells are initially grown as EBs and then a subset of cells expressing VEGF-R2 are separated by flow cytometry. These VEGF-R2 cells are grown on the OP9 cells they gradually differentiate into endothelial cells expressing VE-cadherin and CD31 (PECAM-1). Interestingly, the endothelial cells exhibited two morphological characteristics. On the one hand endothelial cells grew as sheets of cells and on the other hand the cells coalesced into cord-like structures. It was determined that the sheet-like Endothelial cells were of lymphatic origin, whereas the other endothelial cells were more like blood endothelial cells. Two soluble factors made by the OP9 cells that contribute to the differentiation of these cells into lymphatic endothelial cells include Angiopoietin-1 and VEGF-C.

A third method of culturing the murine ES cells into endothelial cells consists of isolating a subpopulation of ES cells that express the VEGF receptor 2 (VEGF-R2) and allowing them to differentiate on an acellular matrix such as type IV collagen [4]. By adding growth factors to a serum free media it was determined that VEGF was a critical factor for differentiating VEGF-R2 expressing ES cells into endothelial cells.

3. Markers of the endothelial lineage

A critical determinant of endothelial differentiation is the identification of selective markers that separate the endothelial lineage from other lineages. Because of the close association between the hematopoietic and the endothelial lineage, the existence of a bipotent cell called the hemangioblast capable of differentiating into either the endothelial or hematopoietic lineages was suggested and identified [5,6]. A commonly used marker to define this cell type is the VEGF receptor 2 (VEGF-R2). Using an embryoid body (EB) model of ES the temporal expression pattern of several endothelial markers was evaluated by PCR and immunohistochemistry [7]. The expression of VEGF-R2 on day three of differentiation preceded the expression of all of the endothelial markers. The expression of PECAM-1, Tie-1, Tie2, and VE-cadherin, followed shortly thereafter on days 4 and 5 of differentiation. Furthermore, the number of cells expressing these EC-specific markers represented a small fraction of the overall number of ES cells that appeared to coalesce into discreet regions of the EBs and by day 12 of differentiation when they formed primitive vascular structures. The number of cells expressing the endothelial marker PECAM-1 was enhanced by adding the growth factor VEGF on day 6 of ES cell differentiation [7]. We have similarly used the embryoid body model to identify a population of VEGF-R2 expressing mouse embryonic stem cells that also express the endothelial marker VE-cadherin and that are distinct from those that express the hematopoietic marker CD41 [8].

The close association between the hematopoietic and endothelial lineages that is seen during ES cell differentiation has also been observed in a variety of different organisms including the mouse, chicken, zebrafish and humans during embryonic development. In the mouse for example, cells of the hematopoietic and endothelial lineages are first observed in the yolk sac in regions called blood islands. In addition to the yolk sac, the generation of blood is first observed in the developing embryo in a region called the aorta-gonad-mesonephros (AGM), in the vitelline and umbilical arteries, and in the allantois/placenta region [9] [10,11]. In the AGM region hematopoietic cells are found in close association with the endothelial wall of the aorta suggesting that these early hematopoietic cells are generated from an early intermediate called the hemogenic endothelium [9,12]. Additional support for the hemogenic endothelium has come from in vitro studies of mouse embryonic stem cell differentiation. Blast colony-forming cells (BL-CFCs) were identified that can give rise to cells of both the endothelial and hematopoietic lineages [5,6]. More recently, studies using time-lapse photography and FACS analysis of differentiating mouse embryonic stem cells, have demonstrated that the hemangioblast generates hematopoietic cells through the formation of a hemogenic endothelium intermediate [13]. In particular, $Tie2^{hi}c-Kit^+CD41^-$ expressing cells were identified as a population of cells that constitute the hemogenic endothelium.

Further differentiation of endothelial cells into cells of arterial, venous, and lymphatic endothelium has also been shown to occur in ES cells and do so in the developing embryo prior to the development of blood flow. The differentiation of embryonic stem cells into arterial endothelial cells is dependent on the presence and concentration of VEGF. When mouse ES cells are cultured in the presence of lower molecular weight isoforms of VEGF (120 and 164) they differentiate into endothelial cells expressing arterial markers [14]. The differentiation of ES cells into arterial versus venous endothelial cells is also dependent on the dose of VEGF. Whereas at low concentration of VEGF (2ng/ml) cultured VEGF-R2 expressing mouse ES cells differentiate into endothelial cells expressing venous EC markers such as neuropilin-2 (NRP2), at higher concentrations of VEGF (50 ng/ml) the same cells will differentiate into EC expressing the arterial markers Ephrin B2 and neuropiin-1 (NRP1) [15]. ES cells have also been used study their differentiation into lymphatic endothelial cells. For example, murine ES cells were aggregated to form EBs and then were cultured in a 3-dimensional collagen matrix for up to 18 days [16]. Treatment with a combination of growth factors including VEGF-C and VEGF-A enhanced the formation of lymphatic endothelial cells in the EBs [17]. An alternative approach of promoting the differentiating ES cell along the lymphatic lineage is to use VEGF-R2 expressing ES cells and to co-culture them with OP9 stromal cells [18]. The differentiation of the VEGF-R2 cells into lymphatic endothelial cells is dependent upon VEGF-C and angiopoietin-1.

4. Signal transduction pathways

A variety of signal transduction pathways have been implicated during the process of endothelial differentiation. At the top of the hierarchy of signal transduction molecules are the hedgehog (HH) family of signaling proteins, which play a number of different roles in determination of cell fate, embryonic patterning, and morphogenesis [19]. HH signaling activates the transcription factor GLI. Inhibition of Indian hedgehog (IHH) during the differentiation of mouse or human ES cells blocks their ability to differentiate along the endothelial and hematopoietic lineages [20] [21]. In addition to IHH, several studies have suggested a role for sonic hedgehog (SHH) in endothelial differentiation. In the absence of SHH, angioblasts fail to form into EC tubes or vascular networks [22]. Administration of SHH was able to promote the differentiation of human multipotent adult progenitor cells into arterial endothelial cells both in vivo and in vitro [23].

Bone morphogenic proteins (BMPs) belong to the TGF-beta family of proteins that are involved in regulating cell proliferation, survival, and differentiation during embryogenesis [24]. In particular, BMP-2 and BMP-4 are known mediators of endothelial function and differentiation during embryogenesis and ES cell differentiation [25,26]. BMP appears to function downstream of the HH proteins during the in vitro differentiation of ES cells along the EC lineage. Inhibition of EC differentiation by blocking the HH pathway can be rescued with BMP-4 [20]. Furthermore, when human ES cells are cultured in the presence of BMP-4, this augments their differentiation along the endothelial lineage [25].

BMPs can also activate a number of downstream signal transduction pathways. For example, the induction of angiogenesis by BMP-2 is dependent upon activation of the canonical and non-canonical WNT pathways [26]. BMPs can also activate the MAP kinase signaling pathways. For example, BMP-4 activation of EC sprouting is dependent upon p38 MAP kinase [27]. Inhibition of EC migration by BMPs is dependent upon the JNK and ERK pathways [28]. In contrast to BMP-2 and BMP-4, two BMPs, BMP-9 and BMP-10 inhibit the growth of endothelial cells and promote endothelial quiescence [29,30]. The role of BMP-9 and BMP-10 in endothelial differentiation has not been studied, however in contrast to other endothelial cells, BMP-9 promotes the proliferation of mouse embryonic-stem cell derived endothelial cells [31].

WNT signaling is involved in processes that determine cell fate, self-renewal of stem cells, polarity, and organogenesis. There are three classical WNT pathways: (1) the canonical or WNT/β-catenin pathway; (2) the planar cell polarity pathway; and (3) the WNT/Ca^{2+} pathway [32]. WNT5A is a mediator of EC proliferation, survival, and differentiation. WNT5A is expressed in the developing vasculature of several organs including the skin, retina, stomach, and liver [33]. WNT5A functions predominantly through the non-canonical WNT pathways. Signaling cascades activated by WNT5A include the protein kinase C (PKC) and c-Jun n-terminal kinase (JNK) pathways [34]. WNT5A can also inhibit the activity of the canonical WNT/β-catenin pathway [35]. WNT5A contributes to the regulation of the differentiation of ES cells along the endothelial lineage [36]. WNT5A deficient ES cells cannot differentiate into endothelial cells. In endothelial cells WNT5A can activate both the canonical and non-canonical WNT pathways. The WNT/Ca^{2+} pathway is the predominant WNT pathway activated in WNT5A deficient ES cells exposed to exogenous WNT5A. A role for WNT signaling has also been evaluated during the differentiation of the hemangioblast in human ES cells [37]. Administration of the WNT inhibitor dickkopf1 markedly inhibited the differentiation of ES cells towards the endothelial or hematopoietic lineages. Likewise, when ES cells were cultured in the presence of WNT1, there was a marked increase in the number of hemangioblast like cells. In contrast, when ES cells were exposed to WNT5A, they did not have the same effect of increasing the number of hemangioblasts, suggesting that WNT5A principally acts at later stages of EC differentiation [38].

5. Transcription factors

A variety of transcription factors are known to play a critical role in cellular differentiation during embryonic development. In particular, selected transcription factors are known to regulate the differentiation of embryonic stem along the endothelial or hematopoietic lineages. As mentioned above, the hemangioblast is a bipotent cell capable of differentiating into either endothelial or hematopoietic cells. The basic helix-loop-helix (HLH) transcription factor SCL (Tal1) has been shown to be critical for blood and endothelial cell development [39]. SCL is expressed early during embryogenesis in hematopoietic and endothelial cells and its disruption in either mouse or zebrafish leads to severe defects in vasculogenesis [40-42]. SCL is also an early marker of the hemangioblast in embryonic stem cells during their differentiation towards the hematopoietic and endothelial lineages [43]. In this model of ES cells were cultured in serum free conditions and sequentially exposed to BMP4, activin A, bFGF, and VEGF. As the mesodermal marker brachyury gradually decreases there is an increase in the expression of SCL together with two other transcription factors Runx1 and Hhex. SCL deficient ES cells are unable to generate either primitive or definitive hematopoietic cells [44]. SCL also appears to be critical for the development of the hemogenic endothelium [13]. SCL deficient ES cells failed to differentiate into Tie2^{hi}c-Kit$^+$CD41$^-$ cells that constitute cells with the capacity to differentiate into hematopoietic and endothelial cells.

Members of the ETS family of transcription factors have also been shown to play a role in the regulation of EC-specific gene expression and EC differentiation. For example, ER71 has been shown to be critical for endothelial differentiation and vascular development in mice and zebrafish [45,46]. In ES cells ER71 is critical for the expression of VEGF-R2 [47]. ER71 appears to induce VEFGF-R2 downstream of BMP, Notch, and Wnt signaling. Another ETS factor that is expressed in the vasculature and regulates hematopoiesis is Fli-1. Fli-1 deficient mice die at embryonic day E12.5 of defective vasculogenesis leading to cerebral hemorrhage [48]. Fli-1 deficient ES cells also exhibit defective hematopoiesis with a marked reduction in the number of blast colony forming cells. In contrast to most other ETS factors we and other groups have shown that the ETS factor ERG exhibits an EC-restricted expression pattern [49-52]. Furthermore, it has also been shown that several EC-restricted genes including VE-cadherin, endoglin, and vWF, are regulated by ERG [53-55]. In addition to its role in regulating EC-restricted genes we have recently shown that ERG is critical effector of EC differentiation of ES cells that appears to be independent of hematopoiesis [56]. ERG was selectively expressed in VEGF-R2$^+$VE-caherin$^+$ cells and not in VEGF-R2$^+$CD41$^+$ cells. Suppression of ERG in ES cells by lentivirally delivery of shRNA resulted in a significant reduction in EC differentiation but not hematopoietic cells.

There are several transcription factors that facilitate the differentiation of ES cells into arterial, venous, and lymphatic endothelial cells. The critical transcription factor that promotes the differentiation of the hemangioblast or VEGF-R2 expressing cells into venous endothelial cells is COUP-TFII [15]. The differentiation of these cells was dependent upon the dose of VEGF. Whereas low doses of VEGF (2-10 ng/ml) induced the differentiation of VEGF-R2 cells into venous endothelial cells expressing high levels of COUP-TFII, high doses of VEGF (50 ng/ml) repressed COUP-TFII levels and induced the differentiation of VEGF-R2 cells into endothelial cells expressing markers of arterial endothelial cells such as Ephrin B2. Transcription factors that are preferentially upregulated in arterial endothelial cells include the HLH factors Hey1 and Hey2. Notch signaling appears to be critical for promoting differentiation of ES cells into arterial endothelial cells. Inhibition of Notch signaling with a gamma secretase inhibitor preferentially leads to the expression of venous EC markers and a repression of arterial markers [15]. An environmental stimulus that promotes the differentiation of ES cells into arterial endothelial cells is hypoxia. Exposure of ES cells to hypoxia was associated with an increase in the expression of the Notch ligand Dll4 and the transcription factors Hey1 and Hey2 [57].

The prototypic transcription factor that regulates the differentiation of ES cells into lymphatic endothelial cells is Prox1. Prox1 expression can be induced by three-dimensional culture of murine ES cells into EBs in collagen matrices in the presence of VEGF-C and VEGF-A [16]. Similarly when VEGF-R2 cells were co-cultured with OP9 cells expression of Prox1 was observed in lymphatic endothelial cells on day 3 [18]. Expression of Prox1 in blood endothelial cell leads expression of lymphatic markers and transdifferentiation into lymphatic endothelial cells [58]. Another transcription factor that regulates the expression of the VEGF-R3, which binds to VEGF-C, is the T box transcription factor Tbx1 [59]. Although Tbx1 is not required for LEC differentiation it is required for the growth and maintenance of lymphatic vessels. A transcription factor that is involved in regulating later stages of lymphatic EC maturation is the forkhead transcription factor Foxc2 [60,61]. Foxc2 was shown to be important for the development of lymphatic valves and controlling interactions between lymphatic endothelial cells and mural cells.

6. Therapeutic implications

One of the ultimate goals of developing culture methods that promote the differentiation of stem cells into endothelial cell is to provide a source of cells for a variety of different therapeutic applications. One obvious application would be to generate new blood vessels or repair existing blood vessels in clinical settings where blood flow is compromised. As an initial proof of concept a population of VEGF-R2 expressing mouse ES cells were injected into chicken embryo hearts. These cells were shown to be able to integrate into the host vasculature and differentiate into two cellular components of the vasculature, endothelial cell and smooth muscle cells [62]. Based on these promising studies embryonic stem cell derived endothelial cell have been used in animal models of human disease to promote angiogenesis and ultimately improve blood flow. For example, murine ES cell derived endothelial cell were injected either intramuscularly or intra-arterially in a hindlimb model of ischemia, and were shown to engraft at the site of ischemia and improve tissue perfusion [63]. One of the concerns of using ES cells for therapeutic purposes is the potential formation of teratomas from undifferentiated ES cells. In the hindlimb ischemia study no teratomas formed when ES cell derived endothelial cell were used compared to their uniform development within two weeks when undifferentiated ES cells were used. A similarly promising study was done using human ES cell (hESC) derived endothelial cells [64]. The hESC derived endothelial cells were shown to engraft into blood vessels at sites of myocardial ischemia using a mouse myocardial infarction model. Together these exciting proof-of-concept studies provide evidence that ES cell derived endothelial cells can be used in a variety of settings to promote blood vessel growth at sites of ischemia. One of the major challenges in using the currently available stem cells as a source of endothelial cells for therapeutic applications is the potential of significant immune responses to the engrafted cells. One potential mechanism of overcoming this hurdle more recently is the development of induced pluripotent stem (iPS) cells in which skin fibroblasts from any individual can be transformed into ES cells by introducing four transcription factors [65]. These iPS cells have subsequently been cultured to promote their differentiation into vascular cells that are very similar to those obtained from human ES cells [66].

7. Acknowledgements

This work was supported by NIH grant PO1 HL76540.

8. References

[1] Evans MJ, Kaufman MH. Establishment in culture of pluripotential cells from mouse embryos. Nature. 1981;292:154-156.

[2] Hwang NS, Varghese S, Elisseeff J. Controlled differentiation of stem cells. Adv Drug Deliv Rev. 2008;60:199-214.

[3] Feraud O, Cao Y, Vittet D. Embryonic stem cell-derived embryoid bodies development in collagen gels recapitulates sprouting angiogenesis. Lab Invest. 2001;81:1669-1681.

[4] Hirashima M, Ogawa M, Nishikawa S, Matsumura K, Kawasaki K, Shibuya M. A chemically defined culture of VEGFR2+ cells derived from embryonic stem cells reveals the role of VEGFR1 in tuning the threshold for VEGF in developing endothelial cells. Blood. 2003;101:2261-2267.

[5] Kennedy M, Firpo M, Choi K, et al. A common precursor for primitive erythropoiesis and definitive haematopoiesis. Nature. 1997;386:488-493.

[6] Choi K, Kennedy M, Kazarov A, Papadimitriou JC, Keller G. A common precursor for hematopoietic and endothelial cells. Development. 1998;125:725-732.

[7] Vittet D, Prandini MH, Berthier R, et al. Embryonic stem cells differentiate in vitro to endothelial cells through successive maturation steps. Blood. 1996;88:3424-3431.

[8] Nikolova-Krstevski V, Bhasin M, Otu HH, Libermann TA, Oettgen P. Gene expression analysis of embryonic stem cells expressing VE-cadherin (CD144) during endothelial differentiation. BMC Genomics. 2008;9:240.

[9] de Bruijn MF, Speck NA, Peeters MC, Dzierzak E. Definitive hematopoietic stem cells first develop within the major arterial regions of the mouse embryo. Embo J. 2000;19:2465-2474.

[10] Rhodes KE, Gekas C, Wang Y, et al. The emergence of hematopoietic stem cells is initiated in the placental vasculature in the absence of circulation. Cell Stem Cell. 2008;2:252-263.

[11] Zeigler BM, Sugiyama D, Chen M, Guo Y, Downs KM, Speck NA. The allantois and chorion, when isolated before circulation or chorio-allantoic fusion, have hematopoietic potential. Development. 2006;133:4183-4192.

[12] Garcia-Porrero JA, Godin IE, Dieterlen-Lievre F. Potential intraembryonic hemogenic sites at pre-liver stages in the mouse. Anat Embryol (Berl). 1995;192:425-435.

[13] Lancrin C, Sroczynska P, Stephenson C, Allen T, Kouskoff V, Lacaud G. The haemangioblast generates haematopoietic cells through a haemogenic endothelium stage. Nature. 2009;457:892-895.

[14] Mukouyama YS, Shin D, Britsch S, Taniguchi M, Anderson DJ. Sensory nerves determine the pattern of arterial differentiation and blood vessel branching in the skin. Cell. 2002;109:693-705.

[15] Lanner F, Sohl M, Farnebo F. Functional arterial and venous fate is determined by graded VEGF signaling and notch status during embryonic stem cell differentiation. Arterioscler Thromb Vasc Biol. 2007;27:487-493.

[16] Kreuger J, Nilsson I, Kerjaschki D, Petrova T, Alitalo K, Claesson-Welsh L. Early lymph vessel development from embryonic stem cells. Arterioscler Thromb Vasc Biol. 2006;26:1073-1078.

[17] Liersch R, Nay F, Lu L, Detmar M. Induction of lymphatic endothelial cell differentiation in embryoid bodies. Blood. 2006;107:1214-1216.

[18] Kono T, Kubo H, Shimazu C, et al. Differentiation of lymphatic endothelial cells from embryonic stem cells on OP9 stromal cells. Arterioscler Thromb Vasc Biol. 2006;26:2070-2076.

[19] Ingham PW. Transducing Hedgehog: the story so far. EMBO J. 1998;17:3505-3511.

[20] Kelly MA, Hirschi KK. Signaling hierarchy regulating human endothelial cell development. Arterioscler Thromb Vasc Biol. 2009;29:718-724.

[21] Maye P, Becker S, Kasameyer E, Byrd N, Grabel L. Indian hedgehog signaling in extraembryonic endoderm and ectoderm differentiation in ES embryoid bodies. Mech Dev. 2000;94:117-132.

[22] Vokes SA, Yatskievych TA, Heimark RL, et al. Hedgehog signaling is essential for endothelial tube formation during vasculogenesis. Development. 2004;131:4371-4380.

[23] Aranguren XL, Luttun A, Clavel C, et al. In vitro and in vivo arterial differentiation of human multipotent adult progenitor cells. Blood. 2007;109:2634-2642.

[24] Chen D, Zhao M, Mundy GR. Bone morphogenetic proteins. Growth Factors. 2004;22:233-241.

[25] Goldman O, Feraud O, Boyer-Di Ponio J, et al. A boost of BMP4 accelerates the commitment of human embryonic stem cells to the endothelial lineage. Stem Cells. 2009;27:1750-1759.

[26] de Jesus Perez VA, Alastalo TP, Wu JC, et al. Bone morphogenetic protein 2 induces pulmonary angiogenesis via Wnt-beta-catenin and Wnt-RhoA-Rac1 pathways. J Cell Biol. 2009;184:83-99.

[27] Zhou Q, Heinke J, Vargas A, et al. ERK signaling is a central regulator for BMP-4 dependent capillary sprouting. Cardiovasc Res. 2007;76:390-399.

[28] David L, Mallet C, Vailhe B, Lamouille S, Feige JJ, Bailly S. Activin receptor-like kinase 1 inhibits human microvascular endothelial cell migration: potential roles for JNK and ERK. J Cell Physiol. 2007;213:484-489.

[29] David L, Mallet C, Mazerbourg S, Feige JJ, Bailly S. Identification of BMP9 and BMP10 as functional activators of the orphan activin receptor-like kinase 1 (ALK1) in endothelial cells. Blood. 2007;109:1953-1961.

[30] Scharpfenecker M, van Dinther M, Liu Z, et al. BMP-9 signals via ALK1 and inhibits bFGF-induced endothelial cell proliferation and VEGF-stimulated angiogenesis. J Cell Sci. 2007;120:964-972.

[31] Suzuki Y, Ohga N, Morishita Y, Hida K, Miyazono K, Watabe T. BMP-9 induces proliferation of multiple types of endothelial cells in vitro and in vivo. J Cell Sci;123:1684-1692.

[32] Komiya Y, Habas R. Wnt signal transduction pathways. Organogenesis. 2008;4:68-75.

[33] Masckauchan TN, Agalliu D, Vorontchikhina M, et al. Wnt5a signaling induces proliferation and survival of endothelial cells in vitro and expression of MMP-1 and Tie-2. Mol Biol Cell. 2006;17:5163-5172.

[34] Wright M, Aikawa M, Szeto W, Papkoff J. Identification of a Wnt-responsive signal transduction pathway in primary endothelial cells. Biochem Biophys Res Commun. 1999;263:384-388.

[35] Weidinger G, Moon RT. When Wnts antagonize Wnts. J Cell Biol. 2003;162:753-755.

[36] Yang DH, Yoon JY, Lee SH, et al. Wnt5a is required for endothelial differentiation of embryonic stem cells and vascularization via pathways involving both Wnt/beta-catenin and protein kinase Calpha. Circ Res. 2009;104:372-379.

[37] Woll PS, Morris JK, Painschab MS, et al. Wnt signaling promotes hematoendothelial cell development from human embryonic stem cells. Blood. 2008;111:122-131.

[38] Kim DJ, Park CS, Yoon JK, Song WK. Differential expression of the Wnt and Frizzled genes in Flk1+ cells derived from mouse ES cells. Cell Biochem Funct. 2008;26:24-32.

[39] Bloor AJ, Sanchez MJ, Green AR, Gottgens B. The role of the stem cell leukemia (SCL) gene in hematopoietic and endothelial lineage specification. J Hematother Stem Cell Res. 2002;11:195-206.

[40] Visvader JE, Fujiwara Y, Orkin SH. Unsuspected role for the T-cell leukemia protein SCL/tal-1 in vascular development. Genes Dev. 1998;12:473-479.

[41] Patterson LJ, Gering M, Patient R. Scl is required for dorsal aorta as well as blood formation in zebrafish embryos. Blood. 2005;105:3502-3511.

[42] Patterson C, Ike C, Willis PWt, Stouffer GA, Willis MS. The bitter end: the ubiquitin-proteasome system and cardiac dysfunction. Circulation. 2007;115:1456-1463.

[43] Pearson S, Sroczynska P, Lacaud G, Kouskoff V. The stepwise specification of embryonic stem cells to hematopoietic fate is driven by sequential exposure to Bmp4, activin A, bFGF and VEGF. Development. 2008;135:1525-1535.

[44] Porcher C, Swat W, Rockwell K, Fujiwara Y, Alt FW, Orkin SH. The T cell leukemia oncoprotein SCL/tal-1 is essential for development of all hematopoietic lineages. Cell. 1996;86:47-57.

[45] Ferdous A, Caprioli A, Iacovino M, et al. Nkx2-5 transactivates the Ets-related protein 71 gene and specifies an endothelial/endocardial fate in the developing embryo. Proc Natl Acad Sci U S A. 2009;106:814-819.

[46] Sumanas S, Lin S. Ets1-related protein is a key regulator of vasculogenesis in zebrafish. PLoS Biol. 2006;4:e10.

[47] Lee D, Park C, Lee H, et al. ER71 acts downstream of BMP, Notch, and Wnt signaling in blood and vessel progenitor specification. Cell Stem Cell. 2008;2:497-507.

[48] Spyropoulos DD, Pharr PN, Lavenburg KR, et al. Hemorrhage, impaired hematopoiesis, and lethality in mouse embryos carrying a targeted disruption of the Fli1 transcription factor. Mol Cell Biol. 2000;20:5643-5652.

[49] Vlaeminck-Guillem V, Carrere S, Dewitte F, Stehelin D, Desbiens X, Duterque-Coquillaud M. The Ets family member Erg gene is expressed in mesodermal tissues and neural crests at fundamental steps during mouse embryogenesis. Mech Dev. 2000;91:331-335.

[50] Baltzinger M, Mager-Heckel AM, Remy P. Xl erg: expression pattern and overexpression during development plead for a role in endothelial cell differentiation. Dev Dyn. 1999;216:420-433.

[51] Hewett PW, Nishi K, Daft EL, Clifford Murray J. Selective expression of erg isoforms in human endothelial cells. Int J Biochem Cell Biol. 2001;33:347-355.

[52] Yuan L, Nikolova-Krstevski V, Zhan Y, et al. Antiinflammatory effects of the ETS factor ERG in endothelial cells are mediated through transcriptional repression of the interleukin-8 gene. Circ Res. 2009;104:1049-1057.

[53] Birdsey GM, Dryden NH, Amsellem V, et al. Transcription factor Erg regulates angiogenesis and endothelial apoptosis through VE-cadherin. Blood. 2008;111:3498-3506.

[54] Liu J, Yuan L, Molema G, et al. Vascular bed-specific regulation of the von Willebrand factor promoter in the heart and skeletal muscle. Blood;117:342-351.

[55] Pimanda JE, Chan WY, Donaldson IJ, Bowen M, Green AR, Gottgens B. Endoglin expression in the endothelium is regulated by Fli-1, Erg, and Elf-1 acting on the promoter and a -8-kb enhancer. Blood. 2006;107:4737-4745.

[56] Nikolova-Krstevski V, Yuan L, Le Bras A, et al. ERG is required for the differentiation of embryonic stem cells along the endothelial lineage. BMC Dev Biol. 2009;9:72.

[57] Diez H, Fischer A, Winkler A, et al. Hypoxia-mediated activation of Dll4-Notch-Hey2 signaling in endothelial progenitor cells and adoption of arterial cell fate. Exp Cell Res. 2007;313:1-9.

[58] Petrova TV, Makinen T, Makela TP, et al. Lymphatic endothelial reprogramming of vascular endothelial cells by the Prox-1 homeobox transcription factor. Embo J. 2002;21:4593-4599.

[59] Chen L, Mupo A, Huynh T, et al. Tbx1 regulates Vegfr3 and is required for lymphatic vessel development. J Cell Biol;189:417-424.

[60] Dagenais SL, Hartsough RL, Erickson RP, Witte MH, Butler MG, Glover TW. Foxc2 is expressed in developing lymphatic vessels and other tissues associated with lymphedema-distichiasis syndrome. Gene Expr Patterns. 2004;4:611-619.

[61] Petrova TV, Karpanen T, Norrmen C, et al. Defective valves and abnormal mural cell recruitment underlie lymphatic vascular failure in lymphedema distichiasis. Nat Med. 2004;10:974-981.

[62] Yamashita J, Itoh H, Hirashima M, et al. Flk1-positive cells derived from embryonic stem cells serve as vascular progenitors. Nature. 2000;408:92-96.

[63] Huang NF, Niiyama H, Peter C, et al. Embryonic stem cell-derived endothelial cells engraft into the ischemic hindlimb and restore perfusion. Arterioscler Thromb Vasc Biol;30:984-991.

[64] Li Z, Wilson KD, Smith B, et al. Functional and transcriptional characterization of human embryonic stem cell-derived endothelial cells for treatment of myocardial infarction. PLoS One. 2009;4:e8443.

[65] Yu J, Vodyanik MA, Smuga-Otto K, et al. Induced pluripotent stem cell lines derived from human somatic cells. Science. 2007;318:1917-1920.

[66] Taura D, Sone M, Homma K, et al. Induction and isolation of vascular cells from human induced pluripotent stem cells--brief report. Arterioscler Thromb Vasc Biol. 2009;29:1100-1103.

Dissecting the Signal Transduction Pathway that Directs Endothelial Differentiation Using Embryonic Stem Cell-Derived Vascular Progenitor Cells

Kyoko Kawasaki[1] and Keiji Miyazawa[2]
[1]Helen Diller Family Comprehensive Cancer Center,
University of California-San Francisco,
[2]Department of Biochemistry, Interdisciplinary Graduate School of
Medicine and Engineering, University of Yamanashi,
[1]USA
[2]Japan

1. Introduction

Blood vessels are essential for embryonic development and tissue homeostasis in adults (Coultas et al., 2005). They supply oxygen and nutrients and remove metabolic waste from tissues. Blood vessels also participate in intercellular communication. Secretion of growth/differentiation factors by blood vessels is essential for liver and pancreas organogenesis (Matsumoto et al., 2001; Lammert et al., 2001). Additionally, developing sympathetic neurons are guided by endothelins secreted by blood vessels (Makita et al., 2008), and liver regeneration in adults is triggered by factors secreted by liver sinusoidal endothelial cells (Ding et al., 2010).

In mice, vascular progenitor cells first develop in the posterior primitive streak in response to fibroblast growth factor-2 (FGF-2) and bone morphogenetic protein 4 (BMP4), and they are marked as vascular endothelial growth factor receptor 2 (VEGFR2)–positive mesodermal cells (Fig. 1; Park et al., 2004; Flamme et al., 1995). These precursor cells are committed for development into the hematopoietic and/or vascular lineage (hemangioblasts or angioblasts), and they migrate into extra-embryonic sites including the yolk sac and allantois, as well as into intra-embryonic sites (Huber et al., 2004; Hiratsuka et al., 2005). In the yolk sac, these progenitors aggregate and form clusters known as blood islands. The outer cells of the blood islands differentiate into endothelial cells, whereas the inner cells give rise to hematopoietic progenitor cells. These cells subsequently form primary capillary plexuses (vasculogenesis). In contrast, intra-embryonic angioblasts do not form a plexus intermediately and directly assembles into the dorsal aorta or cardinal vein. The extra-embryonic primary capillary plexuses then fuse with the intra-embryonic vessels to form a complete vascular network (angiogenesis). Angiopoietins and Tie receptors, along with vascular endothelial growth factor-A (VEGF-A) and Notch, are involved in this process (Thurston et al., 2003). Finally, mural cells that have differentiated in response to transforming growth factor-β (TGF-β) are recruited to nascent vessels by platelet-derived growth factor (PDGF) secreted by endothelial cells (Betsholtz et al., 2005; Lebrin et al., 2005). This entire process ultimately leads to mature blood vessel formation.

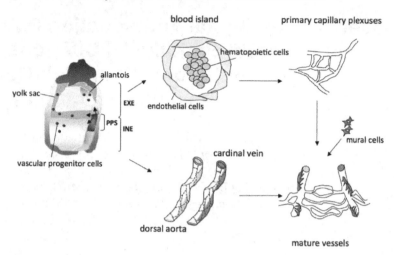

Fig. 1. Blood vessel formation during mouse development. EXE, extra-embryonic ectoderm; INE, intra-embryonic ectoderm; PPS, posterior primitive streak

A number of extracellular signaling molecules are involved in vascular development, some of which, including FGF-2, angiopoietins, PDGF, and VEGF-A, transmit their signals through receptor tyrosine kinases (RTKs). Signal transduction pathways downstream of RTKs have been extensively studied, and most share downstream effector components such as the Ras-mitogen–activated kinase (Ras-MAPK) and the phosphatidylinositol-3' kinase (PI3K) pathways. Intriguingly, these RTKs still transmit distinct signals and play unique roles that drive vascular development. The molecular basis for the observed signaling specificity remains unclear. To better understand this important process, we focused on signaling downstream of VEGFR2, a functional receptor for VEGF-A, using embryonic stem cell–derived VEGFR2+ vascular progenitor cells (Suzuki et al., 2005; Kawasaki et al., 2008; Sase et al., 2009). VEGFR2-null mice demonstrate severe defects in vasculogenesis, and VEGFR2 signaling is thought to play crucial roles in embryonic blood vessel formation (Shalaby et al., 1995; Shalaby et al., 1997; see below for details).

2. Use of differentiating embryonic stem cells for the study of lineage specification

To elucidate the signaling pathways important for the endothelial differentiation of vascular progenitor cells, we employed an *in vitro* vascular differentiation system using mouse embryonic stem cells (ESC) (Hirashima et al., 1999; Yamashita et al., 2000). *In vivo*, vascular progenitor cells must migrate to the correct microenvironment where they receive a cue for endothelial specification and further proliferate. It is challenging to identify the contributions of distinct signaling pathways to each *in vivo* event that occurs during vascular development, but the use of the *in vitro* system has allowed us to focus on the signaling

Dissecting the Signal Transduction Pathway that Directs Endothelial Differentiation Using
Embryonic Stem Cell-Derived Vascular Progenitor Cells

15

events required for endothelial specification by providing well-defined supplements to the culture medium.

We used ESC-derived vascular progenitor cells because it is practically impossible to prepare a sufficient amount of vascular progenitor cells from mouse embryos for biochemical study. In this *in vitro* system, ESCs are differentiated by culture on type IV-collagen–coated dishes in the absence of leukemia inhibitory factor (LIF) for four days, and during this time, mesodermal cells expressing VEGFR2 are induced. VEGFR2[+] cells (comprising 5–10% of the total cell population) are then sorted by magnetic-activated cell sorting (MACS) and used as vascular progenitors. These cells differentiate into α-smooth muscle actin-positive (αSMA[+]) mural cells resembling vascular smooth muscle cells in the presence of PDGF-BB or serum, whereas they differentiate into platelet-endothelial adhesion molecule 1-positive (PECAM1[+]) endothelial cells in response to VEGF-A (Fig. 2; Yamashita et al., 2000; Ema et al., 2003; Watabe et al., 2003). Alteration of the differentiation fate of vascular progenitor cells was also examined by limiting dilution assay. VEGFR2[+] cells were seeded at low density (90–120 cells/cm[2]) and allowed to form single-cell–derived colonies for four days. After immunostaining, the numbers of PECAM1[+] or αSMA[+] colonies, which reflect the fate of differentiation, were counted. In the presence of VEGF-A, endothelial differentiation occurs at the expense of mural differentiation: stimulation with VEGF-A increases PECAM1[+] colonies and decreases αSMA[+] colonies, while the total number of colonies remains constant. Thus, VEGF-A stimulation alters the differentiation fate of vascular progenitor cells.

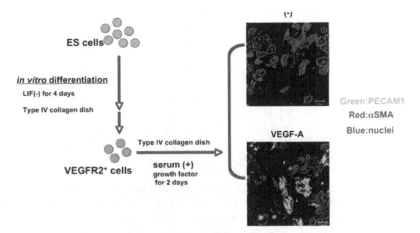

Fig. 2. *In vitro* vascular differentiation system (Yamashita et al., 2000)

This *in vitro* system was originally established using CCE embryonic stem cells. However, we used MGZ-5 cells and MGZRTcH cells because they are more amenable to transgene expression. Accordingly, we first studied MGZ-5 cells expressing genes contained in the pCAGIP vector (Fujikura et al., 2002). MGZ-5 cells express polyoma large T antigen, and this allows the efficient episomal propagation of plasmids with a polyoma origin of replication such as pCAGIP. Thus, transgenes contained within the pCAGIP vector are stably expressed in MGZ-5 cells (supertransfection method, Gassmann et al., 1996). In later experiments, we used MGZRTcH cells derived from MGZ-5 cells (Masui et al., 2005) in which a target gene can be knocked into the *ROSA26* locus by homologous recombination using the Cre-*loxP* system, and gene expression is under the control of tetracycline (Tc) (tet-off system, Masui et al., 2005). Importantly, the *ROSA26* locus is minimally affected by epigenetic silencing during cell differentiation (Zamobrowicz et al., 1997). Therefore, expression of a transgene knocked into this locus can be regulated by Tc during nearly any stage of differentiation.

Using this *in vitro* system, we have successfully pursued two different lines of investigation of vasculogenesis: examination of downstream effectors of VEGFR2 signaling (Section 3) and screening of pharmacological inhibitors (Section 4).

3. VEGFR2 transmits unique signals to induce endothelial differentiation

VEGFR2, also known as Flk1 in mice and KDR in human, is a member of the VEGFR family of RTKs, which contains three members, VEGFGR1-3 (Fig. 3; Shibuya & Claesson–Welsh, 2006). VEGFRs share characteristic structural features: they are composed of seven extracellular immunoglobulin-like domains, a transmembrane region, and an intracellular region with intrinsic tyrosine kinase activity. They have distinct expression profiles and different ligand specificities among VEGF family members.

VEGFR1, also called Flt-1 (fms-like tyrosine kinase 1) is expressed in vascular endothelial cells, hematopoietic stem cells, macrophages, and monocytes. VEGFR2 is expressed in both vascular and lymphatic endothelial cells. VEGFR3, also called Flt-4 (fms-like tyrosine kinase 4), is principally expressed in lymphatic endothelial cells.

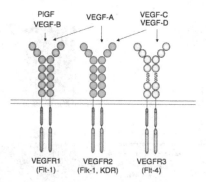

Fig. 3. VEGFR family members and their cognate ligands. The tyrosine kinase domains of VEGFRs are separated by the "kinase insert" of ~60 amino acid residues, a structural feature common to PDGF receptors and FGF receptors. The fifth immunoglobulin-like domain of VEGFR3 has an internal cleavage. The resultant N-terminal and C-terminal polypeptides are linked together by a disulfide bond.

VEGF family members, including VEGF-A, -B, -C, -D and placenta growth factor (PlGF), regulate the development, growth and function of vascular as well as lymphatic endothelial cells (Ferrara et al., 2003). VEGF-A is bound by VEGFR2 and VEGFR1, which transmit signals essential for vasculogenesis and angiogenesis. VEGF-C and VEGF-D are bound by VEGFR2 and VEGFR3 and are both involved in lymphangiogenesis (Karkkainen et al., 2004; Baldwin et al., 2005). PlGF and VEGF-B signal through VEGFR1, and they contribute to pathological angiogenesis (Carmeliet et al., 2001; Mould et al., 2003) and endothelial fatty acid uptake (Hagberg et al., 2010).

Dissecting the Signal Transduction Pathway that Directs Endothelial Differentiation Using
Embryonic Stem Cell-Derived Vascular Progenitor Cells

17

3.1 Essential role of VEGFR2 during vasculogenesis

Individual knock-out mice lacking VEGFR1, VEGFR2, or VEGFR3 all demonstrate vascular defects. VEGFR1-deficient mice exhibit disorganized vasculature secondary to endothelial cell overgrowth (Fong et al., 1995). VEGFR3 knockout mice have defects in vascular remodeling and develop fluid accumulations in the pericardial sac (Dumont et al., 1998). Blood vessel formation occurs in VEGFR1$^{-/-}$ and VEGFR3$^{-/-}$ mice. VEGFR1 and VEGFR3 are thus indispensable for angiogenesis but not vasculogenesis. In contrast, VEGFR2 plays essential roles during vasculogenesis. It is first expressed in the vascular progenitor cells at the posterior primitive streak. VEGFR2-deficient mice die *in utero* between 8.5 and 9.5 d.p.c. due to lack of organized blood vessels and hematopoietic cells. VEGFR2 signaling is required for the formation of blood islands at extraembryonic sites (Shalaby et al., 1995), where vascular endothelial cells and hematopoietic cells differentiate to form primary plexuses. In the absence of VEGFR2 signaling, vascular progenitor cells fail to migrate to extraembryonic sites from the posterior primitive streak (Shalaby et al., 1997). In the embryo proper, VEGFR2 signaling is required for endothelial specification of the vascular progenitor cells (Shalaby et al., 1997). Potential endothelial precursor cells are located at the correct anatomical niche, but they fail to complete the differentiation pathway. The identified roles of VEGFR2 signaling in vascular development *in vivo* include promoting the proliferation, migration, and differentiation of progenitor cells. Additionally, VEGF-A$^{+/-}$ mice have defects in vascular development (Carmeliet te a., 1996; Ferrara et al., 1996), but VEGF-C$^{-/-}$ mice and VEGF-D$^{-/-}$ mice exhibit lymphatic defects (Karkkainen et al., 2004; Baldwin et al., 2005). Therefore, the VEGF-A/VEGFR2 axis appears to be essential for vasculogenesis.

Because VEGFR2$^+$ mesodermal cells can give rise to lineages other than endothelial and hematopoietic cells, including vascular mural cells, skeletal muscle cells, and cardiomyocytes (Motoike et al., 2003; Ema et al., 2006), differentiation of VEGFR2$^+$ cells should be appropriately specified. We examined the nature of this unique and specific signaling.

3.2 VEGFR2, but not VEGFR3, directs endothelial differentiation

Although VEGFRs differ in their ligand-binding properties, their intracellular domains share structural similarities. However, the signaling properties of VEGFRs remain incompletely understood.

VEGF-A, which initiates signaling from both VEGFR1 and VEGFR2, promotes the differentiation of endothelial cells from ESC-derived VEGFR2$^+$ cells, whereas PlGF, a specific ligand for VEGFR1, fails to induce endothelial differentiation despite VEGFR1 expression by precursor cells (Yamashita et al., 2000). Thus, VEGFR1 signaling does not direct endothelial differentiation. We then examined the ability of VEGFR3 to induce endothelial differentiation (Suzuki et al., 2005). While VEGFR3 is not expressed by VEGFR2$^+$ vascular progenitor cells, we ectopically expressed VEGFR3 to examine whether VEGFR3 signaling induces endothelial cell differentiation.

3.2.1 VEGFR3 fails to induce endothelial differentiation

VEGFR3 cDNA was introduced into MGZ-5 ES cells using the supertransfection technique followed by drug selection (Gassmann et al., 1996). VEGFR2$^+$ vascular progenitor cells were then collected from the transfected cells after *in vitro* differentiation (Suzuki et al., 2005).

These cells differentiated into PECAM1+ endothelial cells in response to VEGF-C stimulation. Although VEGF-C is bound by both VEGFR2 and VEGFR3, it does not promote endothelial differentiation through endogenous VEGFR2 signaling, because it failed to induce endothelial differentiation of mock-transfected cells. We next examined the effect of VEGF-C(C152S), a mutant that selectively stimulates VEGFR3 (Kirkin et al., 2001). This mutant did not induce endothelial differentiation, but it caused vascular progenitor cell differentiation into mural cells (Suzuki et al., 2005). Thus, VEGFR3 signaling alone is not sufficient to induce endothelial differentiation. It remains possible that VEGF-C induces endothelial differentiation through heterodimer formation between ectopic VEGFR3 and endogenous VEGFR2 in these experimental conditions. Collectively, these findings indicate that VEGFR2 has unique properties among VEGFR family members even in this *in vitro* system.

3.2.2 The intracellular domain of VEGFR2 can transmit signals for endothelial differentiation

We next examined the intracellular events downstream of VEGFR2 that are required for endothelial differentiation. For this purpose, we constructed a chimeric receptor (denoted R32) that is composed of the extracellular and the transmembrane domains of VEGFR3 fused with the intracellular domain of VEGFR2 (Fig. 4; Sase et al., 2009). We then established ES cell lines expressing either R32 or VEGFR3 under the control of the Tc-regulated promoter in MGZRTcH cells (denoted Tc-R32 and Tc-VEGFR3, respectively).

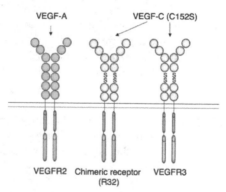

Fig. 4. Schematic structure of the chimeric receptor R32

VEGFR2+ vascular progenitor cells prepared from these cell lines differentiated into PECAM1+ cells following VEGF-A stimulation, indicating that these cell lines retain their ability to differentiate into endothelial cells. However, VEGFR2+ cells derived from Tc-R32, but not Tc-VEGFR3, differentiated into PECAM1+ cells upon stimulation with VEGF-C(C152S). The PECAM1+ cells were also positive for other endothelial markers (VE-cadherin, CD34, and endoglin) and appeared to be endothelial cells. Therefore, the differences in phenotypes between VEGFR2+ cells derived from Tc-R32 and Tc-VEGFR3 cells are due to intrinsic properties of the intracellular domains of VEGFR2 and VEGFR3. The intracellular domain of VEGFR2 is sufficient to direct endothelial differentiation of ESC-derived vascular progenitor cells.

Dissecting the Signal Transduction Pathway that Directs Endothelial Differentiation Using
Embryonic Stem Cell-Derived Vascular Progenitor Cells

19

3.2.3 Tyrosine 1175 of human VEGFR2 is required for endothelial specification of vascular progenitor cells and endothelial cell survival

The role of signal transduction pathways downstream of VEGFR2 for cell proliferation, migration and survival have been well explored in mature endothelial cells. Five tyrosine residues (Y951, Y1054, Y1059, Y1175, and Y1214) have been identified in the intracellular domain of VEGFR2 as major phosphorylation sites (Matsumoto et al., 2005). Y1054 and Y1059 are located in the activation loop of the kinase domain and are required for the activation of intrinsic kinase activity. The remaining tyrosine residues are located outside of the kinase domain and are required for recruitment of downstream effectors. Phosphorylation of Y1175 leads to phospholipase Cγ-activation, followed by protein kinase C (PKC) β-mediated Raf activation to induce cell proliferation (Takahashi et al., 2000). Y1175 is also involved in the activation of the PI3 kinase pathway through the adaptor protein Shb (Welch et al., 1994). In contrast, phosphorylation of Y951 leads to cell migration and actin stress fiber organization through interactions with T cell specific adaptor (TSAd) (Matsumoto et al., 2005). Phosphorylation of Y1214 is also implicated in actin stress fiber remodeling through the p38 mitogen activated kinase pathway (Lamalice et al., 2004). Y951 and Y1175 are unique tyrosine residues in VEGFR2, whereas Y1214 is conserved in VEGFR2 and VEGFR3.

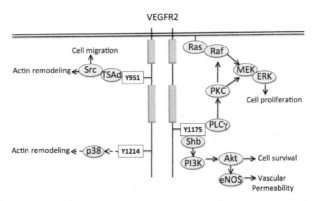

Fig. 5. Signal transduction downstream of VEGFR2

Y1173 in mouse VEGFR2 (corresponding to Y1175 in humans) is indispensable for blood vessel formation *in vivo* (Sakurai et al., 2005). VEGFR2 Y1173F knock-in mice died between E8.5 and E9.5, similar to VEGFR2-null mice. In Y1173F knock-in mice, VEGFR2+ vascular progenitor cells failed to migrate into the yolk sac to form blood islands, and, because vasculogenesis was aborted and progenitor cells did not receive specification signals, it remained unclear whether Y1173 is also important for endothelial specification of vascular progenitor cells. Therefore, we addressed this question using the *in vitro* differentiation system.

3.2.3.1 Tyrosine 1175 of human VEGFR2 is required for endothelial differentiation

To examine the roles of individual tyrosine residues in the induction of endothelial differentiation, we constructed three mutants of the R32 chimeric receptor (R32Y951F, R32Y1175F, and R32Y1214F) in which the indicated tyrosine residues were mutated to phenylalanine. After confirming the ability of these mutants to activate effective signals, we established MGZRTcH ES cell lines expressing these mutant receptors (Tc-R32Y951F, Tc-R32Y1175F, and Tc-R32Y1214F). VEGFR2⁺ vascular progenitor cells were prepared from these cell lines and examined for endothelial differentiation in the presence of VEGF-C(C152S) (Sase et al., 2009).

VEGFR2⁺ cells derived from Tc-R32Y951F and Tc-R32Y1214F differentiated into endothelial cells following treatment with VEGF-C(C152S) whereas those from Tc-R32Y1175F failed to do so. To exclude the possibility that signals associated with residues Y951 and Y1214 could compensate for one another to promote endothelial differentiation, we also established a cell line expressing a double mutant, Tc-R32Y951/1214F. VEGFR2⁺ cells derived from this cell line retained their ability to undergo endothelial differentiation. These findings indicate that signaling from Y1175 plays a central role in the endothelial differentiation of vascular progenitor cells, but residues Y951 and Y1214 are dispensable for this function.

In this *in vitro* differentiation system, endothelial cells appear only when vascular progenitor cells are successfully specified into endothelial cells and when the differentiated endothelial cells are able to survive and proliferate (Fig. 6, top panel). Endothelial cells are unable to survive in the presence of serum alone, and they typically require growth factors such as VEGF-A or FGFs for survival and/or proliferation. We investigated whether signaling from Y1175 plays a role in specification, survival, or both processes.

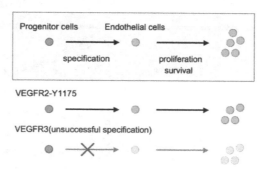

Fig. 6. VEGFR signaling and endothelial differentiation

3.2.3.2 Tyrosine 1175 of human VEGFR2 is required for endothelial survival

We first performed an endothelial survival assay (Fig. 7) with Tc-R32, Tc-R32Y1175F, and Tc-VEGFR3. ESC-derived VEGFR2⁺ cells were cultured with VEGF-A in serum-free medium for two days to induce mature endothelial cells, and the endothelial cells were then cultured in serum-free medium with or without VEGF-C(C152S) to activate the chimeric receptors.

The number of endothelial cells cultured in the absence of VEGF-C(C152S) was considerably decreased within 12 h. VEGF-C(C152S)–induced signaling from R32 led to a significant recovery in the number of cells, but VEGF-C(C152S) treatment of cells expressing R32Y1175 failed to do so. Thus, Y1175 is involved in the transmission of survival signals to endothelial cells. As described in 3.2.1, VEGFR3 signaling is not sufficient for inducing endothelial differentiation from VEGFR2⁺ vascular progenitor cells. However, VEGFR3 signaling increased the survival of ESC-derived endothelial cells. We also found that LY294002, an inhibitor of PI3K, abrogated the effects of VEGFR3 on endothelial survival. These findings suggest that VEGFR3 signaling promotes endothelial survival despite its inability to direct endothelial specification (Fig. 6).

Dissecting the Signal Transduction Pathway that Directs Endothelial Differentiation Using
Embryonic Stem Cell-Derived Vascular Progenitor Cells

21

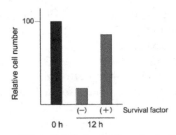

Fig. 7. Endothelial survival assay. When ESC-derived endothelial cells are cultured in serum-free medium, the cell number largely decreases within 12 h, while in the presence of an appropriate survival factor, the cell number is maintained.

3.2.3.3 Tyrosine 1175 of human VEGFR2 is required for endothelial specification

We next examined the involvement of signaling from Y1175 in the endothelial specification of vascular progenitor cells. Because R32Y1175F failed to transmit appropriate survival signals, we supplemented the cell cultures with a low dose of FGF-2 (0.5 ng/ml) to promote endothelial cell survival. VEGFR2+ cells derived from Tc-R32Y1175F failed to differentiate into endothelial cells upon stimulation with VEGF-C(C152S) although those derived from Tc-R32 successfully underwent differentiation. Thus, human VEGFR2 Y1175 is essential for the induction of endothelial cells from vascular progenitor cells through both specification of VEGFR2+ cells and their subsequent survival (Fig. 6).

3.2.4 The VEGFR2-Y1175-PLCγ1 pathway is indispensable for endothelial specification

In mature endothelial cells, Y1175 of human VEGFR2 primarily transmits cell proliferation signals through the recruitment of PLCγ and cell survival signals through the recruitment of Shb (Fig. 5). Intriguingly, PLCγ1 deficient mice are embryonically lethal secondary to a lack of vasculogenesis and erythrogenesis despite the presence of hemangioblasts (Liao et al., 2002). Thus, PLCγ1 may be involved in the specification of vascular progenitor cells and/or subsequent survival of endothelial cells. We hypothesized that R32Y1175F failed to induce endothelial differentiation because it does not activate PLCγ1.

3.2.4.1 Knockdown of PLCγ1 attenuated endothelial differentiation

To elucidate the function of PLCγ1 in endothelial differentiation, we established a stable ES cell line in which expression of PLCγ1 can be knocked down by expression of pre-miRNA under the control of Tc (Tc-miRNA-PLCγ1) (Sase et al., 2009). We used this system to perform gene silencing studies because we had difficulty introducing siRNA oligonucleotides to VEGFR2+ vascular progenitor cells; we were able to easily introduce them into ES cells or differentiated endothelial cells, however (Kawasaki et al., 2008). It is likely that differentiating ES cells may be resistant to transfection at certain stages of development.

Expression of the miRNA targeting PLCγ1 resulted in a modest decrease in PLCγ1 protein expression and decreased appearance of endothelial cells, indicating that PLCγ1 signaling is required for endothelial differentiation.

3.2.4.2 Constitutively active PLCγ1 induces endothelial specification

We next constructed a constitutively active form of PLCγ1, PalmPLCγ1, in which a sequence for myristoylation and palmitoylation was added to its N-terminus. This mutant protein is constitutively localized at the plasma membrane. We then established a stable ES cell line harboring Tc-regulatable PalmPLCγ1 (Tc-PalmPLCγ1) or a negative control cell line (Tc-empty) and examined the differentiation of VEGFR2+ cells derived from these cell lines.

The induced expression of PalmPLCγ1 did not lead to the appearance of PECAM1+ cells from VEGFR2+ progenitor cells, and, after performing an endothelial survival assay, we found that PalmPLCγ1 did not transmit signals for cell survival in ESC-derived endothelial cells. We next examined endothelial differentiation of VEGFR2+ cells in the presence of a low dose of FGF-2 to support survival of endothelial cells. Stimulation with PalmPLCγ1 plus FGF-2 reconstituted signaling for endothelial differentiation although stimulation with only FGF-2 did not affect the number of differentiated endothelial cells. PalmPLCγ1-expressing progenitor cells treated with FGF-2 became positive for PECAM1, VE-cadherin, CD34, and endoglin, and these findings indicate that PLCγ1 signaling is involved in the endothelial specification of vascular progenitor cells but not in the survival of differentiated endothelial cells (Fig. 8). Consistent with this, VEGFR3, which transmits signals for endothelial survival but not endothelial specification, failed to activate PLCγ1 (Sase et al., 2009).

At present, the signaling pathways downstream of Y1175 that mediate survival of endothelial cells remain to be elucidated. However, Shb may be a good candidate for a signaling effector because it activates the PI3K pathway.

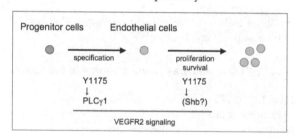

Fig. 8. Signaling from VEGFR2-Y1175 for induction of endothelial cells *in vitro*

4. Ras signaling specifies endothelial lineage

In addition to the chimeric receptor approach described above, we also used various pharmacological inhibitors to study endothelial differentiation (Kawasaki et al., 2008), and we found that temporally regulated Ras signaling plays a crucial role in endothelial specification downstream of PLCγ1.

4.1 A farnesyltransferase inhibitor, FTI-277, inhibits VEGF-A–induced endothelial differentiation of ESC-derived VEGFR2+ cells

To determine the signaling components involved in VEGF-A–induced endothelial differentiation from vascular progenitor cells, we screened various low molecular weight compounds targeting signaling molecules for their ability to inhibit endothelial differentiation *in vitro*. Among the compounds tested, we found that the farnesyltransferase inhibitor FTI-277 (Lerner et al., 1995) selectively affects endothelial differentiation. FTI-277 interferes with the farnesylation of small G proteins and their subsequent association with the plasma membrane, thus abrogating their signaling functions. FTI-277 inhibited the appearance of VEGF-A–induced PECAM1+ cells, but that of αSMA+ was not. The effect of

Dissecting the Signal Transduction Pathway that Directs Endothelial Differentiation Using
Embryonic Stem Cell-Derived Vascular Progenitor Cells

23

FTI-277 was also confirmed in a limiting dilution assay. In the presence of FTI-277, the number of PECAM1+ colonies was decreased while αSMA+ colonies were increased. Importantly, the total number of derived colonies was not significantly changed. These findings indicate that FTI-277 specifically inhibits the endothelial differentiation of ESC-derived VEGFR2+ cells.

We next performed an *ex vivo* whole-embryo culture assay to confirm the effects of FTI-277 on vascular development in a mouse embryo (Fig. 9; Kawasaki et al., 2008). Concepti at embryonic day 6.75 (E 6.75) were picked out from the uteri of pregnant mice and cultured *in vitro* for three days, and, in the absence of further manipulation, PECAM1+ blood vessels formed in the yolk sac during this time. However, FTI-277 treatment led to a reduced number of PECAM1+ vessels, but the overall development of the yolk sac was not affected. Quantitative RT-PCR analysis also indicated that PECAM1 expression was decreased in the presence of FTI-277, while the expression of αSMA was not affected. These findings suggest that FTI-277 selectively suppresses vascular development. Importantly, endothelial differentiation induced by constitutively active PalmPLCγ1 plus FGF-2 was inhibited by FTI-277, indicating that FTI-277 targets signaling pathway(s) downstream of PLCγ1.

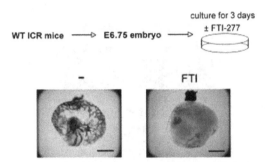

Fig. 9. FTI-277 inhibited *ex vivo* yolk sac vascularization (Kawasaki et al., 2008. Originally published *in Journal of Cell Biology*. doi: 10.1083/jcb.200709127). E6.75 concepti were picked out and cultured with or without FTI-277 (10 μM) for three days and whole-mount stained for PECAM1.

4.2 Loss of H-Ras attenuates endothelial differentiation of VEGFR2+ cells *in vitro*

Because the principal targets of FTI-277 include H-Ras, we hypothesized that H-Ras signaling could be involved in the VEGF-A–induced endothelial differentiation of vascular progenitor cells. To examine this possibility, we established an ES cell line based on MGZRTcH cells in which a pre-miRNA sequence targeting H-Ras is expressed under the control of Tc (Tc-miR-H-Ras). In Tc-miR-H-Ras cells, expression of endogenous H-Ras was efficiently knocked down in the absence of Tc (Tet-off system). A limiting dilution assay was performed using Tc-miR-H-Ras–derived VEGFR2+ cells in the presence or absence of Tc. In the absence of Tc (H-Ras knocked-down condition), the number of VEGF-A–induced PECAM1+ colonies was decreased while the number of αSMA+ colonies was increased compared to cells grown in the presence of Tc (PECAM1:αSMA=51.6%:48.4% to 36.8%:63.2%). These findings suggest that H-Ras plays a role in the endothelial differentiation of VEGFR2+ progenitor cells.

4.3 Loss of H-Ras attenuates endothelial differentiation in mouse embryos

To examine the importance of H-Ras signaling during vascular development *in vivo*, we investigated the vascular phenotype of H-*ras* knockout mice. Because heterozygous H-*ras*+/- mice produced homozygous H-*ras*-/- offspring in the expected Mendelian ratio as previously reported (Ise et al., 2000), we focused on the vascular phenotype during early development. There were no clear differences in the vascular phenotypes of wild-type (WT) and H-*ras*+/- embryos. Vascular anomalies were found in the brain of 73% of H-*ras*-/- embryos examined at E9.5 although they contained similar numbers of somites as their WT littermates (Fig. 10; Kawasaki et al., 2008).

We next double-stained the cephalic region of the embryos for PECAM1 and VEGFR2, the earliest marker of endothelial cell differentiation. In H-*ras*+/- embryos, numerous complex vascular networks were stained for both PECAM1 and VEGFR2, but vascular structures positive for either PECAM1 or VEGFR2 were strikingly reduced in H-*ras*-/- embryos. However, these defects were transient because no abnormalities were apparent in E10.5 H-*ras*-/- embryos. Collectively, these data suggest that H-Ras signaling is involved in the *in vivo* differentiation of endothelial cells although it is not indispensable.

+/-   -/-

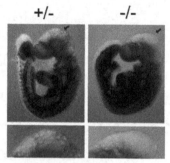

Fig. 10. Whole-mount PECAM1 staining of E9.5 H-*ras*+/- and H-*ras*-/- mice (Kawasaki et al., 2008. Originally published *in Journal of Cell Biology*. doi: 10.1083/jcb.200709127). Magnifications of the area marked with arrows in the top are shown in the bottom.

4.4 A constitutively active G12V mutant of H-Ras induces PECAM1+ cells from VEGFR2+ progenitor cells

We next established an ES cell line carrying a constitutively active form of H-Ras (Tc-H-Ras[G12V]) under the control of Tc, and we examined the differentiation of VEGFR2+ cells derived from this cell line. When H-Ras[G12V] expression was suppressed by Tc treatment, the appearance of PECAM1+ cells was VEGF-A–dependent. However, expression of H-Ras[G12V] led to the VEGF-A–independent induction of PECAM1+ cells. These PECAM1+ cells were also positive for other endothelial markers including CD34 and endoglin, and they incorporated AcLDL. Additionally, the aggregated VEGFR2+ cells derived from Tc-H-Ras[G12V] cells formed tube-like structures even in the absence of VEGF-A when cultured in type I collagen gel for seven days, indicating that vascular formation by VEGFR2+ cells is dependent on H-Ras signaling. Furthermore, Tc-H-Ras[G12V] cells formed vascular structures when subcutaneously injected with Matrigel into the abdominal region of mice, dependent upon the expression of H-Ras[G12V]. These findings suggest that active Ras induces the differentiation of cells with characteristics of endothelial cells from VEGFR2+

Dissecting the Signal Transduction Pathway that Directs Endothelial Differentiation Using
Embryonic Stem Cell-Derived Vascular Progenitor Cells

25

progenitor cells (Kawasaki et al., 2008). Additionally, data from a limiting dilution assay showed that expression of H-Ras[G12V] led to endothelial differentiation at the expense of mural differentiation. Thus, the fate of cell differentiation was altered by Ras signaling. Although Ras signaling induces the expression of VEGF-A (Rak et al., 1995; Gruger et al., 1995), Ras-induced endothelial differentiation was not dependent on autocrine stimulation by induced VEGF-A. Endothelial differentiation by H-Ras[G12V] proceeded normally in the presence of SU5614, an inhibitor of VEGFR2 kinase (Spiekermann et al., 2002), or VEGFR1 (Flt1)-Fc chimeric protein which competes with VEGFR2 for binding to VEGF-A. Collectively, these findings suggest that differentiation depends on intracellular Ras signaling.

4.5 Signaling for endothelial differentiation is mediated through the Ras-Erk pathway

Ras proteins activate both the Raf/MEK/Erk and the PI3K/Akt pathways. To determine the signaling pathway(s) that mediate Ras-induced endothelial differentiation, we established ES cell lines in which H-Ras effector mutants H-Ras[G12V, T35S] or H-Ras[G12V, Y40C] can be inducibly expressed. The effector mutants H-Ras[G12V, T35S] and H-Ras[G12V, Y40C] preferentially activate the Raf/MEK/Erk and PI3K/Akt pathways, respectively (Joneson et al., 1996). When H-Ras[G12V, T35S] was expressed, PECAM1[+] colonies increased in number, while αSMA[+] colonies were decreased as determined by limiting dilution assay. In contrast, when H-Ras[G12V, Y40C] was expressed, the numbers of PECAM1[+] colonies and αSMA[+] colonies were unchanged. These findings suggest that the Ras-PI3K pathway does not affect the determination of cell fate, and we concluded that the Ras-Erk pathway specifies the endothelial fate of VEGFR2[+] progenitor cells.

4.6 Kinetics of Ras activation by VEGF-A

Ras proteins are activated by extracellular stimuli including hormones, cytokines and growth factors. ESC-derived VEGFR2[+] cells differentiate into endothelial cells upon stimulation with VEGF-A, but not upon stimulation with PDGF-BB, a known activator of Ras signaling. Thus, the activation statuses of Ras are different between that downsteam of VEGFR2 and that downstream of PDGF receptors.

We examined the effects of FTI-277 treatment at different time points after VEGF-A stimulation. FTI-277 inhibited endothelial differentiation even when added 3 h after VEGF-A stimulation, indicating that Ras activation later than 3 h after stimulation plays a role in endothelial differentiation. We hypothesized that the specificity of Ras signaling induced by VEGFR2 may be attributed to the timing of Ras activation, and we investigated the window within which Ras is specifically activated by VEGF-A, focusing on the period later than 3 h after VEGF-A stimulation.

We examined the levels of phosphorylation of Erk, a downstream effector of Ras, 3–12 h after stimulation with VEGF-A. Erk phosphorylation peaked at 6 h and 9 h after stimulation, suggesting that Ras could be activated with a similar time course. We next examined the activation of Ras in cells stimulated with VEGF-A or PDGF-BB for 6 h, and the patterns of Ras activation in response to VEGF-A or PDGF-BB were markedly different. At 6 h after stimulation, VEGF-A caused intense activation of Ras and Erk, whereas PDGF-BB failed to activate both Ras and Erk. At 5 min after stimulation, both VEGF-A and PDGF-BB induced activation of Ras and Erk although to different extents. Activation of Ras and Erk by VEGF-A was also observed at 9 h, but not at 3 h after stimulation (Fig. 11). Importantly, phosphorylation of Erk around 6 h after VEGF-A stimulation was sensitive to FTI-277. Activation of the Ras-Erk pathway 6–9 h after stimulation with VEGF-A thus appears to direct endothelial differentiation of VEGFR2+ progenitor cells. These findings provide mechanistic insights into signaling events required for cell specification through widely-shared effector molecules.

4.7 VEGF-A–specific Ras activation precedes the expression of endothelial markers
We finally examined whether the expression of vascular markers is induced after the delayed activation of the Ras-Erk pathway during *in vitro* differentiation of vascular progenitor cells. The mRNA expression of the endothelial markers PECAM1 and VE-cadherin increased from 12 h after VEGF-A stimulation. Intriguingly, the expression of VEGFR2 in VEGF-A–stimulated cells was similar to that seen in non-stimulated cells up to 6 h after treatment. However, at time points later than 12 h after stimulation, VEGFR2 expression was up-regulated in VEGF-A–stimulated cells, but it was down-regulated in non-stimulated cells. These observations suggest that specification to endothelial lineage occurs between 6–12 h after stimulation with VEGF-A, and this is preceded by the delayed activation of Ras (Fig. 11). We conclude that VEGF-A stimulation of VEGFR2+ vascular progenitor cells specifically induces Ras-Erk activation around 6–9 h after stimulation, and this event in turn specifies endothelial differentiation.

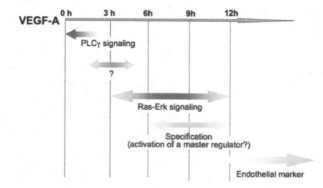

Fig. 11. Kinetics of endothelial differentiation of vascular progenitor cells after VEGF-A stimulation. The link between PLCγ and Ras-Erk (the second double-headed arrow) remains to be elucidated.

5. Unsolved questions in signaling for endothelial differentiation

The development of multicellular organisms requires the orchestrated interactions of a wide variety of cells, including growth, migration, and differentiation. Extracellular factors as well as intracellular signaling molecules are involved in the regulation of cellular processes during development. Each signaling molecule appears to have defined functions that are dependent upon the appropriate cellular context.

VEGFR2 signaling plays a central role in *de novo* blood vessel formation. In an *in vitro* embryoid body culture system, VEGFR2-/- ES cells still give rise to endothelial cells with low efficiency (Schuh et al., 1999). This may be due to an effects of FGF-2 included in the culture

Dissecting the Signal Transduction Pathway that Directs Endothelial Differentiation Using
Embryonic Stem Cell-Derived Vascular Progenitor Cells

27

medium (Schuh et al., 1999), because FGF-2 induces endothelial differentiation of ESC-derived VEGFR2+ cells to a modest extent (Kano et al., 2005). VEGFR2 signaling appears to be the primary pathway for controlling endothelial specification with high efficiency, although it is not the sole pathway capable of mediating these effects. We found that activation of the Ras-Erk pathway 6–9 h after stimulation with VEGF-A plays a critical role in endothelial specification of vascular progenitor cells. The mechanism(s) regulating the delayed activation of Ras and the downstream signaling of the Ras-Erk pathway are the next questions to be solved.

5.1 Upstream and downstream of the delayed Ras activation induced by VEGF-A

In ESC-derived VEGFR2+ progenitor cells, the PKC-dependent pathway (Fig. 5) appears to be activated early, since phosphorylation of Erk was notably increased while activation of Ras was modest 5 min after VEGF-A stimulation (Kawasaki et al., 2008). In contrast, the Ras pathway strongly induced Erk phosphorylation 6–9 h after stimulation, a finding supported by the inhibition of Erk phosphorylation by FTI-277. The mechanism(s) controlling the delayed activation of Ras remain unclear. At present, we only know that PLCγ1 lies upstream of the delayed Ras activation. It is possible that Ras activation is mediated through the transcriptional induction of some signaling molecules and/or activation of other signaling receptor(s). It is also important to identify transcription factors that are phosphorylated by Erk to better understand the signaling specificity of early and late Erk activation. VEGFR2+ cells develop into mural cells in the absence of growth factor, and mural differentiation may be the default fate of VEGFR2+ cells. During the differentiation of vascular progenitor cells, induction of mural markers is delayed compared to the induction of endothelial markers by VEGF-A: expression of αSMA was increased at 24 h while PECAM1 became expressed from 12 h after stimulation. It appears likely that VEGFR2+ cells in which the delayed Ras-Erk signaling is activated before the determination of cell fate to mural cells are differentiated into endothelial cells. However, it remains possible that VEGF-A signaling merely suppresses mural differentiation, thus altering the default differentiation fate. Alternatively, it is possible that VEGF-A signaling not only induces endothelial differentiation but also suppresses mural differentiation.

Although Ras appears to be activated downstream of PLCγ1 in vascular progenitor cells after stimulation with VEGF-A, constitutively active Ras transmits sufficient signals for full endothelial differentiation while constitutively active PLCγ1 transmits signals only for endothelial specification. This discrepancy remains unexplored. It is likely that constitutively active effector molecules may transmit artificial signals. In particular, G12V mutants of Ras proteins are resistant to intrinsic negative regulation through hydrolysis of GTP. H-Ras[G12V] may constitutively send strong signals that are sufficient to fully induce endothelial differentiation.

5.2 Phenotypes of H-Ras knockout mice

We examined vascular formation in H-ras-/- mice, and vascular anomalies were found in the brain of 73% of E9.5 H-ras-/- embryos. However, there were no obvious abnormalities in E10.5 H-ras-/- embryos, consistent with the previous report that H-ras knockout mice are born and grow normally (Ise et al., 2000). These findings suggest that H-ras-/- embryos catch up for the delay in vascular formation in the cephalic region until E10.5. It is possible that expression of other Ras family members, N-Ras and K-Ras, is upregulated, and these proteins may compensate for the loss of H-Ras (Ise et al., 2000). Alternatively, a reduction of endothelial differentiation in the absence of H-Ras may be permissive for embryonic development. Compensatory growth of differentiated endothelial cells may offset the reduction in endothelial differentiation. It appears likely that N-Ras and K-Ras are also involved in endothelial specification because treatment with FTI-277 or knockdown of H-Ras failed to completely inhibit endothelial specification induced by VEGF-A in the *in vitro* vascular differentiation system.

5.3 Towards more efficient differentiation of endothelial cells

In recent years, revascularization therapy using endothelial progenitor cells (EPCs) has been studied for the treatment of ischemic disorders and arteriosclerosis. In this therapy, EPCs implanted at sites of disease form new vascular structures. Identification of the signaling pathways required for endothelial differentiation could provide valuable information for establishing a highly efficient endothelial differentiation system. This would be a boon to the field of regenerative medicine.

The efficiency of endothelial differentiation of vascular progenitor cells *in vitro* remains ~50%. Differentiating ES cells actively proliferate, indicating that they are going through cell cycles. Recent work revealed that Ras can efficiently transmit signals during G1 phase but not during G1/S or S/G2 (Sakaue–Sawano et al., 2008). Signals for endothelial specification are likely successfully transmitted in vascular progenitor cells at G1 phase (Fig. 12). Manipulations that control the cell cycle status may improve the efficiency of specification of vascular progenitor cells to endothelial cells, which is transmitted principally through Ras proteins.

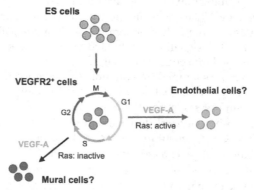

Fig. 12. Possible cell cycle–dependent signaling for endothelial differentiation through Ras activation

Modulation of the VEGFR2 signaling pathway at the level of receptor–ligand interaction may also improve the efficiency of endothelial differentiation *in vitro*. Recently, protein kinase A was found to induce expression of VEGFR2 and its co-receptor neuropilin-1, thus enhancing vascular progenitor potential (Yamamizu et al., 2009).

6. Conclusions

Vascular endothelial growth factor 2 (VEGFR2) is a critical signaling component controlling many aspects of vasculogenesis during embryonic development, including proliferation,

Dissecting the Signal Transduction Pathway that Directs Endothelial Differentiation Using
Embryonic Stem Cell-Derived Vascular Progenitor Cells

29

migration, and endothelial differentiation of vascular progenitor cells. However, the signaling pathways specifying endothelial differentiation downstream of VEGFR2 are poorly understood. We investigated these signaling pathways using an *in vitro* endothelial differentiation system (Kawasaki et al., 2008; Sase et al., 2009). Using a variety of different approaches including chimeric receptors, gene silencing, gain-of-function mutants, and pharmacological inhibitors, we dissected the signal transduction pathway that directs endothelial differentiation (Fig. 13). In response to VEGF-A stimulation, VEGFR2 transmits signals for specification of vascular progenitor cells and survival of endothelial cells through Y1175. PLCγ1, a downstream effector that is recruited to phosphorylated Y1175, relays endothelial specification signals. Activation of H-Ras that occurs at a delayed phase after VEGF-A stimulation triggers endothelial specification. The unique activation of signaling molecules downstream of VEGFR2/PLCγ/Ras is essential for transmitting signals controlling endothelial specification. At the present time, the link between PLCγ1 and H-Ras remains to be identified. Shb, another downstream effector recruited to phosphorylated Y1175, may be involved in the survival of endothelial cells through activation of the PI3K pathway. VEGFR3 lacks the ability to induce endothelial specification, and this may be due to its inability to activate PLCγ1, although it activates the PI3K pathway to support endothelial cell survival. It has previously been shown that Y1175 signaling is indispensable for migration of vascular progenitor cells to the site of their differentiation (Sakurai et al., 2005). Therefore, Y1175 of VEGFR2 appears to be a central node transmitting signals required for endothelial differentiation including migration, specification, and subsequent cell survival.

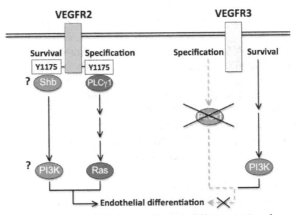

Fig. 13. Signal transduction pathways for endothelial differentiation from VEGFR2

7. Acknowledgement

This work was done when the authors worked in the Department of Molecular Pathology, Graduate School of Medicine, University of Tokyo. We thank co-workers in the laboratory; Prof. Kohei Miyazono for giving us so much advice and great encouragement. Dr. Hiroyuki Suzuki and Dr. Hitoshi Sase for their scientific contributions. Mr. Kazuyuki Morishita and Ms. Keiko Yuki for their skilled technical assistance. Dr. Tetsuro Watabe for valuable advises.

8. References

Baldwin, M.E., Halford, M.M., Roufail, S., Williams, R.A., Hibbs, M.L., Grail, D., Kubo, H., Stacker, S.A., and Achen, M.G. (2005) Vascular endothelial growth factor D is dispensable for development of the lymphatic system. *Mol. Cell. Biol.* 25, 2441-2449

Betsholtz, C., Lindblom, P. and Gerhardt, H. (2005) Role of pericytes in vascular morphogenesis. *EXS* 94, 115-125

Carmeliet, P., Ferreira, V., Breier, G., Pollefeyt, S., Kieckens, L., Gertsenstein, M., Fahrig, M., Vandenhoeck, A., Harpal, K., Eberhardt, C., Declercq, C., Pawling, J., Moons, L., Collen, D., Risau, W., ans Nagy, A. (1996) Abnormal blood vessel development and lethality in embryos lacking a single VEGF allele. *Nature* 380, 435-439

Carmeliet, P., Moons, L., Luttun, A., Vincenti, V., Compernolle, V., De Mol, M., Wu, Y., Bono, F., Devy, L., Beck, H., Scholz, D., Acker, T., DiPalma, T., Dewerchin, M., Noel, A., Stalmans, I., Barra, A., Blacher, S., Vandendriessche, T., Ponten, A., Eriksson, U., Plate, K.H., Foidart, J.M., Schaper, W., Charnock-Jones, D.S., Hicklin, D.J., Herbert, J.M., Collen, D., and Persico, M.G. (2001) Synergism between vascular endothelial growth factor and placental growth factor contributes to angiogenesis and plasma extravasation in pathological conditions. *Nat. Med.* 7, 575-583

Coultas, L., Chawengsaksophak, K., and Rossant, J. (2005) Endothelial cells and VEGF in vascular development. *Nature* 438, 937-945

Ding, B.S., Nolan, D.J., Butler, J.M., James, D., Babazadeh, A.O., Rosenwaks, Z., Mittal, V., Kobayashi, H., Shido, K., Lyden, D., Sato, T.N., Rabbany, S.Y., and Rafii, S. (2010) Inductive angiocrine signals from sinusoidal endothelium are required for liver regeneration. *Nature* 468, 310-315

Dumont, D. J., Fong, G. H., Puri, M. C., Gradwohl, G., Alitalo, K., Breitman, M. L. (1998) Cardiovascular failure in mouse embryos deficient in VEGF receptor-3. *Science* 282, 946-949

Ema, M., Faloon, P., Zhang, W.J., Hirashima, M., Reid, T., Stanford, W.L., Orkin, S., Choi, K., and Rossant, J. (2003) Combinatorial effects of *Flk1* and *Tal1* on vascular and hematopietic development in the mouse. *Genes Dev.* 17, 380-393

Ema, M., Takahashi, S., and Rossant, J. (2006) Deletion of the selection cassette, but not *cis*-acting elements, in targeted *Flk1-lacZ* allele reveals *Flk1* expression in multipotent mesodermal progenitors. *Blood* 107, 111-117

Ferguson III, J.E., Kelley, R.W., and Patterson, C. (2005) Mechanisms of endothelial differentiation in embryonic vasculogenesis. *Arterioscler. Thromb. Vasc. Biol.* 25, 2246-2254

Ferrara, N., Carver-Moore, K., Chen, H., Dowd, M., Lu, L., O'Shea, K.S., Powell-Braxton, L., Hillan, K.J., and Moore, M.W. (1996) Heterozygous embryonic lethality induced by targeted inactivation of the VEGF gene. *Nature* 380, 439-442

Ferrara, N., Gerber, H.P., and LeCouter, J. (2003) The biology of VEGF and its receptors. *Nat. Med.* 9, 669-676

Flamme, I., Breier, G., and Risau, W. (1995) Vascular endothelial growth factor (VEGF) and VEGF receptor 2 (flk-1) are expressed during vasculogenesis and vascular differentiation in the quail embryo. *Dev. Biol.* 169, 699-712

Fong, G. H., Rossant, J., Gertsenstein, M., and Breitman, M. L. (1995) Role of the Flt-1 receptor tyrosine kinase in regulating the assembly of vascular endothelium. *Nature* 376, 66-70

Dissecting the Signal Transduction Pathway that Directs Endothelial Differentiation Using
Embryonic Stem Cell-Derived Vascular Progenitor Cells

31

Fujikura, J., Yamato, E., Yonemura, S., Hosoda, K., Masui, S., Nakao, K., Miyazaki, J.-i., and
Niwa, H. (2002) Differentiation of embryonic stem cells is induced by GATA
factors. *Genes Dev.* 16, 784-789

Gassmann, M., Donoho, G., and Berg, P. (1995) Maintenance of an extrachromosomal
plasmid vector in mouse embryonic stem cells. *Proc. Natl. Acad. Sci. USA* 92, 1292-
1296

Gruger, S., Finkenzeller, G., Weindel, K., Barleon, B., and Marmé, D. (1995) Both v-Ha-Ras
and v-Raf stimulate expression of the vascular endothelial growth factor in NIH
3T3 cells. *J. Biol. Chem.* 270, 25915-25919

Hagberg, C.E., Falkevall, A., Wang, X., Larsson, E., Huusko, J., Nilsson, I., van Meeteren,
L.A., Samen, E., Lu, L., Vanwildemeersch, M., Klar, J., Genove, G., Pietras, K.,
Stone-Elander, S., Claesson-Welsh, L., Ylä-Herttuala, S., Lindahl, P., and Eriksson,
U. (2010) Vascular endothelial growth factor B controls endothelial fatty acid
uptake. *Nature* 464, 917-921

Hirashima, M., Kataoka, H., Nishikawa, S., Matsuyoshi, N., and Nishikawa, SI. (1999)
Maturation of embryonic stem cells into endothelial cells in an in vitro model of
angiogenesis. *Blood* 93, 1253-1263

Hiratsuka, S., Kataoka, Y., Nakao, K., Nakamura, K., Morikawa, S., Tanaka, S., Katsuki, M.,
Maru, Y., and Shibuya, M. (2005) Vascular endothelial growth factor A (VEGF-A) is
involved in guidance of VEGF receptor-positive cells to the anterior portion of early
embryos. *Mol. Cell. Biol.* 25, 355-363

Huber, T.L., Kouskoff, V., Joerg Fehling, H., Palis, J., and Keller, G. (2004) Haemangioblast
commitment is initiated in the primitive streak of the mouse embryo. *Nature* 432,
625-630

Ise, K., Nakamura, K., Nakao, K., Shimizu, S., Harada, H., Ichise, T., Miyoshi, J., Gondo, Y.,
Ishikawa, T., Aiba, A., and Katsuki, M. (2000) Targeted deletion of the H-*ras* gene
decreases tumor formation in mouse skin carcinogenesis. *Oncogene* 19, 2951-2956

Joneson, T., White, M.A., Wigler, M.H., and Bar-Sagi, D. (1996) Stimulation of membrane
ruffling and MAP kinase activation by distinct effectors of RAS. *Science* 271, 810-812

Karkkainen, M.J., Haiko, P., Sainio, K., Partanen, J., Taipale, J., Petrova, T. V., Jeltsch, M.,
Jackson, D. G., Talikka, M., Rauvala, H., Betsholtz, C., and Alitalo, K. (2004)
Vascular endothelial growth factor C is required for sprouting of the first lymphatic
vessels from embryonic veins. *Nat. Immunol.* 5, 74-80

Kano, M.R., Morishita, Y., Iwata, C., Iwasaka, S., Watabe, T., Ouchi, Y., Miyazono, K., and
Miyazawa, K. (2005) VEGF-A and FGF-2 synergistically promote neoangiogenesis
through enhancement of endogenous PDGF-B-PDGFRβ signaling. *J. Cell Sci.* 118,
3759-3768

Kawasaki, K., Watabe, T., Sase, H., Hirashima, M., Koide, H., Morishita, Y., Yuki, K.,
Sasaoka, T., Suda, T., Katsuki, M., Miyazono, K., and Miyazawa, K. (2008) Ras
signaling specifies endothelial differentiation of VEGFR2+ vascular progenitor cells.
J. Cell Biol. 181, 131-141

Kirkin, V., Mazitschek, R., Krishnan, J., Steffen, A., Waltenberger, J., Pepper, M.S., Giannis,
A., and Sleeman, J.P. (2001) Characterization of indolinones which preferentially
inhibit VEGF-C- and VEGF-D-induced activation of VEGFR-3 rather than VEGFR-
2. *Eur. J. Biochem.* 268, 5530-5540

Lamalice, L., Houle, F., Jourdan, G., and Hout, J. (2004) Phosphorylation of tyrosine 1214 on VEGFR2 is required for VEGF-induced activation of cdc42 upstream of SAPK/p38. *Oncogene* 23, 434-445

Lammert, E., Cleaver, O., and Melton, D. (2001) Induction of pancreatic differentiation by signals from blood vessels. *Science* 294, 564-567

Lebrin, F., Deckers M., Bertolino, P. and Ten Dijke, P. (2005) TGF-β receptor function in the endothelium. *Cardiovasc. Res.* 65, 599-608

Lerner, E.C., Qian, Y., Blaskovich, M.A., Fossum, R.D., Vogt, A., Sun, J., Cox, A.D., Der, C.J., Hamilton, A.D., and Sebti, S.M. (1995) Ras *CAAX* peptidemimetic FTI-277 selectively blocks oncogenic Ras signaling by inducing cytoplasmic accumulation of inactive Ras-Raf complexes. *J. Biol. Chem.* 270, 26802-26806

Liao, H.J., Kume, T., McKay, C., Xu, M.J., Ihle, J.N., and Carpenter, G. (2002) Absence of erythrogenesis and vasculogenesis in *plcg1*-deficient mice. *J. Biol. Chem.* 277, 9335-9341

Makita, T., Sucov, H.M., Gariepy, C.E., Yanagisawa, M., and Ginty, D.D. (2008) Endothelins are vascular-derived axonal guidance cues for developing sympathetic neurons. *Nature* 452, 759-763

Masui, S., Shimosato, D., Toyooka, Y., Yagi, R., Takahashi, K., and Niwa, H. (2005) An efficient system to establish multiple embryonic stem cell lines carrying an inducible expression unit. *Nucleic Acids Res.* 33, e43

Matsumoto, K., Yoshitomi, H., Rossant, J., and Zaret, K.S. (2001) Liver organogenesis promoted by endothelial cells prior to vascular function. *Science* 294, 559-563

Matsumoto, T., Bohman, S., Dixelius, J., Berge, T., Dimberg, A., Magnusson, P., Wang, L., Wikner, C., Qi, J.H., Wernstedt, C., Wu, J., Bruheim, S., Mugishima, H., Mukhopadhyay, D., Spurkland, A.,and Claesson-Welsh, L. (2005) VEGF receptor-2 Y951 signaling and a role for the adaptor mulecule TSAd in tumor angiogenesis. *EMBO J.* 24, 2342-2353

Motoike, T., Markham, D.W., Rossant, J., and Sato, T.N. (2003) Evidence for novel fate of Flk1+ progenitor: contribution to muscle lineage. *Genesis* 35, 153-159

Mould, A.W., Tonks, I.D., Cahill, M.M., Pettit, A.R., Thomas, R., Hayward, N.K., and Kay, G.F. (2003) *Vegfb* gene knockout mice display reduced pathology and synovial angiogenesis in both antigen-induced and collagen-induced models of arthritis. *Arthritis Rheum.* 48, 2660-2669

Park, C., Afrikanova, I., Chung, Y.S., Zhang, W.J., Arentson, E., Fong, G., Rosendahl, A and Choi, K. (2004) A hierarchical order of factors in the generation of FLK1- and SCL-expressing hematopoietic and endothelial progenitors from embryonic stem cells. *Development* 131, 2749-2762

Rak, J., Mitsuhashi, Y., Bayko, L., Filmus, J., Shirasawa, S., Sasazuki, T., and Kerbel, R.S. (1995) Mutant *ras* oncogenes upregulate VEGF/VPF expression: Implications for induction and inhibition of tumor angiogenesis. *Cancer Res.* 55, 4575-4580

Sakaue-Sawano, A., Kurokawa, H., Morimura, T., Hanyu, A., Hama, H., Osawa, H., Kashiwagi, S., Fukami, K., Miyata, T., Miyoshi, H., Imamura, T., Ogawa, M., Masai, H., and Miyawaki, A. (2008) Visualizing apatiotemporal dynamics of multicellular cell-cycle pregression. *Cell* 312, 487-498

Dissecting the Signal Transduction Pathway that Directs Endothelial Differentiation Using
Embryonic Stem Cell-Derived Vascular Progenitor Cells

33

Sakurai, Y., Ohgimoto, K., Kataoka, Y., Yoshida, N., and Shibuya, M. (2005) Essential role of Flk-1 (VEGF receptor 2) tyrosine residue 1173 in vasculogenesis in mice. *Proc Natl Acad Sci USA* 102, 1076-1081

Sase, H., Watabe, T., Kawasaki, K., Miyazono, K., and Miyazawa, K. (2009) VEGFR2-PLCγ1 axis is essential for endothelial specification of VEGFR2+ vascular progenitor cells. *J. Cell Sci.* 122, 3303-3311

Schuh, A.C., Faloon, P., Hu, Q.-L., Bhimani, M., and Choi, K. (1999) In vitro hematopoietic and endothelial potential of *flk-1-/-* embryonic stemcells and embryos. *Proc. Natl. Acad. Sci. USA* 96, 2159-2164

Shalaby, F., Rossant, J., Yamaguchi, T.P., Gertsenstein, M., Wu, X.F., Breitman, M.L, and Schuh, A.C. (1995) Failure of blood-island formation and vasculogenesis in Flk-1-deficient mice. *Nature* 376, 62-66

Shalaby, F., Ho, J., Stanford, W.L., Fischer, K.D., Schuh, A.C., Schwartz, L., Bernstein, A., and Rossant, J. (1997) A requirement for Flk1 in primitive and definitive hematopoiesis and vasculogenesis. *Cell* 89, 981-990

Shibuya, M., and Claesson-Welsh, L. (2006) Signal transduction by VEGF receptors in regulation of angiogenesis and lymphangiogenesis. *Exp. Cell Res.* 312, 549-560

Spiekermann, K., Faber, F., Voswinckel, R., and Hiddemann, W. (2002) The protein tyrosine kinase inhibitor SU5614 inhibits VEGF-induced endothelial cell sprouting and induces growth arrest and apoptosis by inhibition of c-kit in AML cells. *Exp. Hematol.* 30, 767-773

Suzuki, H., Watabe, T., Kato, M., Miyazawa, K., and Miyazono, K. (2005) Roles of vascular endothelial growth factor receptor 3 signaling in differentiation of mouse embryonic stem cell-derived vascular progenitor cells into endothelial cells. *Blood* 105, 2372-2379

Takahashi, T., Ueno, H., and Shibuya, M. (1999) VEGF activates proteins kinase C-dependent, but Ras-independent Raf-MEK-MAP kinase pathway for DNA synthesis in primary endothelial cells. *Oncogene* 18, 2221-2230

Takahashi, T., Yamaguchi, S., Chida, K., and Shibuya, M. (2001) A single autophosphorylation site on KDR/Flk-1 is essential for VEGF-A-dependent activation of PLC-γ and DNA synthesis in vascular endothelial cells. *EMBO J.* 20, 2768-2778

Thurston, G. (2003) Role of angiopietins and Tie receptor tyrosine kinase in angiogenesis and lymphangiogenesis. *Cell Tissue Res.* 314, 61-68

Watabe, T., Nishihara, A., Mishima, K., Yamashita, J., Shimizu, K., Miyazawa, K., Nishikawa, S., and Miyazono, K. (2003) TGF-β receptor kinase inhibitor enhances growth and integrity of embryonic stem cell-derived endothelial cells. *J. Cell Biol.* 163, 1303-1311

Welsh, M., Mares., J., Karlsson, T., Lavergne, C., Bréant, B., and Claesson-Welsh, L. (1994) Shb is a ubiquitously expressed Src homology 2 protein. *Oncogene* 9, 19-27

Yamamizu, K., Kawasaki, K., Katayama, S., Watabe, T., and Yamashita, J.K. (2009) Enhancement of vascular progenitor potential by protein kinase A through dual induction of Flk-1 and Neuropilin-1. *Blood* 114, 3707-3716

Yamashita, J., Itoh, H., Hirashima, M., Ogawa, M., Nishikawa, S., Yurugi, T., Naito, M., Nakao, K., and Nishikawa, S. (2000) Flk-1 positive cells derived from embryonic stem cells serves as vascular progenitors. *Nature* 408, 92-96

Zambrowicz, B.P., Imamoto, A., Fiering, S., Herzenberg, L.A., Kerr, W.G., Soriano, P. (1997) Disruption of overlapping transcripts in the *ROSA* β geo 26 gene trap strain leads to widespread expression of β-galactosidase in mouse embryos and hematopoietic cells. *Proc.Natl. Acad. Sci. USA* 94, 3789-3794

Part 2

Hepatic Differentiation

3

Hepatic Differentiation of Human Embryonic and Induced Pluripotent Stem Cells for Regenerative Medicine

Toshio Miki

Eli and Edythe Broad Center for Regenerative Medicine and Stem Cell Research at USC
Department of Biochemistry and Molecular Biology, Keck School of Medicine
University of Southern California, Los Angeles
USA

1. Introduction

A hepatocyte is one of the most desired cells for regenerative medicine as well as for pharmaco-toxicological testing. Hepatocytes, the parenchymal cells of the liver, possess a wide range of functions, including protein synthesis/storage, detoxification, transformation of carbohydrates, synthesis of cholesterol, bile salts and phospholipids, as well as the excretion of exogenous and endogenous substances (Blouin et al 1977).

The various functions of the liver are essential for the maintenance of the human body and liver failure is often only treatable by organ liver transplantation (OLT). The shortage of donated organs, however, limits this treatment option available to patients. Since the Model for End-Stage Liver Disease and Pediatric End-Stage Liver Disease (MELD/PELD) liver allocation system was introduced in February 2002, the usage of borderline-quality donated livers for OLT has increased (Freeman et al 2002). As a result, the number of patients on waiting lists for OLT has stabilized; however, more than 15,000 patients await OLT annually in the United of States alone (Thuluvath et al 2010).

Hepatocyte transplantation (HT), a cell-replacement therapy for liver disease, could decrease the number of the patients on the waiting list. HT is particularly useful for metabolic liver diseases that do not require whole organ replacement but rather a partial restoration of specific liver metabolic functions (Fox et al 1998, Strom et al 1997). The feasibility and the therapeutic efficacy of HT have been demonstrated in several clinical trials (Strom et al 2006). However, the limited availability of human hepatocytes due to organ shortage prohibits the provision of this promising therapy to patients as a standard option. Human hepatocytes can be isolated from cadaveric livers that are donated but not suitable for OLT (Strom et al 1982). The number of unused donated livers has decreased since the MELD liver allocation system was initiated. This dilemma has led to an urgent demand for developing stem cell-derived functional human hepatocytes as an alternative. Stem cell-derived hepatocytes could also be utilized in artificial liver bio-devices for patients with acute liver failure who may not need the OLT (Gerlach et al 2010, Gerlach et al 2008, Soto-Gutierrez et al 2006a). An unlimited supply of stem cell-derived hepatocytes could facilitate the development of these cell-based therapies for treatment of life-threatening liver diseases.

Moreover, these stem cell-derived hepatocytes could be utilized not only for therapeutic applications but also for pharmaco-toxicological testing (Davila et al 2004). It is anticipated that stem cell-derived hepatocytes will be important as *in vitro* tools for testing drug safety, thereby significantly facilitating drug development. Toxicity assessment for drug development could be conducted with phenotypically and genotypically standardized human hepatocytes. In this regard, genetically homogeneous stem cell-derived hepatocytes would be superior to primary human hepatocytes. Human stem cell-derived hepatocytes would be particularly useful for conducting some infectious disease research as well. As a case in point, hepatocytes derived from animals have been demonstrated to not be useful for the study of human hepatitis virus biology such as HCV (Cai et al 2007).

A number of different stem/progenitor cells have been proposed as an alternative cell source for generation of functional hepatocytes – these include fetal hepatocytes (Suzuki et al 2000), adult hepatic progenitor/stem (epithelial) cells (Alison & Sarraf 1998), bone-marrow derived-stem cells (Gilchrist & Plevris 2010), and adipose-derived stem cells (Schaffler & Buchler 2007). Although the biological potential of fetal hepatocytes and adult hepatic progenitor cells is promising, ethical issues and limited availability hampers development for use in the clinic. Relatively small numbers of stem/progenitor cells would be insufficient for use to generate stem cell-derived hepatocytes in the clinic, particularly for HT, as HT recipients require transplantations of more than a billion cells at a time (Fox et al 1998). Some reports claimed that there was hepatic differentiation of mesenchymal stem cells from adipose tissue or bone marrow. However, the differentiation to functional hepatocytes, remains controversial (Goodell 2003, Wagers & Weissman 2004). Further research efforts are required to gain consensus for utilizing these adult stem cell-derived hepatocytes in the clinic.

To date, pluripotent stem cells are the most realistic candidate for the generation of stem cell-derived hepatocytes. Pluripotent stem cells possess nearly unlimited self-renewal capability *in vitro* and are able to differentiate into all three germ layers. Human embryonic stem cells (hESCs) are derived from blastocysts (Thomson et al 1998), and several protocols have been published for the differentiation of hESCs to functional hepatocytes. Additionally, recent breakthroughs in the field of induced pluripotent stem (iPS) cell technology (Takahashi & Yamanaka 2006) have provided yet another promising source to generate stem cell-derived hepatocytes. The human iPS cells may overcome the ethical concerns of utilizing blastocyst-derived pluripotent stem cell and may provide patient specific immunotype cells so as to avoid the lifelong use of immunosuppressants (Takahashi et al 2007). Disease-specific iPS cells, derived from patients who suffer from various congenital liver diseases, such as alpha1-antitrypsin deficiency, familial hypercholesterolemia, and glycogen storage disease, are anticipated to become important tools for studying the mechanisms underlying the pathogenesis of these diseases and investigations of new treatments (Ghodsizadeh et al 2010). Moreover, human iPS-derived hepatocytes would be an unlimited source for materials that are genetically homogeneous for conducting consistent pharmaco-toxicological evaluations. For example, an iPS-derived hepatocyte library could be established based upon single-nucleotide polymorphisms (SNPs) in drug metabolizing enzymes (eg. cytochrome P450s), and this could enable evaluation of drug metabolism with specific SNP-type hepatocytes. These data could be utilized to design personalized therapies for future "made-to-order" medicine (Medine et al 2010).

In this chapter, we describe the developmental progression from a pluripotent stem cell state to hepatocytes and provide an overview of protocols for hepatic differentiation of pluripotent stem cells. Enrichment strategies of functional hepatocytes and functional evaluation methodologies are also discussed.

2. Lessons from liver development

A reasonable approach to induce hepatic differentiation from pluripotent stem cells is to recapitulate actual embryonic developmental events *in vitro*. Liver development occurs through a series of cell-to-cell interactions between the embryonic endoderm and its nearby mesoderm (Duncan 2003, Zaret 1996). A number of genes and signaling pathways that are involved in this process have been identified (Lemaigre & Zaret 2004). Understanding the molecular pathways controlling hepatogenesis is essential in designing protocols for inducing hepatic differentiation *in vitro*. Although our knowledge of embryonic liver development is based on studies from non-human embryos, it is anticipated that the fundamental processes are similar if not identical to those in human liver development. Studies from mouse, chicken, zebrafish and Xenopus have shown that much of hepatogenesis is evolutionarily conserved (Roberts 2000, Tian & Meng 2006). Numerous signals are required at each step of hepatogenic development (Lemaigre & Zaret 2004, Zhao & Duncan 2005). Here, we review these sequential events – we have divided them into four stages to highlight the crucial cues at each stage for a better understanding of hepatic differentiation protocols that will be described in subsequent sections.

2.1 Stage 1. Toward definitive endoderm

The earliest event of organogenesis during mouse embryonic development is gastrulation. At this phase (ED6.5-7.5), the definitive endoderm layer is formed from mesendoderm lineage cells (Tada et al 2005). The process begins with the migration of Brachyury (T) positive cells through the anterior region of the primitive streak and through the Node, located at the anterior-most position of the streak (Vincent et al 2003). It has been shown that signaling by a member of the transforming growth factor (TGF)-β superfamily, specifically Nodal, initiates both endoderm and mesoderm formation (Vincent et al 2003). The epidermal growth factor family molecule, Cripto-1/FRL1/cryptic, plays a central role as a co-receptor for Nodal. Nodal/ALK signaling in conjunction with Cripto contributes to generate endoderm precursor cells and for the subsequent specification of definitive endoderm (DE) (Strizzi et al 2005). The duration and magnitude of Nodal signaling influence the specification of mesoderm or endoderm. The physical position of cells relative to the Node also seems to control this specification. Exposure to longer and higher levels of Nodal signaling induce endoderm specification, whereas lower stimulation of Nodal signaling promotes differentiation into the mesoderm (Schier 2003). Nodal signaling targets a core group of endoderm transcription factors genes expression including Sox17, Foxa2 (HNF3β) (Shen 2007).

2.2 Stage 2. Influence from cardiogenic mesodermal cells and septum transversum mesenchyme

Following gastrulation, the definitive endoderm is patterned along the A-P axis into foregut, midgut and hindgut progenitor domains (Dessimoz et al 2006). Morphogenesis forms foregut and hindgut pockets as the endodermal cup is transformed into a gut tube. At ED8 the definitive endoderm cells occupy a portion of the ventral foregut adjacent to the heart. Signaling cues from cardiogenic mesodermal cells such as fibroblast growth factors (FGFs) (Jung et al 1999) and cues from the septum transversum mesenchyme (STM), such as bone morphogenic proteins 2 and 4 (BMP2, BMP4) are essential to direct cell fate to a hepatic lineage (Rossi et al 2001). It has been demonstrated that mouse embryonic foregut explants express albumin when co-cultured with cardiac mesoderm (Calmont et al 2006, Rossi et al 2001). Studies using explant systems have shown that the cardiac mesoderm can be replaced by exogenous FGF1 or FGF2 supplementation (Jung et al 1999). BMP signaling is required, but not sufficient, for hepatic induction in explants (Rossi et al 2001).

2.3 Stage 3. Hepatoblast proliferation

The domain that eventually becomes the liver moves to the midgut, and the liver diverticulum forms by ED9 (Rifkind et al 1969). By ED9.5, the basal lamina breaks down and hepatoblasts delaminate and migrate into the STM. The liver diverticulum expands into a pronounced liver bud by ED10. The liver bud then undergoes tremendous growth and becomes the major site of fetal hematopoiesis. The massive proliferation and protection from apoptosis are regulated by paracrine signals from adjacent mesenchyme. These signals are including the FGFs, BMPs, Wnts, and the TGFβ signaling pathways. Hepatocyte Growth Factor (HGF) signaling is also required for hepatoblast migration and proliferation (Birchmeier et al 2003).

Although Wnt/β-catenin signaling appears to repress liver fate during earlier endoderm patterning stages of development, β-catenin has the opposite effect and promotes hepatic growth in the liver bud at this stage (ED10) (McLin et al 2007, Micsenyi et al 2004, Monga et al 2003). Immunohistochemical studies showed TGF-β3 expression in the liver bud mesenchyme at ED13.5 (Pelton et al 1991). Similarly, Stenvers *et al* showed a predominant expression of the TGF-β receptor III (TbetaRIII) mRNA in liver at midgestation. They also demonstrated that TbetaRIII gene disruption induced apoptosis in the liver at ED13.5 (Stenvers et al 2003).

2.4 Stage 4. A bifurcation point to hepatocyte or cholangiocyte

The differentiation of bi-potential hepatoblasts into hepatocytes or cholangiocytes begins around ED13 of mouse development. Hepatoblasts, adjacent to the portal vein, transform into cuboidal cells, which eventually forms the intrahepatic bile ducts during the prenatal period through the ductal plate remodeling process (Lemaigre 2003, Raynaud et al 2011), while other hepatoblasts gradually differentiate into mature hepatocytes. It has been shown that oncostatin M (OSM) promotes hepatic maturation (Kamiya et al 2001) During this phase, the liver bud transitions from a hematopoietic organ to a metabolic organ. Coexisting hematopoietic cells also play a significant role in the hepatic maturation process. For example, OSM is released from the hematopoietic cells and activates a JAK/Stat3 signaling pathway via the gp130 receptor (Ito et al 2000, Kamiya et al 1999), and intrahepatic structures are organized by ED15. The final maturation of the liver is a gradual process and continues into the postnatal period. Many hepatic enzymes such as cytochrome P450s shift from a fetal form to a mature form during the postnatal period.

3. Hepatic differentiation of pluripotent stem cells

Currently hepatic differentiation strategies from pluripotent stem cells can be classified into three approaches; 1) via formation of spontaneous embryoid body (EB), 2) co-culture with supporter cells, and 3) directed hepatic differentiation via stepwise stimulation by defined growth factors.

3.1 Embryoid body formation and spontaneous hepatic differentiation

Mouse ESCs aggregate in suspension to form spheroid clumps of cells called embryoid bodies (EBs). Removal of leukemia inhibitory factor (LIF) induces spontaneous differentiation into three germ layers (Itskovitz-Eldor et al 2000). Chinzei *et al* reported that AFP and albumin gene expressions were detected in EBs after 9 days and 12 days, respectively, without additional exogenous growth factors (Chinzei et al 2002). However, the spontaneous differentiation of hepatocytes in EBs is inefficient (usually under 10%) and is highly cell line dependent (Lavon & Benvenisty 2005, Schwartz et al 2005, Shirahashi et al 2004). To increase the ratio of hepatic cells in the EBs, differentiation can be directed by exposure to exogenous growth factors. Hamazaki and colleagues demonstrated that the combination and consecutive supplementation of FGF, HGF, OSM, and dexamethasone efficiently induced hepatic differentiation (Hamazaki et al 2001). In regards to human ESCs, hepatic induction using the EB formation approach was reported by Schuldiner and colleagues (Schuldiner et al 2000). These studies with EB formation provided evidence that mouse and human pluripotent stem cells were able to differentiate to the hepatic lineage *in vitro*. The 3D structure of EBs has an advantage over the 2D culture system in further inducing functional maturation. However, the uncontrolled heterogeneous cell populations in EBs and the variation in size and morphology prohibit further clinical applications.

3.2 Co-culture of pluripotent stem cells with supporter cells

Another approach for hepatic differentiation is providing *in vivo*-like supplements including cytokines, growth factors, and extracellular matrixes. These elements can be provided by co-culturing appropriate supporter cells, such as hepatic mesenchymal cells. A co-culture strategy for hepatic differentiation was first applied using Thy1-positive mesenchymal cells derived from mouse fetal liver (Ishii et al 2005). An enhanced green fluorescent protein (EGFP)-AFP labeling system was used to isolate hepatic lineage committed ES-derived cells, which were subsequently co-cultured with the Thy1 positive mesenchymal cells. Several late-phase hepatic markers such as tyrosine amino transferase, tryptophan 2,3-dioxygenase, and glucose-6-phosphatase were expressed in the co-cultured ES-derived hepatocytes. Fair et al reported that co-cultured mESCs with chick embryonic cardiac mesoderm cells expressed mesendoderm genes, Sox17α, HNF3β, GATA4, after 24 hours (Fair et al 2003). They also demonstrated that the xenogeneic cell-to-cell contact between mESCs and the chick cells, apart from providing cytokines/growth factors, may also provide signals via direct cell-to-cell interaction. In contrast, Saito et al demonstrated that diffusible factors from mouse fetal liver-derived cells were sufficient to stimulate hepatic differentiation of cynomolgus monkey ES cells (Saito et al 2006). They also demonstrated that induction of hepatic differentiation utilizing the co-culture system was faster than chemical/growth factor induction. Soto-Gutierrez et al combined a co-culture system of human liver nonparenchymal cell lines with growth factors. This protocol resulted in the successful derivation of 70% albumin positive cells from mESCs (Soto-Gutierrez et al 2007). These data indicate the feasibility of the co-culture system for inducing hepatic differentiation from pluripotent stem cells. However, it might be difficult to reproduce hepatic differentiation by co-culturing with primary cells as the quality and the secreted factors are uncertain. Moreover, the contamination of the supporter cells and the difficulty in the scale-up of hepatocyte production are issues that hamper clinical applications.

3.3 Guided hepatic differentiation with specific factors

The *in vitro* developmental capability of ES cells has been shown with spontaneous differentiation with EB formation. The co-culture studies indicate that exogenous signals could induce hepatic differentiation. As described in section 2, extensive developmental biology studies have uncovered the pathways controlling hepatogenesis. To mimic the sequential stimulation of *in vivo* hepatogenesis, various combinations of stepwise growth factor stimulation strategies have been tested.

The critical first step is to efficiently induce definitive endoderm (DE) commitment of ESCs. Based on researches of mesendoderm and definitive endoderm differentiation in rodent and Xenopus, it was reasonable to expect that a high concentration of Nodal is key to the induction of definitive endoderm differentiation (Schier 2003). In most studies, a high dose of Activin A was used as a substitute for Nodal. Activin shares the same receptors (ActRII and ALK4) with Nodal but does not require the association of Cripto to initiate the Nodal/Smad2 signaling pathway (Strizzi et al 2005). After a few days of Activin treatment, most of the ES cells express definitive endoderm genes (Sox17 and Foxa2), while mesoderm, pluripotency and the extraembryonic endoderm genes are down regulated (D'Amour et al 2005, Kubo et al 2004). Further studies indicate that generation of hESC-DE requires two conditions: signaling by Activin/Nodal family members and the release from inhibitory signals generated by PI3K through insulin/IGF (McLean et al 2007). In this approach, using a high-density monolayer culture, pluripotent stem cells are cultured in a feeder cell-free system and mesendoderm differentiation is induced by a defined serum-free medium, supplemented with high-dose of Activin A (e.g. 100ng/ml) (Yoshie et al 2010).

The signaling pathways regulating foregut formation can be recapitulated in cell culture by the addition of specific growth factors such as FGFs and BMPs. A number of groups have used this combination to generate hepatic cells (Dan & Yeoh 2008, Ochiya et al 2009). The endoderm specification stage is followed by HGF stimulation to expand the hepatoblast population (LaBrecque 1994). Hepatic maturation is normally regulated and promoted by some combination of OSM and Dexamethasone. (Agarwal et al 2008, Baharvand et al 2008, Cai et al 2007, Soto-Gutierrez et al 2006b, Teratani et al 2005).

Hay and colleagues introduced a similar stepwise induction concept, except using chemicals to induce hepatic differentiation in ES and iPS cells (Hay et al 2008a, Hay et al 2008b, Sullivan et al 2010). A combination of Activin A and the histone deacetylase inhibitors (HDI), sodium butyrate, were utilized for the definitive endoderm induction and 1% DMSO for further hepatic specification (Hay et al 2008b). Although the effect of butyrate for inducing differentiation has been known for a long time (Leder & Leder 1975), the role of HDI in the hepatic differentiation process was not totally elucidated. McLean showed that a combination of Activin and a PI3K inhibitor is more efficient to induce DE differentiation (McLean et al 2007). Recent progress on studies in signal transduction pathways has led researchers to control not only the initiation of signal transduction by adding exogenous growth factors, but also the regulation of intracellular signaling to induce hepatic differentiation in a more precise and efficient manner. Touboul et al used the PI3K inhibitor, LY294002, for DE induction and activin receptor-like kinase (ALK) 5 inhibitor, SB431542, for hepatic specification. Currently, these protocols still require combinations with recombinant growth factors. Since mass production of these recombinant proteins is cost prohibitive, a totally defined chemical protocol would be ideal for a large-scale hepatocyte production.

Although hepatic differentiation protocols are now more sophisticated, fully differentiated stem cell-derived hepatocytes that possess identical hepatic functions to primary adult hepatocytes have yet to be produced. Using a unique primary hepatocyte culture system, Michalopoulos's group demonstrated that a combination of dexamethasone, HGF, and EGF was required for formation of liver-like tissue. Dexamethasone induces expression of both

HNF4α and C/EBP-α, essential transcription factors for hepatocyte differentiation, while HGF and EGF induce members of the TGF-β family and HNF6β, which are essential for maintenance of hepatic functions (Michalopoulos et al 2003). Although this unique culture system has not been tested with stem cell-derived hepatic cells, this combination and culture system may be essential to achieve further hepatic maturation.

4. Enrichment strategies of stem cell derived hepatocytes

Despite utilizing these well-designed differentiation protocols on mouse and human ES cells, hepatic induction from pluripotent stem cells results in mixtures with non-hepatic cells. Generally speaking, in the areas of stem cell-derived cell studies, there has not been a differentiation protocol that is able to induce 100% of this desired target cells based upon current technologies. This is one of the issues that is hindering further clinical development. Particularly in the use of pluripotent stem cells, contamination with undifferentiated cells is one of the biggest concerns due to their tumorigenic potential (Ben-David & Benvenisty 2011, Dressel et al 2008). Therefore, further investigations will be necessary to obtain clinically applicable stem cell-derived hepatocytes. One of the approaches is to develop techniques that allow for isolation and purification of specific hepatic subtypes.

For basic research, it is common to use genetic selection techniques. Under this strategy, undifferentiated pluripotent stem cells are genetically modified to carry either a reporter gene, usually a green fluorescence protein (EGFP) gene or an antibiotic resistance gene under the transcriptional control of a hepatic-promoter such as alpha-fetoprotein (Yin et al 2002). The transgenic cells are then induced to differentiate and subsequently selected based on the activation of the hepatocyte-specific promoter. The major disadvantage of this approach is the risks associated with the genetic modification which may lead to insertional oncogenesis. In addition, these transcriptional markers are also common to immature hepatocytes. It is, therefore difficult to designate one gene as a definitive single marker of hepatic differentiation.

An endogenously expressed surface marker, asialoglycoprotein receptor (ASGPR), has been proposed as a cell surface marker for functional hepatocytes (Li et al 2008, Treichel et al 1995). Recent studies have utilized ASGPR to identify mature hepatic cells from a mixed population of fetal hepatocytes (Ring et al 2010). ASGPR is a transmembrane hepatocellular surface carbohydrate binding glycoprotein that lacks terminal sialic acid residues (=asialoglycoproteins). Characterization of the ASGPR has revealed its functional role in the binding, internalization and transport of a wide range of glycoproteins in a selective manner via the process of receptor-mediated endocytosis. The expression of the ASGPR has been clinically correlated to loss of hepatic functions in liver diseases associated with cancer, viral hepatitis, and cirrhosis. Basma et al enriched hESC-derived hepatic cells using the ASGPR marker (Basma et al 2009). Although the G6Pase, albumin, and TAT mRNA expressions were dramatically improved by this enrichment step, mRNA expression of both Oct4 and AFP were still detectable. This data indicates that a single enrichment step could not completely eliminate the undifferentiated stem cell or the progenitor cell contamination.

Kumashiro et al used a silica-based colloidal medium (Percoll) and PECAM-1 antibodies to separate mESCs-derived hepatocytes from Oct4 positive undifferentiated cells. The ES-derived hepatocytes were transplanted into the CCl4-injured mouse liver and this led to improved liver function. Importantly, unlike unselected ES-derived hepatocytes, the enriched ES-derived hepatocytes did not develop teratomas in the recipients' liver (Kumashiro et al 2005).

Conclusively, the hepatic enrichment studies demonstrate the advantages of selecting hepatic cells from mixed ES-derived cell population. However, there is to date, no single standard technology to achieve sufficient hepatocyte enrichment or non-hepatic cell exclusion. The influence of other cell types on hepatic differentiation is one aspect that requires further studies. Non-hepatic cells such as cholangiocyte contamination may have a positive influence for further maturation in stem cell-derived hepatic cells. For future clinical applications, genetic modification of stem cell will not be acceptable. Although the ASGPR enrichment protocol is promising, the need for a large quantity of antibody remains a substantial financial burden for large-scale production of stem cell-derived hepatocytes. Thus, additional investigations are needed to find novel strategies to enrich clinically viable stem cell-derived hepatocytes.

5. Characteristics of pluripotent stem cell derived hepatocytes

One of the difficulties for stem cell research is the interpretation of *in vitro* data on the extent of terminal differentiation. Since human primary hepatocytes lose their hepatic functions *in vitro* within a week after their isolation, it is clearly a challenge to induce full maturation status equivalent to that of adult hepatocytes in stem cell-derived hepatocytes *in vitro*. With this in mind, the *in vitro* evaluation for hepatic differentiation has to be undertaken very carefully using multi-pronged approaches. The evaluation should be conducted at 1) the transcription level, 2) the translation level, 3) performing biochemical (*in vitro*) functional tests, as well as 4) *in vivo* functional assays.

5.1 Transcriptional evaluation. Hepatic marker genes expression

Many genes have been proposed as hepatocyte-specific genes. The most commonly cited genes are; albumin, alpha-fetoprotein (AFP), cytokeratin-18, glucose-6-phosphatase (G6P), phosphoenolpyruvate carboxykinase (PEPCK), alpha-1-antitrypsin (A1AT), bilirubin, uridine diphosphate-glucuronosyltransferase, coagulation factor VII. However, some of these are also expressed in other tissues such as extra-embryonic yolk sac. AFP, for example, is expressed in both the liver and the yolk sac. Therefore, AFP expression needs to be demonstrated along with definitive endoderm marker genes, Sox17 and CXCR4. Transcriptome studies on mouse liver development have revealed that the expression patterns of these hepatic markers are dramatically altered during hepatogenesis. For instance, Jochheim et al. demonstrated that HNF4α gene expression peaked on ED11.5 and decreased until ED13.5, after which, it gradually increased but its levels were not as high as at ED11.5 (Jochheim et al 2003). Therefore, quantitative RT-PCR data must be carefully interpreted, as a downregulation of HNF4α mRNA expression could still be an indication of increased hepatocyte maturation. Genes encoding cytochrome P-450 (CYP)-7A1, bilirubin, uridine diphosphate-glucuronosyltransferase, coagulation factor VII, and asialoglycoprotein receptors are considered late phase hepatic marker genes and are not expressed in the yolk sac. Therefore, these genes could be useful as markers for mature hepatocytes. In contrast, G6P, CYP3A4 and PEPCK are also deemed late-phase marker genes, however, their expression is not liver specific. CYP7A1 is a member of the cytochrome P450 superfamily of enzymes. This liver specific endoplasmic reticulum membrane protein is involved in the cholesterol catabolic pathway, which converts cholesterol to bile acids. Other CYP enzymes are responsible for oxidative metabolism of most therapeutic drugs. Therefore, it is important to demonstrate the expression of these genes in the stem cell-derived hepatic cells for drug testing. Among the CYP enzymes, 3A4, 1A2, 2C19, 2D6, are dominant players for drug metabolism in human liver.

Ideally the gene expression levels in stem cell-derived hepatic cell at the end of the differentiation protocol should be comparable to that of an adult hepatocyte. Concurrently, evaluations for non-hepatocyte specific genes to determine the extent of differentiation to specific hepatic lineage should also be performed.

With regards to the development of drug metabolizing enzymes such as CYP genes, both the pattern and the level of expressions are important. Many metabolic and detoxifying enzymes are expressed at significant levels only after birth. Therefore, the gene expression ratio of the fetal form to the adult form could be used as a determinant of the status of hepatic maturation. For example, fetal liver cells express CYP3A7, a fetal form of CYP3A4. Higher 3A4/3A7 ratio indicates increased hepatic maturation of stem cell-derived hepatic cells (Ek et al 2007, Miki et al 2011).

5.2 Translational evaluation. Hepatic marker proteins expression

Gene expression does not necessarily translate to protein production and activity. Using a hepatic differentiation protocol, Hay et al demonstrated that Oct4 protein was undetectable after the second day, while Oct4 mRNA remains detectable until day 11 of the protocol. Along the same vein, albumin mRNA expression was observed at day 11 but albumin protein was detected only starting at day 15 (Hay et al 2008b). Therefore, immunohistochemistry and/or Western blot analyses must be performed to verify the expression of key proteins at the end of any differentiation protocol. AFP, Albumin, A1AT, and cytokeratins (8, 18, 19) are common proteins that were used in many reports. As mentioned in section 4, some cell surface marker proteins (e.g. ASGPR) are also important.

5.3 Biochemical functional assay

Demonstration of albumin production and secretion from stem cell-derived hepatic cells is the gold standard assay to demonstrate functional protein synthesis. In the human body, albumin is the most abundant protein in serum and is produced specifically by the liver. Therefore, serum albumin has been used as an indicator to evaluate liver function in a clinical setting. Although albumin production and secretion are essential, it is however insufficient to use this as a marker for stem cell-derived hepatic cells. It has been shown the albumin gene is expressed at a relatively early stage of hepatogenesis, and furthermore, visceral endoderm cells such as yolk sac cells also produce albumin (Meehan et al 1984). Therefore, albumin production from stem cell-derived hepatic cells must be further supported through a combination of other assays.

The ability to metabolize ammonia is also a standard assay to evaluate hepatic detoxification function. *In vivo*, ammonia is a metabolic product generated from dietary amino acids, and 80-90% of ammonia is converted into urea by hepatocytes through the urea cycle. To test this function *in vitro*, excess amount of ammonium chloride is added to the culture medium (ammonia challenge). Ammonia clearance or urea production can then be measured as functional readout of the assay. Since precise parameter adjustment for measuring ammonia level in culture media is difficult, the standard protocol is measuring urea concentration in the supernatant via the enzymatic urease method. A pitfall in this assay is the possibility of arginase leakage from damaged cells due to the excess ammonium chloride, which could produce urea independently from the urea cycle activity. Therefore, the acquisition of urea metabolism function should be further confirmed by the expression of key enzymes in the urea cycle, such as arginase I (ARG1), argininosuccinate lyase (ASL), argininosuccinate synthetase 1 (ASS1), carbamoyl-phosphate synthetase 1 (CPS1), and ornithine carbamoyltransferase (OTC) (Mavri-Damelin et al 2008, Miki et al 2011).

To meet the demand for pharmaco-toxicological applications, demonstration of activities of xenobiotic-metabolizing phase I and phase II enzymes and phase III transporters must be satisfied (Xu et al 2005). To evaluate phase I activities, CYP-dependent monooxygenase activity assays; 7-ethoxycoumarin-O-deethylase (ECOD assay) (Lubet et al 1985), 7-ethoxyresorufin-O-deethylase (EROD assay), and specific oxidation of testosterone are commonly used. In measuring phase II activities, glucuronosyltransferase activity and sulfotransferase activity toward p-nitrophenol, and glutathione S-transferase activity are commonly used. Functional assays for phase III transporters have yet to be standardized. Measurement of fluorescent protein conjugated bile acid could be useful to evaluate one of the phase III transporters, i.e. the bile salt export pump (BSEP/ABCB11), for activity in stem cell-derived hepatocytes (Yamaguchi et al 2010).

5.4 *In vivo* analysis

These *in vitro* hepatic functional assays are essential and useful. However, the most definitive proof for the functionality of stem cell-derived hepatic cells would be the demonstration of hepatic engraftment *in vivo* using animal models (Soto-Gutierrez et al 2006a, Yamamoto et al 2003). It would be ideal if stem cell-derived hepatic cells could improve survival rates in lethal disease models. Transgenic mouse models of congenital liver diseases would be candidates for such assays. The fumarylacetoacetate hydrolase (FAH) deficiency mouse model (Lagasse et al 2000) and urokinase-type plasminogen activator-transgenic SCID mice (Tateno et al 2004) have been previously and provide a means to test stem cell-derived hepatocytes in a liver transplantation setting. Unfortunately such animal models are not widely available and also require significant technical expertise to perform hepatocyte transplantation in neonatal animals.

Nevertheless, whether human or rodent, primary hepatocytes tend to lose their differentiated characteristics in culture. One question that arises is whether the stem cell-derived hepatic cells have to be fully differentiated *in vitro*. It is anticipated that stem cell-derived hepatic progenitor cells spontaneously differentiate to fully mature hepatocytes in their correct endogenous environment. Once hepatic lineage commitment is confirmed, stem cell-derived hepatic progenitor cells could be an acceptable source for cell replacement therapy. The endogenous mouse liver environment is suitable to test this hypothesis. It is therefore extremely important to establish standard animal models that are easy to experiment with, and also widely available for stem cell-derived hepatic cell transplantation.

6. Conclusion and future perspectives

Hepatic differentiation is a sequential dynamic event that involves various types of cells and complex signaling networks. Although the signaling pathways and growth factors that are involved in definitive endoderm specification have been well documented, only portions of the mechanisms involved in the human hepatogenic development have been defined. Therefore, the goal of inducing directed differentiation of pluripotent stem cells toward hepatocytes remains a big challenge. A number of differentiation protocols have been described to generate hepatocytes from pluripotent stem cells. Collectively, various hepatic differentiation studies demonstrate how the exposure of various growth factors to pluripotent stem cells, with the appropriate timing and doses, is essential for directing the differentiation process from early mesendoderm via definitive endoderm towards more functionally mature hepatocytes. Based on the recent advances in the field of developmental biology, hepatic differentiation protocols have been modified to provide more than 70% albumin positive cells from mESCs (Soto-Gutierrez et al 2007) and 35% of ASGPR positive cells from hESCs (Touboul et al 2010). It appears that iPS cells possess a similar capacity to hES cells to generate hepatocytes using similar differentiation protocols (Sullivan et al 2010). It must be noted that the stem cell-derived hepatocytes described to date generally exhibit fetal hepatocyte-like gene expression profiles and immature functional characteristics compared to authentic adult primary hepatocytes. Recent finding suggested that a 3D dynamic bioreactor culture system which provides an *in vivo*-like culture environment induced teratoma-like multi-directional differentiation of human ESCs (Gerlach et al 2010). When a hepatic differentiation protocol was applied in this system, the 3D dynamic culture system induced further hepatic maturation, including tissue-like structure formation (Miki et al 2011). Although the superiority of the culture conditions in the 3D dynamic culture system has been clearly demonstrated, it is difficult to determine which parameters are critical for this advantage in hepatic maturation. Using matrigel or collagen gel, it has been shown that static 3D culture conditions prolong hepatic function of primary hepatocytes (Kono et al 1997). It has been proposed that the 3D structure allows more physiological cell-to-cell interactions, and induces polarity in hepatocytes (Haouzi et al 2005). Baharvand et al demonstrated that hESCs are more efficiently differentiated to hepatic cells under static 3D culture conditions than conventional 2D culture conditions (Baharvand et al 2008).

Dynamic culture conditions are, not surprisingly, more advantageous than static culture conditions (Vinci et al 2011). Unlike static cultures, the dynamic culture system provides continuous and gradual medium change under controlled oxygen tension and temperature. Taken together, the dynamic 3D culture system can provide a more physiological and homeostatic environment that could be favorable for stem cell-derived hepatocyte maturation. The continuous supply of fresh medium via nano-size porous hollow fibers also provides micro steady flow around the cells (Gerlach et al 2010) and low shear stress that could further stimulate maturation signals through sensory systems (e.g. cilia) on the polarized hepatic cells (Decaens et al 2008). Furthermore, it is noteworthy that in the human body, the liver passively but dynamically moves with the movements of diaphragm. In addition to the oxygen concentration in the blood flow, such movement could be a factor to induce rapid postnatal hepatic maturation events such as cytochrome isotype switching from CYP3A7 to 3A4.

As reviewed, the current differentiation protocols demonstrated the feasibility of hepatic cell production from pluripotent stem cells. Further optimization will be required to better define hepatic differentiation protocols and improved culture conditions to obtain fully differentiated functional hepatocytes *in vitro*. On the other hand, for cell replacement therapy applications, such *in vitro* full maturation may not be essential. Both fetal and adult hepatocytes demonstrated bilirubin conjugating activity in the Gunn rat after cell transplantation (Borel-Rinkes et al 1992). Hepatic progenitor cells could mature in the endogenous hepatic environment and thereby provide therapeutic effects to patients. The direction of research for this goal will be generating hepatic lineage committed cells *in vitro*, establishing an appropriate enrichment protocol, and critically evaluating the efficacy and safety of these cells in animal models.

In conclusion, the promise of pluripotent stem cells for the generation of hepatocytes and with further investigations will eventually lead us to a more in-depth understanding of mechanisms of hepatogenesis and hepatic maturation. The widespread utility of pluripotent stem cell-derived functional hepatocytes for basic research and pharmaceutical applications, could also become a reality. In the future, stem cell-derived hepatocytes are anticipated to have an enormous impact on the treatment of liver disease.

7. References

Agarwal S, Holton KL, Lanza R. 2008. Efficient differentiation of functional hepatocytes from human embryonic stem cells. *Stem Cells* 26: 1117-27

Alison M, Sarraf C. 1998. Hepatic stem cells. *J Hepatol* 29: 676-82

Baharvand H, Hashemi SM, Shahsavani M. 2008. Differentiation of human embryonic stem cells into functional hepatocyte-like cells in a serum-free adherent culture condition. *Differentiation* 76: 465-77

Basma H, Soto-Gutierrez A, Yannam GR, Liu L, Ito R, et al. 2009. Differentiation and transplantation of human embryonic stem cell-derived hepatocytes. *Gastroenterology* 136: 990-9

Ben-David U, Benvenisty N. 2011. The tumorigenicity of human embryonic and induced pluripotent stem cells. *Nat Rev Cancer* 11: 268-77

Birchmeier C, Birchmeier W, Gherardi E, Vande Woude GF. 2003. Met, metastasis, motility and more. *Nat Rev Mol Cell Biol* 4: 915-25

Blouin A, Bolender RP, Weibel ER. 1977. Distribution of organelles and membranes between hepatocytes and nonhepatocytes in the rat liver parenchyma. A stereological study. *J Cell Biol* 72: 441-55

Borel-Rinkes IH, Bijma AM, Kappers WA, Sinaasappel M, Hoek FJ, et al. 1992. Evidence of metabolic activity of adult and fetal rat hepatocytes transplanted into solid supports. *Transplantation* 54: 210-4

Cai J, Zhao Y, Liu Y, Ye F, Song Z, et al. 2007. Directed differentiation of human embryonic stem cells into functional hepatic cells. *Hepatology* 45: 1229-39

Calmont A, Wandzioch E, Tremblay KD, Minowada G, Kaestner KH, et al. 2006. An FGF response pathway that mediates hepatic gene induction in embryonic endoderm cells. *Dev Cell* 11: 339-48

Chinzei R, Tanaka Y, Shimizu-Saito K, Hara Y, Kakinuma S, et al. 2002. Embryoid-body cells derived from a mouse embryonic stem cell line show differentiation into functional hepatocytes. *Hepatology* 36: 22-9

D'Amour KA, Agulnick AD, Eliazer S, Kelly OG, Kroon E, Baetge EE. 2005. Efficient differentiation of human embryonic stem cells to definitive endoderm. *Nat Biotechnol* 23: 1534-41

Dan YY, Yeoh GC. 2008. Liver stem cells: a scientific and clinical perspective. *J Gastroenterol Hepatol* 23: 687-98

Davila JC, Cezar GG, Thiede M, Strom S, Miki T, Trosko J. 2004. Use and application of stem cells in toxicology. *Toxicol Sci* 79: 214-23

Decaens C, Durand M, Grosse B, Cassio D. 2008. Which in vitro models could be best used to study hepatocyte polarity? *Biol Cell* 100: 387-98

Dessimoz J, Opoka R, Kordich JJ, Grapin-Botton A, Wells JM. 2006. FGF signaling is necessary for establishing gut tube domains along the anterior-posterior axis in vivo. *Mech Dev* 123: 42-55

Dressel R, Schindehutte J, Kuhlmann T, Elsner L, Novota P, et al. 2008. The tumorigenicity of mouse embryonic stem cells and in vitro differentiated neuronal cells is controlled by the recipients' immune response. *PLoS One* 3: e2622

Duncan SA. 2003. Mechanisms controlling early development of the liver. *Mech Dev* 120: 19-33

Ek M, Soderdahl T, Kuppers-Munther B, Edsbagge J, Andersson TB, et al. 2007. Expression of drug metabolizing enzymes in hepatocyte-like cells derived from human embryonic stem cells. *Biochem Pharmacol* 74: 496-503

Fair JH, Cairns BA, Lapaglia M, Wang J, Meyer AA, et al. 2003. Induction of hepatic differentiation in embryonic stem cells by co-culture with embryonic cardiac mesoderm. *Surgery* 134: 189-96

Fox IJ, Chowdhury JR, Kaufman SS, Goertzen TC, Chowdhury NR, et al. 1998. Treatment of the Crigler-Najjar syndrome type I with hepatocyte transplantation. *N Engl J Med* 338: 1422-6

Freeman RB, Jr., Wiesner RH, Harper A, McDiarmid SV, Lake J, et al. 2002. The new liver allocation system: moving toward evidence-based transplantation policy. *Liver Transpl* 8: 851-8

Gerlach JC, Hout M, Edsbagge J, Bjorquist P, Lubberstedt M, et al. 2010. Dynamic 3D culture promotes spontaneous embryonic stem cell differentiation in vitro. *Tissue Eng Part C Methods* 16: 115-21

Gerlach JC, Zeilinger K, Patzer Ii JF. 2008. Bioartificial liver systems: why, what, whither? *Regen Med* 3: 575-95

Ghodsizadeh A, Taei A, Totonchi M, Seifinejad A, Gourabi H, et al. 2010. Generation of liver disease-specific induced pluripotent stem cells along with efficient differentiation to functional hepatocyte-like cells. *Stem Cell Rev* 6: 622-32

Gilchrist ES, Plevris JN. 2010. Bone marrow-derived stem cells in liver repair: 10 years down the line. *Liver Transpl* 16: 118-29

Goodell MA. 2003. Stem-cell "plasticity": befuddled by the muddle. *Curr Opin Hematol* 10: 208-13

Hamazaki T, Iiboshi Y, Oka M, Papst PJ, Meacham AM, et al. 2001. Hepatic maturation in differentiating embryonic stem cells in vitro. *FEBS Lett* 497: 15-9

Haouzi D, Baghdiguian S, Granier G, Travo P, Mangeat P, Hibner U. 2005. Three-dimensional polarization sensitizes hepatocytes to Fas/CD95 apoptotic signalling. *J Cell Sci* 118: 2763-73

Hay DC, Fletcher J, Payne C, Terrace JD, Gallagher RC, et al. 2008a. Highly efficient differentiation of hESCs to functional hepatic endoderm requires ActivinA and Wnt3α signaling. *Proc Natl Acad Sci U S A* 105: 12301-6

Hay DC, Zhao D, Fletcher J, Hewitt ZA, McLean D, et al. 2008b. Efficient differentiation of hepatocytes from human embryonic stem cells exhibiting markers recapitulating liver development in vivo. *Stem Cells* 26: 894-902

Ishii T, Yasuchika K, Fujii H, Hoppo T, Baba S, et al. 2005. In vitro differentiation and maturation of mouse embryonic stem cells into hepatocytes. *Exp Cell Res* 309: 68-77

Ito Y, Matsui T, Kamiya A, Kinoshita T, Miyajima A. 2000. Retroviral gene transfer of signaling molecules into murine fetal hepatocytes defines distinct roles for the STAT3 and ras pathways during hepatic development. *Hepatology* 32: 1370-6

Itskovitz-Eldor J, Schuldiner M, Karsenti D, Eden A, Yanuka O, et al. 2000. Differentiation of human embryonic stem cells into embryoid bodies compromising the three embryonic germ layers. *Mol Med* 6: 88-95

Jochheim A, Cieslak A, Hillemann T, Cantz T, Scharf J, et al. 2003. Multi-stage analysis of differential gene expression in BALB/C mouse liver development by high-density microarrays. *Differentiation* 71: 62-72

Jung J, Zheng M, Goldfarb M, Zaret KS. 1999. Initiation of mammalian liver development from endoderm by fibroblast growth factors. *Science* 284: 1998-2003

Kamiya A, Kinoshita T, Ito Y, Matsui T, Morikawa Y, et al. 1999. Fetal liver development requires a paracrine action of oncostatin M through the gp130 signal transducer. *Embo J* 18: 2127-36

Kamiya A, Kinoshita T, Miyajima A. 2001. Oncostatin M and hepatocyte growth factor induce hepatic maturation via distinct signaling pathways. *FEBS Lett* 492: 90-4

Kono Y, Yang S, Roberts EA. 1997. Extended primary culture of human hepatocytes in a collagen gel sandwich system. *In Vitro Cell Dev Biol Anim* 33: 467-72

Kubo A, Shinozaki K, Shannon JM, Kouskoff V, Kennedy M, et al. 2004. Development of definitive endoderm from embryonic stem cells in culture. *Development* 131: 1651-62

Kumashiro Y, Asahina K, Ozeki R, Shimizu-Saito K, Tanaka Y, et al. 2005. Enrichment of hepatocytes differentiated from mouse embryonic stem cells as a transplantable source. *Transplantation* 79: 550-7

LaBrecque D. 1994. Liver regeneration: a picture emerges from the puzzle. *Am J Gastroenterol* 89: S86-96

Lagasse E, Connors H, Al-Dhalimy M, Reitsma M, Dohse M, et al. 2000. Purified hematopoietic stem cells can differentiate into hepatocytes in vivo. *Nat Med* 6: 1229-34

Lavon N, Benvenisty N. 2005. Study of hepatocyte differentiation using embryonic stem cells. *J Cell Biochem* 96: 1193-202

Leder A, Leder P. 1975. Butyric acid, a potent inducer of erythroid differentiation in cultured erythroleukemic cells. *Cell* 5: 319-22

Lemaigre F, Zaret KS. 2004. Liver development update: new embryo models, cell lineage control, and morphogenesis. *Curr Opin Genet Dev* 14: 582-90

Lemaigre FP. 2003. Development of the biliary tract. *Mech Dev* 120: 81-7

Li Y, Huang G, Diakur J, Wiebe LI. 2008. Targeted delivery of macromolecular drugs: asialoglycoprotein receptor (ASGPR) expression by selected hepatoma cell lines used in antiviral drug development. *Curr Drug Deliv* 5: 299-302

Lubet RA, Mayer RT, Cameron JW, Nims RW, Burke MD, et al. 1985. Dealkylation of pentoxyresorufin: a rapid and sensitive assay for measuring induction of cytochrome(s) P-450 by phenobarbital and other xenobiotics in the rat. *Arch Biochem Biophys* 238: 43-8

Mavri-Damelin D, Damelin LH, Eaton S, Rees M, Selden C, Hodgson HJ. 2008. Cells for bioartificial liver devices: the human hepatoma-derived cell line C3A produces urea but does not detoxify ammonia. *Biotechnol Bioeng* 99: 644-51

McLean AB, D'Amour KA, Jones KL, Krishnamoorthy M, Kulik MJ, et al. 2007. Activin a efficiently specifies definitive endoderm from human embryonic stem cells only when phosphatidylinositol 3-kinase signaling is suppressed. *Stem Cells* 25: 29-38

McLin VA, Rankin SA, Zorn AM. 2007. Repression of Wnt/beta-catenin signaling in the anterior endoderm is essential for liver and pancreas development. *Development* 134: 2207-17

Medine CN, Greenhough S, Hay DC. 2010. Role of stem-cell-derived hepatic endoderm in human drug discovery. *Biochem Soc Trans* 38: 1033-6

Meehan RR, Barlow DP, Hill RE, Hogan BL, Hastie ND. 1984. Pattern of serum protein gene expression in mouse visceral yolk sac and foetal liver. *Embo J* 3: 1881-5

Michalopoulos GK, Bowen WC, Mule K, Luo J. 2003. HGF-, EGF-, and dexamethasone-induced gene expression patterns during formation of tissue in hepatic organoid cultures. *Gene Expr* 11: 55-75

Micsenyi A, Tan X, Sneddon T, Luo JH, Michalopoulos GK, Monga SP. 2004. Beta-catenin is temporally regulated during normal liver development. *Gastroenterology* 126: 1134-46

Miki T, Ring A, Gerlach J. 2011. Hepatic differentiation of human embryonic stem cells is promoted by three-dimensional dynamic perfusion culture conditions. *Tissue Eng Part C Methods* 17: 557-68

Monga SP, Monga HK, Tan X, Mule K, Pediaditakis P, Michalopoulos GK. 2003. Beta-catenin antisense studies in embryonic liver cultures: role in proliferation, apoptosis, and lineage specification. *Gastroenterology* 124: 202-16

Ochiya T, Yamamoto Y, Banas A. 2009. Commitment of stem cells into functional hepatocytes. *Differentiation*

Pelton RW, Saxena B, Jones M, Moses HL, Gold LI. 1991. Immunohistochemical localization of TGF beta 1, TGF beta 2, and TGF beta 3 in the mouse embryo: expression patterns suggest multiple roles during embryonic development. *J Cell Biol* 115: 1091-105

Raynaud P, Carpentier R, Antoniou A, Lemaigre FP. 2011. Biliary differentiation and bile duct morphogenesis in development and disease. *Int J Biochem Cell Biol* 43: 245-56

Rifkind RA, Chui D, Epler H. 1969. An ultrastructural study of early morphogenetic events during the establishment of fetal hepatic erythropoiesis. *J Cell Biol* 40: 343-65

Ring A, Gerlach J, Peters G, Pazin BJ, Minervini CF, et al. 2010. Hepatic Maturation of Human Fetal Hepatocytes in Four-Compartment Three-Dimensional Perfusion Culture. *Tissue Eng Part C Methods*

Roberts DJ. 2000. Molecular mechanisms of development of the gastrointestinal tract. *Dev Dyn* 219: 109-20

Rossi JM, Dunn NR, Hogan BL, Zaret KS. 2001. Distinct mesodermal signals, including BMPs from the septum transversum mesenchyme, are required in combination for hepatogenesis from the endoderm. *Genes Dev* 15: 1998-2009

Saito K, Yoshikawa M, Ouji Y, Moriya K, Nishiofuku M, et al. 2006. Promoted differentiation of cynomolgus monkey ES cells into hepatocyte-like cells by co-culture with mouse fetal liver-derived cells. *World J Gastroenterol* 12: 6818-27

Schaffler A, Buchler C. 2007. Concise review: adipose tissue-derived stromal cells--basic and clinical implications for novel cell-based therapies. *Stem Cells* 25: 818-27

Schier AF. 2003. Nodal signaling in vertebrate development. *Annu Rev Cell Dev Biol* 19: 589-621

Schuldiner M, Yanuka O, Itskovitz-Eldor J, Melton DA, Benvenisty N. 2000. Effects of eight growth factors on the differentiation of cells derived from human embryonic stem cells. *Proc Natl Acad Sci U S A* 97: 11307-12

Schwartz RE, Linehan JL, Painschab MS, Hu WS, Verfaillie CM, Kaufman DS. 2005. Defined conditions for development of functional hepatic cells from human embryonic stem cells. *Stem Cells Dev* 14: 643-55

Shen MM. 2007. Nodal signaling: developmental roles and regulation. *Development* 134: 1023-34

Shirahashi H, Wu J, Yamamoto N, Catana A, Wege H, et al. 2004. Differentiation of human and mouse embryonic stem cells along a hepatocyte lineage. *Cell Transplant* 13: 197-211

Soto-Gutierrez A, Kobayashi N, Rivas-Carrillo JD, Navarro-Alvarez N, Zhao D, et al. 2006a. Reversal of mouse hepatic failure using an implanted liver-assist device containing ES cell-derived hepatocytes. *Nat Biotechnol* 24: 1412-9

Soto-Gutierrez A, Navarro-Alvarez N, Rivas-Carrillo JD, Chen Y, Yamatsuji T, et al. 2006b. Differentiation of human embryonic stem cells to hepatocytes using deleted variant of HGF and poly-amino-urethane-coated nonwoven polytetrafluoroethylene fabric. *Cell Transplant* 15: 335-41

Soto-Gutierrez A, Navarro-Alvarez N, Zhao D, Rivas-Carrillo JD, Lebkowski J, et al. 2007. Differentiation of mouse embryonic stem cells to hepatocyte-like cells by co-culture with human liver nonparenchymal cell lines. *Nat Protoc* 2: 347-56

Stenvers KL, Tursky ML, Harder KW, Kountouri N, Amatayakul-Chantler S, et al. 2003. Heart and liver defects and reduced transforming growth factor beta2 sensitivity in transforming growth factor beta type III receptor-deficient embryos. *Mol Cell Biol* 23: 4371-85

Strizzi L, Bianco C, Normanno N, Salomon D. 2005. Cripto-1: a multifunctional modulator during embryogenesis and oncogenesis. *Oncogene* 24: 5731-41

Strom SC, Bruzzone P, Cai H, Ellis E, Lehmann T, et al. 2006. Hepatocyte transplantation: clinical experience and potential for future use. *Cell Transplant* 15 Suppl 1: S105-10

Strom SC, Fisher RA, Thompson MT, Sanyal AJ, Cole PE, et al. 1997. Hepatocyte transplantation as a bridge to orthotopic liver transplantation in terminal liver failure. *Transplantation* 63: 559-69.

Strom SC, Jirtle RL, Jones RS, Novicki DL, Rosenberg MR, et al. 1982. Isolation, culture, and transplantation of human hepatocytes. *J Natl Cancer Inst* 68: 771-8

Sullivan GJ, Hay DC, Park IH, Fletcher J, Hannoun Z, et al. 2010. Generation of functional human hepatic endoderm from human induced pluripotent stem cells. *Hepatology* 51: 329-35

Suzuki A, Zheng Y, Kondo R, Kusakabe M, Takada Y, et al. 2000. Flow-cytometric separation and enrichment of hepatic progenitor cells in the developing mouse liver. *Hepatology* 32: 1230-9

Tada S, Era T, Furusawa C, Sakurai H, Nishikawa S, et al. 2005. Characterization of mesendoderm: a diverging point of the definitive endoderm and mesoderm in embryonic stem cell differentiation culture. *Development* 132: 4363-74

Takahashi K, Tanabe K, Ohnuki M, Narita M, Ichisaka T, et al. 2007. Induction of pluripotent stem cells from adult human fibroblasts by defined factors. *Cell* 131: 861-72

Takahashi K, Yamanaka S. 2006. Induction of pluripotent stem cells from mouse embryonic and adult fibroblast cultures by defined factors. *Cell* 126: 663-76

Tateno C, Yoshizane Y, Saito N, Kataoka M, Utoh R, et al. 2004. Near completely humanized liver in mice shows human-type metabolic responses to drugs. *Am J Pathol* 165: 901-12

Teratani T, Yamamoto H, Aoyagi K, Sasaki H, Asari A, et al. 2005. Direct hepatic fate specification from mouse embryonic stem cells. *Hepatology*

Thomson JA, Itskovitz-Eldor J, Shapiro SS, Waknitz MA, Swiergiel JJ, et al. 1998. Embryonic stem cell lines derived from human blastocysts. *Science* 282: 1145-7.

Thuluvath PJ, Guidinger MK, Fung JJ, Johnson LB, Rayhill SC, Pelletier SJ. 2010. Liver transplantation in the United States, 1999-2008. *Am J Transplant* 10: 1003-19

Tian T, Meng AM. 2006. Nodal signals pattern vertebrate embryos. *Cell Mol Life Sci* 63: 672-85

Touboul T, Hannan NR, Corbineau S, Martinez A, Martinet C, et al. 2010. Generation of functional hepatocytes from human embryonic stem cells under chemically defined conditions that recapitulate liver development. *Hepatology* 51: 1754-65

Treichel U, Schreiter T, Meyer zum Buschenfelde KH, Stockert RJ. 1995. High-yield purification and characterization of human asialoglycoprotein receptor. *Protein Expr Purif* 6: 251-5

Vincent SD, Dunn NR, Hayashi S, Norris DP, Robertson EJ. 2003. Cell fate decisions within the mouse organizer are governed by graded Nodal signals. *Genes Dev* 17: 1646-62

Vinci B, Duret C, Klieber S, Gerbal-Chaloin S, Sa-Cunha A, et al. 2011. Modular bioreactor for primary human hepatocyte culture: Medium flow stimulates expression and activity of detoxification genes. *Biotechnol J* 6: 554-64

Wagers AJ, Weissman IL. 2004. Plasticity of adult stem cells. *Cell* 116: 639-48

Xu C, Li CY, Kong AN. 2005. Induction of phase I, II and III drug metabolism/transport by xenobiotics. *Arch Pharm Res* 28: 249-68

Yamaguchi K, Murai T, Yabuuchi H, Hui SP, Kurosawa T. 2010. Measurement of bile salt export pump transport activities using a fluorescent bile acid derivative. *Drug Metab Pharmacokinet* 25: 214-9

Yamamoto H, Quinn G, Asari A, Yamanokuchi H, Teratani T, et al. 2003. Differentiation of embryonic stem cells into hepatocytes: biological functions and therapeutic application. *Hepatology* 37: 983-93

Yin Y, Lim YK, Salto-Tellez M, Ng SC, Lin CS, Lim SK. 2002. AFP(+), ESC-derived cells
        engraft and differentiate into hepatocytes in vivo. *Stem Cells* 20: 338-46
Yoshie S, Shirasawa S, Yokoyama T, Kanoh Y, Takei S, et al. 2010. Lanford medium
        induces high quality hepatic lineage cell differentiation directly from mouse
        embryonic stem cell-derived mesendoderm. *Biochem Biophys Res Commun* 391:
        1477-82
Zaret KS. 1996. Molecular genetics of early liver development. *Annu Rev Physiol* 58: 231-51
Zhao R, Duncan SA. 2005. Embryonic development of the liver. *Hepatology* 41: 956-67

4

Stem Cells for HUMAN Hepatic Tissue Engineering

N.I. Nativ[1], M.A. Ghodbane[1], T.J. Maguire[1],
F. Berthiaume[1] and M.L. Yarmush[1,2]

[1]Department of Biomedical Engineering, Rutgers University, Piscataway, NJ
[2]Center for Engineering in Medicine, Massachusetts General Hospital
USA

1. Introduction

1.1 Clinical implications

End-stage liver disease is a life-threatening condition for which the only effective medical treatment available to date is orthotropic liver transplantation. Other approaches are needed because of the severe shortage of donors. These alternatives include cell transplantation and extracorporeal bioartificial livers. Since adult hepatocytes do not readily proliferate in culture, and healthy human livers are used to meet transplantation needs and are therefore not available for other purposes, a major challenge for these cell-based therapies is to identify a reliable hepatocyte source[1]. In the case of extracorporeal devices, many have suggested the use of animal sources (e.g. rat and pig), where immunoisolation may be possible. This is not likely to be a viable option for cell implantable modalities since these implants must be vascularized to function properly, and as a result would be exposed to xenogeneic immune rejection[2]. An increasingly plausible approach is the use of hepatocytes derived from embryonic stem cells (ESCs), as recent studies – reviewed in greater detail below – show that it is possible to differentiate ESCs into hepatocyte-like cells with high yields. Furthermore, recent developments with induced pluripotent stem cells (iPSCs) suggest that many of the procedures used to differentiate ESCs could be used on iPSCs, thus making it possible to derive patient-specific syngeneic hepatocytes. Besides therapeutic applications, hepatocytes derived from human ESCs can be used for a variety of other applications, such as toxicity drug screening, where the use of human cells is much preferred compared to animal cells that often vary in sensitivity and metabolism of xenobiotics and drugs.

1.2 Industrial implications

One of the fundamental challenges facing the development of new chemical entities within the pharmaceutical industry is the extrapolation of key in vivo parameters from in vitro cell culture assays and animal studies. Development of microscale devices and screening assays incorporating primary human cells can potentially provide better, faster and more efficient prediction of in vivo toxicity and clinical drug performance[3]. With this goal in mind, large strides have been made in the area of microfluidics to provide in vitro surrogates that are designed to mimic the physiological architecture and dynamics. Current embodiments of this synergy cover various microelectromechanical (MEMs) devices that contain hepatocytes, for use in drug metabolism screening and toxicology assessment.

1.3 Liver function and structure

The liver, a key metabolic and detoxification center, contains parenchymal cells called hepatocytes (70%) and various nonparenchymal cell types such as sinusoidal endothelial cells, stellate (fat-storing, Ito) cells, Kupffer cells, and cholangiocytes (bile duct cells). Hepatocytes are responsible for most liver-specific functions, including albumin synthesis, detoxification of ammonia into urea and glutamine, bile and cholesterol production [4]. The liver is also critical for maintaining circulating glucose levels via gluconeogenesis during fasting. A large array of enzymes is responsible for the detoxification of organic compounds, either endogenous (such as many hormones) or exogenous (drugs and toxins) via two sequential mechanisms described as Phase I and Phase II biotransformations. There is an extensive body of literature that has shown that controlling environmental parameters, in other words the culture conditions, which consist of the type of substrate used, spatial orientation of the cultured cells, addition of growth factors, and the combinatorial effects of these parameters, is critically important to induce and maintain a high level of hepatocellular viability and function[5]. The functional and structural complexity of the liver organ has been very difficult to reproduce ex vivo in hepatocyte culture systems. Some of these challenges have been partially met using novel cell culture approaches as well as microfabrication techniques that can emulate the size scales of the liver sinusoid. While all of these studies describe various techniques to boost in vitro hepatocyte function, they do not resolve the limited access to primary hepatocytes, which do not proliferate to any significant degree outside of the liver[1]. This is crucial because despite modifications in the culture environment, large numbers of mature hepatocytes are needed, and yet, are not available, for clinical applicability. Herein, we focus primarily on the challenge of securing a sufficient supply of high functioning hepatocytes for clinical and industrial applications using a stem cell differentiation platform.

1.4 Adult stem cells

To address cell source issues more effectively, research into alternate hepatocyte precursor populations has been conducted. Unlike differentiated cells, hepatoblasts are not only capable of expressing differentiated function, but are also able to self-renew. A few hepatoblasts have been identified that have the capacity to differentiate into mature hepatocytes and include bipotential precursors for hepatocytes and biliary cells, and hematopoietic stem cells [6].

In scenarios following severe hepatic injury, liver regeneration is attributed to a potential stem cell compartment located within the smallest branches of the intrahepatic biliary tree, which gives rise to the bipotential cells known as oval cells [7]; [8]. Oval cells are characterized as small cells with a high nucleus-to-cytoplasm ratio, oval shaped nucleus, and the ability to express markers of both fetal hepatocytes and biliary cells [9]; [10]. Oval cells have been shown to require growth factors such as transforming growth factor alpha (TGFα), epidermal growth factor (EGF), and hepatocyte growth factor (HGF) for progression through the cell cycle as well and subsequent differentiation toward mature hepatocytes [11]. Despite the large number of observations describing liver growth processes driven by oval cell proliferation and differentiation into hepatocytes, oval cells are difficult to isolate and the molecular mechanisms behind these processes must still be elucidated.

Hematopoietic stem cells (HSCs) have also been induced to differentiate along hepatocyte specific pathways. For example, one experimental system utilized HSC transplantation to alleviate liver disease in fumarylacetoacetate hydrolase (FAH) deficient mice [12]. FAH deficiency leads to liver dysfunction and eventual lethality. Following HSC transplantation, liver function was reconstituted. However, it is unclear whether the HSCs or HSC progeny that repopulated the liver. In addition, the mechanism that induces differentiation toward mature hepatocytes is unclear.

Despite the fact that hepatoblasts exhibit the potential to provide a renewable hepatocyte cell source, these cells are hard to isolate and exist in very low numbers [13]. In addition, the full efficacy of utilizing these precursor cells is questionable, since the long-term functional stability of hepatocytes obtained from these systems has yet to be assessed.

2. Embryonic stem cells and induced pluripotent stem cells

There are multiple stem cell starting paths for hepatocytes: 1. ESCs, 2. iPSCs, 3. Endoderm precursors and 4. Hepatic stem cells. However, due to their robust nature and large body of literature, we will focus on the first two. Furthermore these two cell types are readily abundant and have a higher proliferative capacity, thereby providing a strong potential starting point for the aforementioned applications.

2.0.1 Embryonic stem cells (ES cells)

Embryonic stem cells, derived from the inner cell mass of the blastocyst [14], have been proposed as another potential source for the generation of mature hepatocytes. ES cells are pluripotent and can be induced to differentiate into any cell type. When cultured in the presence of an anti-differentiation agent such as leukemia inhibitory factor (LIF) and with or without a feeder layer, these cells can proliferate while maintaining pluripotency [15]. Upon removal of the anti-differentiation agent, ES cells begin to spontaneously differentiate.

2.0.2 Induced pluripotent stem cells (iPS cells)

A new area of research has developed in recent years, majorly in part due to the legislative restrictions certain countries have placed on ES cell research. One area that has shown strong advancement is the area of induced pluripotent stem cells (iPS cells). iPS cells are the result of reprogramming somatic cells to a pluripotent state which resemble ES cells with respect to morphology, proliferation (self- renewal), surface antigens, gene expression, epigenetic status of pluripotent cell-specific genes, epigenomics and telomerase activity [16, 17]. Human iPS cells' autologous nature offers several advantages over human ES cells in regards to potential patient specific therapeutics, the study of disease state, study of developmental processes, drug discovery as well as drug toxicity on differentiated hepatocytes while avoiding the ethical issues associated with isolation and the usage of human ES cells as illustrated in Figure 1.

Yamanaka coined the term induced pluripotent stem cells in 2006 while inducing a pluripotent state in mouse somatic cells by direct reprogramming [16]. The same year, his lab demonstrated the generation of induced pluripotent stem cells from adult human

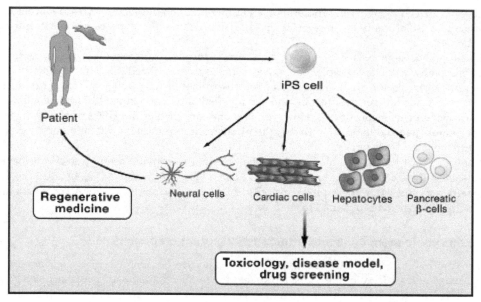

Fig. 1. **Applications of IPS Cell Technology**
Patient-derived iPS cells can produce various somatic cells with the same genetic
information as the patient. These cells could be used to construct disease models and to
screen for effective and safe drugs, as well as to treat patients through cell transplantation
therapy. (Figure taken from [20], figure 1)

fibroblasts by retroviral transfection of four factors: Oct3/4, Sox2, c-Myc and Klf4 [16, 18].
Since then, others have generated human iPS cells using different combination of factors
while preserving Oct3/4 and Sox2 as the core factors needed for pluripotency
reprogramming while Oct3/4 is the most important[19, 20]. The main risk associated with
the use of human iPS derived cells for transplantation is directly influenced by the iPS
generation methods which may involve risk of DNA modification (gene deletion, viral gene
incorporating into the human genome and gene expression alterations) which may lead to
insertional mutations that will affect iPS function, differentiation potential and
tumorigenesis [20, 21]. The human iPS cells generated by the Yamanaka group, for example,
had more than 20 retroviral integration sites in total which may increase tumor formation
[16, 18]. That risk has accelerated the search for new methods for generating clinically safer
iPS cells such as the use of non-integrating episomal vectors or the use of molecules that
promote or enhance reprogramming of somatic cells to iPS cells to improve reprogramming
efficiency and reduce genomic alterations due to viral integration [21, 22].

2.0.3 Induced pluripotent stem cells are similar, but not identical to embryonic stem cells

Although iPS cells share similar features with ES cells as mentioned above, they are not
identical. The reprogramming process does not involve genetic transformation but rather an
epigenomic one. Lister et al. have shown that iPSCs are not identical to ESCs with respect to
epigenomic profile by profiling whole-genome DNA methylation at single-base resolution

in five human iPSC lines, along with methylomes of ES cells, somatic cells, and differentiated iPSCs and ES cells [17]. In addition, iPSCs maintain some epigenomic features which resemble the somatic cell they have been generated from [17]. Cell memory based on epigenomics may suggest that, for example, iPSCs which were generated from primary hepatocytes as a somatic cell source will yield more or better functioning iPSC derived hepatocytes compared to those generated from iPSCs which were generated from fibroblasts as a somatic cell source. These discrepancies between human ES and iPS cells led to the question of what is the difference between the two stem cell types in regards to pluripotency and differentiation potential? And what is the best method to assess it? The ultimate test for pluripotency in the mouse system is the generation of a chimeric mouse which was successfully generated by blastocyst microinjection of mouse ES and iPS cells. Obviously, this test is not applicable to human ES and iPS cells and, therefore, other methods are being used to determine the pluripotency of the cells such as teratoma formation. As in the case of human ES cells, human iPS cells have the potential to differentiate to any of the three germ layers and form teratomas when transplanted subcutaneously into a severe combined immunodefficient (SCID) mouse [16, 18]. Unfortunately, teratoma formation does not guarantee full reprogramming as many mouse ES cell-like cell lines form teratomas but fail to produce germline chimeras [20]. The ultimate method to assess the differentiation potential of human ES and iPS cells to mature and functional hepatocytes is to compare the two with respect to mature hepatocytes gene and protein expression profiles, as well as metabolic activity, drug clearance, glycogen storage, urea and albumin synthesis and secretion while using the same differentiation method.

In addition to the functionality of the differentiated hepatocytes, the efficiency of the process is of high importance due to the potential of human ESCs and iPSCs to differentiate spontaneously into cells from the three germ layers. Complete differentiation of stem cells in vitro is especially important when used for cell based therapies. Heterogeneous populations at the end of the differentiation process composed of differentiated cells as well as stem cells may lead to teratoma formation at the site of transplantation as well at other locations to which the cells migrated.

2.1 Traditional embryonic stem cell and induced pluripotent stem cell differentiation paradigms

Many paradigms currently exist to specifically direct the differentiation of embryonic stem cells toward a hepatocyte lineage in vitro, while utilizing the knowledge of embryological pathways occurring in vivo during normal liver development. This process involves numerous stages and is influenced by cytokines as well as cell-matrix interactions in a temporal and spatial manner. When developing new paradigms for direct differentiation of human ES and iPS cells into mature and functional hepatocytes in vitro with high efficiency, one must refer to the developmental process of the liver during embryonic development.

2.1.1 Hepatocyte differentiation during embryogenesis

The main stages are illustrated in Figure 2A. In the first phase, ES cells differentiate to endodermal cells. ES and iPS cells are pluripotent and therefore can give rise to any of the three germ layers: ectoderm, mesoderm and endoderm where the latter, more specifically the anterior- ventral definitive endoderm, give rise to the cells of the liver. The expression of

Wnt signaling inhibitors in the anterior endoderm represses the Wnt/β catenin pathway and was shown to be required for liver specification in the endoderm [23]. Signaling by the transforming growth factor beta (TGFβ) growth factor Nodal at relatively high concentrations initiates endoderm formation. Nodal signaling stimulates the expression of a core group of endoderm transcription factors including the HMG domain DNA-binding factor Sox17 and the fork head domain proteins Foxa1–3 (HNF3a/β/γ) which in turn regulate a cascade of genes committing cells to the endoderm lineage [24]. FoxA2 and GATA4 serve as transcription factors for the alb1 gene which encodes for serum albumin and appear early in the pre-liver hepatic domain of ventral foregut endoderm and later in liver [25, 26].

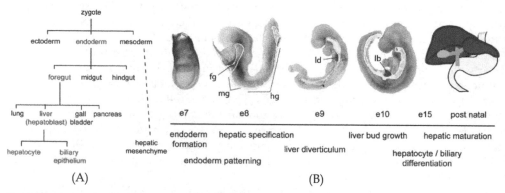

Fig. 2. **Embryonic development of the liver.**
(A) Development of the liver is illustrated from the standpoint of cellular differentiation (red) from uncommitted endoderm to functional adult hepatocytes and biliary epithelium.
(B) The schematic shows mouse embryos at different stages of development with the endoderm tissue highlighted in yellow, the liver in red, and the gall bladder in green. The major developmental events are listed below. The endoderm germ layer is formed during gastrulation (e6.5-e7.5). Throughout gastrulation and early somite stages of development (e7-e8.5) the endoderm is patterned along the A-P axis into foregut (fg) midgut (mg) and hindgut (hg) progenitor domains. Morphogenesis forms foregut and hindgut pockets as the endodermal cup is transformed into a gut tube. By e8.5 hepatic fate specified in a portion of the ventral foregut endoderm adjacent to the heart. As the embryo grows the endoderm forms a gut tube and the liver domain moves to the midgut. The liver diverticulum (ld) forms by e9 and expands into an obvious liver bud (lb) by e10. The liver grows, and by e15 hepatoblasts are differentiating into hepatocyte and biliary cells. Final maturation of the liver is gradual and continues into the postnatal period.
(Figure taken from[74], figures 1 and 2)

In the second phase, we see the differentiation from definitive to hepatic endoderm. The onset of liver development is characterized by the commitment of midgut endoderm to become liver through interactions with cardiac mesoderm which secrete fibroblast growth factors (FGFs) [27]. FGFs signaling in the foregut endoderm activated the MAPK pathway is necessary for initiation and stabilization of hepatic differentiation [28]. Bone morphogenetic proteins (BMPs) (BMP2, BMP4, BMP5, and BMP7) signaling from the septum transversum mesenchyme also contributes to hepatic gene induction in the endoderm [29-32]. Wnt signaling along this stage is suppressed but is required in the following stage where the hepatic endoderm outgrows into the liver bud[23]. In addition, HNF3β and activin A signaling are involved in the process of the specification from endodermal stem cells toward the hepatic epithelial lineages as indicated in Figures 2 and 3 [31, 32]. Under the influence of these signals, endodermal cells (the liver bud) migrate from the ventral foregut into the extracellular matrix (ECM) rich septum traversum, forming the primordial hepatoblasts. This migration is accompanied by major remodeling of the extracellular matrix surrounding the hepatic cells. Some investigators have tried to induce this process in vitro by differentiating ES and iPS cells using various types and configurations of ECM [33].

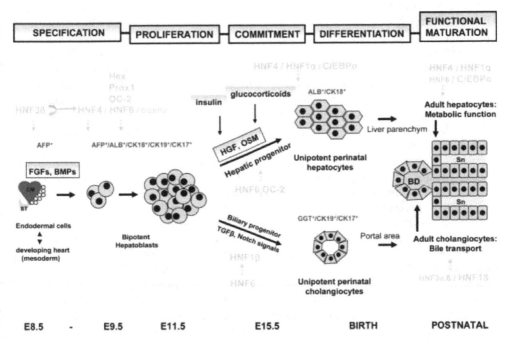

Fig. 3. **Schematic presentation of fetal liver development.** The establishment of a fully functional liver architecture is not accomplished before postnatal stages and follows upon a sequential array of tightly regulated intra- and extracellular signaling pathways, including liver-enriched transcription factors (LETFs) and growth factors, cytokines, glucocorticoids and hormones, respectively. To distinguish the level of expression and/or regulating role among diverse LETFs, different letter sizes are used. Abbreviations: ALB, albumin; AFP, alpha-fetoprotein, BMP, bone morphogenic proteins; C/EBP, CCAAT enhancer binding protein; CK, cytokeratin; CM, cardiogenic mesoderm; E, embryonic day in rodent liver development; FGF, fibroblast growth factors; GGT, c-glutamyltransferase; HGF, hepatocyte growth factor; HNF, hepatocyte nuclear factor; OC-2, Onecut transcription factor; ST, septum transversum; TGF, transforming growth factor. (Figure taken from[31], figure 2)

In the third phase, the liver primordium is induced to invade the septum transversum, giving rise to fetal hepatocytes (primordial hepatoblasts) which are bi-potent and may proliferate of later differentiate into hepatocytes and cholangiocytes (biliary cells). Markers of hepatoblasts inherent in this phase are GATA4, HNF4alpha, HNF6, hepatic alpha-fetoprotein [AFP], albumin [ALB], and biliary cytokeratin (CK 17/CK19) [29, 30, 32].

Hematopoietic stem cells (HSCs) colonize the liver bud, thereby emitting a growth signal for the liver. Hematopoietic tissue and hepatoplasts subsequently release additional growth factors to further develop both tissues. Hepatoblasts continue to proliferate and start expressing placental alkaline phosphatase, intermediate filament proteins (cytokeratins CK14, CK8, and CK18), c-glutamyltransferase, and later also alpha1-antitrypsin, glutathione S-transferase P, C/EBPα, lactate dehydrogenase, and muscle pyruvate kinase [29-32].

At this stage three cell populations exist: (a) hepatocyte-committed cells that exclusively express hepatocyte markers, such as AFP and ALB, (b) cholangiocyte-committed progenitor cells, expressing biliary cell markers such as CK19, and (c) a bipotential hepatoblast population, expressing both hepatic and biliary markers. Bipotential hepatoblasts then proceed through a series of maturation steps which entail proliferation, cellular growth, and functional maturation. These final in vivo steps are induced by various extracellular signals such as: (1) dexamethasone, which induces albumin production and downregulates alpha-fetal protein production; (2) transforming growth factor beta, which inhibits hepatocyte proliferation and increases albumin production; (3) oncostatin M, mostly produced by HSCs, which induces tight cell-cell contacts, necessary for maximum differentiated hepatocyte function, maintenance of albumin production, and upregulation of other various hepatocyte functions; (4) HGF, excreted by mesenchymal cells or nonparenchymal liver cells, antagonizes the latter process, resulting in support of growth and differentiation of the fetal hepatocytes. The hormone insulin synergistically promotes this effect [27, 29, 31].

In parallel, the percentage of bipotent cells is markedly reduced. At this point, although cells continue to proliferate, most of them are unipotent and irreversibly committed to either the hepatic or cholangic lineage [29-32]. Complete functional hepatic maturation ultimately takes place after birth upon coassistance of HGF, produced by the surrounding nonparenchymal liver cells (sinusoidal, stellate, and endothelial cells) [27, 31]. About half of the active genes tested in the liver are bound by the transcription factor HNF4 alpha and it is suggested that it directly regulates hepatic genes and is an important transcription factor during the differentiation process of ES and iPS cells into mature hepatocytes [34, 35].

It is important to mention that mouse iPS cells exhibit full potential for fetal liver development in embryos derived solely from mouse iPS cells by tetraploid complementation compared to wild-type embryos as indicated by similar levels of hepatocyte marker mRNA and liver specific cell type protein expression levels. In addition, liver Hematoxylin and Eosin (H&E) stained sections presented a similarity in liver morphology between the two [36].

2.1.2 Induction of ES and iPS cell differentiation into hepatocyte-like cells in vitro

The resultant paradigms, taking these cues into account, can thus be broadly grouped in terms of temporal regulation through cytokine addition or spatial regulation using various extracellular matrix configurations. Various configurations for generating hepatocyte-like cells in vitro involve culturing human ES and iPS cells on extra cellular matrix and inducing differentiation with hepatocyte development stage specific factors in order to maximize the yield of cells at each stage which will determine the overall differentiation yield of the process.

As mentioned above, the first step involves the differentiation of pluripotent human ES into endodermal cells and most differentiation paradigms utilize Activin A which mimics Nodal signaling. At the end of this stage, most of the cells lost the expression of the pluripotent marker Oct4 while concomitantly gaining strong expression of definitive endoderm (DE) transcription factors Sox17, FoxA2 as well as GATA4 [36-38]. The later steps of differentiation induce endodermal like cells to differentiate into mature and fully functional hepatocytes while utilizing different ECMs and various factors for about 15 additional days [36-38].

The human ES cells exhibited a similar differentiation efficiency as human iPS cells while using the same differentiation procedure (about 81% albumin positive cells) as well as similar hepatocyte mRNA fingerprints [36] . In addition, cell properties of primary human hepatocytes such as albumin and urea secretion, as well as cytochrome CYP450 activity were similar in vitro between hepatocyte-like cells generated from human ES as well as those generated from human iPS cells, although lower compared to primary isolated hepatocytes (10 fold difference for urea and albumin secretion and 30 fold difference for CYP450 isozyme activities after phenobarbital induction) [38]. While comparing the expression of a series of genes encoding phase I and phase II hepatic enzymes between cadaveric liver samples and hepatocyte-like cells, it was indicated that the level of mRNA was similar between the ES and iPS derived hepatocyte-like cells while lower compared with adult liver samples in most cases [36]. This may indicate that differentiated cells are not mature enough and this step of the differentiation procedure demands further optimization [36, 38].

Human ES and iPS cell derived hepatocytes were shown to contribute to the liver parenchyma in vivo and were stained positive for albumin 7 days after their injection to the right lateral liver lobe of newborn mice, which exemplifies the potential of human iPS cells in regenerative medicine therapeutics [36].

2.2 Differentiation paradigms utilizing tissue engineering

A key requirement for effective tissue engineering is the cellular environment that allows the cells to maintain the functional capacity observed in the in vivo environment. Often the environment mimics some critical aspects of the in vivo setting through proper control of the materials and mechanical properties as well as the chemical milieu.

A consideration with tissue-engineered constructs is the presence of exogenous chemical and mechanical stimuli such as soluble growth and differentiation factors as well as mechanical forces (e.g., cyclic mechanical loading, fluid shear).

2.2.1 Matrix configuration

Culturing cells in various controlled three-dimensional (3D) environments has proven to be a successful differentiation technique. This is thought to be a result of mimicking the *in vivo* histoarchitecture of liver, incorporating cell-matrix interactions as well as soluble cues. Several ECMs are present in liver development. One study compared the effect of using type 1 collagen, fibronectin, laminin, and Matrigel™ on directing hepatic differentiation. Cells were cultured for 7 days in embyoid bodies (EBs) before being transferred to one of the substrates. This mimics to some extent the liver development stage where endodermal cells migrate into the ECM rich septum transversum. Type I collagen was shown to cause the greatest increase in liver specific genes, with Matrigel™ also showing a beneficial effect[39].

Therefore, one research group utilized a collagen scaffold as a 3D network for hepatic differentiation. Mouse ES cells were cultured in an EB configuration and implanted into a collagen scaffold and cultured in media containing aFGF, HGF, oncostatin M, dexamethasone, and insulin transferrin sodium selenite (ITS). Cells cultured in the 3D configuration showed gene expression of AFP, ALB, glucose 6-phosphate (G6P) and tyrosine aminotransferase (TAT) after 6 days in cultures as opposed to 12 days in an EB configuration alone. However, these cells stained positive for albumin protein, but not for the CK-18 protein. Following implantation into the median lobe of the liver of a nude mouse for 14 days, the cells stained positive for both CK-18 and albumin proteins. This result signifies that cells were not completely matured by the in vitro protocol [40]. While this study showed the advantages of 3D culture, most studies fail to demonstrate a genetic or functional advantage relative to standard monolayer differentiation protocols. Other groups have used 3D cultures to provide a configuration suitable for direct implantation, eliminating the need to remove cells from culture by using biodegradable and/or biocompatible materials. For example, one group used a polyurethane foam spheroid culture to direct differentiation of mouse ES cells. Embryoid bodies were inoculated into a block of polyurethane foam (PUF) to induce the formation of spheroids in the pores of the scaffold. Induction of hepatic differentiation was accomplished by supplementing the media with aFGF, HGF, oncostatin D, dexamethasone, and ITS. Analysis of gene expression showed the expression of endoderm markers transthyretin (TTR) and AFP as well as hepatocyte specific albumin, arginase, and tryptophan 2,3-dioxygenase (TDO) expression. Notably, ES cell derived hepatocyte like cells demonstrated ammonia clearance and albumin secretion rates within the range, albeit on the low end, of those seen for primary rat hepatocytes seeded in the PUF scaffold. However, this method of differentiation is lengthy and immature endoderm markers were still present at the end of the 30 day protocol[41]. Biodegradable polymer scaffolds have also shown to be an effective three-dimensional environment for hepatic differentiation. One study allowed ES cells to form EBs for 5 days before being mixed them with Matrigel™. The cell suspension was then seeded into a rigid polymer network comprised of poly-L-lactic acid (PLLA) and polyglycolic acid (PGA). The cells formed spheroids along the polymer fibers and were cultured for 20 days with dexamethasone, dimethyl sulfoxide (DMSO), FGF4, HGF, oncostatin M, and ITS. After the culture period, the cells showed expression of AFP, ALB, G6P, TTR, and CK-18 and the ability to secrete albumin, uptake low-density lipoprotein (LDL) and store glycogen [42].

Encapsulation of ES cells in alginate has been explored as a method for the control of hepatic differentiation. The capsules allow the diffusion of nutrient, oxygen, and growth factors into the capsules while sequestering the cells. This technique has been widely used in the past to induce stem cell differentiation and maintain hepatocyte function, making it an ideal candidate for controlled hepatic differentiation. For instance, one group encapsulated 5-day-old embryoid bodies derived from mouse ES cells in a 2% alginate solution. The media was supplemented with aFGF, HGF, oncostatin M, dexamethasone, and ITS, similar to those factors previously used by other research groups. RT-PCR analysis determined that this methods results in the expression of endoderm (AFP) and hepato-specific (ALB, Cyp7A1, TAT, TTR, and CK18) genes. The cells produced albumin and urea, but only with growth factor supplementation. If one takes a closer look at the temporal addition of growth factors in these systems, several similarities exist. FGF is usually added at early time points in order to promote differentiation of definitive endodermal cells into hepatic endoderm cells. This is almost always followed by HGF supplementation, mimicking signaling from the mesenchyme which promotes growth and differentiation of fetal hepatocytes. Lastly, oncostatin M, dexamethasone, and ITS are added, as these factors are known to promote hepatocyte maturation. Sequential supplementation therefore mimics in vivo development. In addition, ES cells are allowed to form embryoid bodies prior to being cultured in a 3D environment. This allows the formation cell-cell interactions known to increase hepatocyte function during development. Although these aforementioned methods yield hepatocyte-like cells from a functional perspective, growth factors are expensive and therefore these approaches are not amendable to scale up for clinical application.

A different approach is the use of cellular encapsulation to control lineage commitment and final maturation of murine ES cells. The novelty of this method lies in the fact that no growth factor supplementation is required to direct hepatic differentiation. This was accomplished through the manipulation cell seeding density and alginate concentration. These two variables dictate the size of cellular aggregates that form within the capsule which in turn direct differentiation. It was found that a 2.0% w/v alginate concentration and a $5x10^6$ cells/mL seeding density were the optimal parameters for hepatic differentiation [43, 44]. Genetic analysis showed the expression of a variety of Cyp450s as well as CK-18. In addition, albumin and urea secretion as well as glycogen storage were shown and reached a maximum around day 20 in culture. This method demonstrates a way to obtain a high yield of hepatocyte-like cells through inducing cell-cell interactions known to upregulate hepatocyte function during development, thus eliminating the need for growth factor supplementation. In addition, the cells can be recovered from the capsule through depolymerization without effecting cell viability. Scalability is also significant, as generating large numbers of cells would simply involve producing large batches of capsules. With all these advantages taken into consideration, this technique is amenable to the mass production of hepatocyte like cells and thus has the potential for clinical utility.

2.2.2 Coculture

A co-culture of ES cells with another cell type present during hepatic development or in the adult liver cell has been shown to induce hepatic differentiation. The supporting cell type directs the ES cells towards the hepatic lineage by introducing cues resulting from soluble factors, cell-cell interactions, or a combination of the two. Thus, this approach is performed by separating the cells with a porous membrane or with the cells in direct contact with one another. Both methods have been shown to induce hepatic differentiation of embryonic stem cells with careful choice of feeder layers. In fact, investigators often develop their own cell lines optimized to drive hepatic differentiation. For example, one group first developed a protocol to differentiate endoderm cells by culturing the cells on Matrigel™ and supplementing the media with activin A and HGF [45]. The endoderm cells were separated by fluorescence-activated cell sorting (FACS), made possible by the transfection of enhanced GFP (EGFP) under the control of an AFP promoter. The purified cells were then further exposed to a co-culture with MLSgt20 cells, a cell line cloned from fetal murine stromal cells experimentally shown to promote hepatic differentiation in ES cells [46]. Combining the results of the two studies, the AFP positive endoderm cells were contact co-cultured with the MLSgt20 cells. The co-cultured cells expressed markers for both immature (GATA4, AFP) and mature (Alb, TAT, TO, CYP3a4/7) hepatocytes at the end of the culture period. The cells also showed the ability to clear ammonia and store glycogen. However, gene expression was not identical to that of adult human liver hepatocytes [47]. A drawback of contact co-culture is that the hepatocyte like cells must be separated from the supporting cell type after the culture period. To eliminate the need for purification of differentiated cells, one group co-cultured three human liver non-parenchymal cell lines with ES cells using a transwell membrane. Mouse ES cells containing a GFP gene with and albumin promoter were cultured in suspension for 2 days to facilitate embryoid body formation. The EBs were then cultured on a poly-amino-urethane (PAU) coated non-woven polytetrafluoroethylene (PTFE) fabric that allowed the cells to adhere. The media was supplemented with basic FGF and activin A for 3 days. The ES cells were then co-cultured in Matrigel layered transwells with the human cells lines growth-arrested with mitomycin C. Cholangiocytes, liver endothelial, and hepatic stellate cell lines were chosen due to their secretion of soluble factors that have shown to be important for liver regeneration. Cholangiocytes generate IL-6 and TNF-α, liver endothelial cells produce FGF4 and vascular endothelial growth factor (VEGF) and hepatic stellate cells produce HGF. The cells were co-cultured with media supplementation of dHGF and DMSO for 8 days and dexamethasone for the final 3 days of culture. The differentiated GFP positive cells were separated by cell sorting and showed a yield of 70%. These cells expressed both hepatocyte markers as well as endoderm markers, demonstrating that the cells were not fully mature. They also stained positive for albumin and GFP, secreted albumin, and metabolized ammonia, lidocaine, and diazepam. However, albumin secretion and metabolic activity occurred at lower levels than primary mouse hepatocytes[48]. Another example of a non-contact co-culture was demonstrated using cynomolgus monkey ES cells with mouse fetal liver-derived cells to simulate the environment of the developing liver. The ES cells lost pluripotent markers and expressed AFP, ALB, CYP7A1, and HNF4α, an important transcription factor for mature hepatocytes. The cells also stained positively for AFP, albumin, alpha1AT, and HNF4α, as well as for Hep Par 1, an anti-hepatocyte antibody. Functional analysis also showed glycogen storage through Periodic acid-Schiff (PAS) staining as well as ammonia clearance[49].

While the aforementioned co-culture systems utilize non-parenchymal cells or fetal liver cells as a support cell type, the use of hepatocytes as the feeder cell type in co-culture differentiation schemes has also been attempted. Moore et al. examined the effects of co-cultivated hepatocytes on the hepatospecific differentiation of murine ES cells[50]. Hepatocytes co-cultured with cadherin-expressing ES cells markedly enhanced ES cell differentiation toward the hepatic lineage, as demonstrated by hepatic-like cuboidal morphology, heightened gene expression of the late maturation marker G6P in relation to the early marker AFP, and the intracellular localization of albumin. The effect was mediated by cadherin, since it was reversed through E-cadherin blockage and inhibited in control ES cells with reduced cadherin expression. Direct contact co-cultures of hepatocytes and ES cells maximally promoted ES cell commitment towards hepato-differentiation. This study showed that both soluble signaling and cell-cell interaction creates a synergistic effect that drives hepatic differentiation.

Cho et al. developed another co-culture method with hepatocytes[51]. A collagen gel was formed on tissue culture dishes and primary rat hepatocytes were plated after gelation. A thick collagen layer was then deposited on top of the hepatocytes. We have previously shown that this collagen sandwich hepatocyte culture maintains hepatocyte function in vitro. Murine ES cells were then seeded on the thick collagen layer and cultured in this configuration for 10 days. At this stage, the ES cells were removed from the collagen layer by dispase treatment while leaving the collagen sandwiched hepatocytes intact. RT-PCR demonstrated the presence of endoderm markers Foxa2, Sox17, and AFP and the absence of mesoderm and ectoderm markers. The presence of Foxa2 and AFP were confirmed by immunostaining, and flow cytometry showed that they were expressed in 95% of cells. In addition, the cells proliferated and stopped expressing Oct4, a marker for pluripotency. These results showed that mouse ES cells cultured on top of collagen-sandwiched hepatocytes differentiated and proliferated into a uniform and homogeneous cell population of endoderm-like cells. However, the endoderm cells did not express albumin, signifying that they had not yet committed to the hepatic lineage. To further mature the cells, they were co-cultured for 20 days with fibroblasts due to the in vivo interactions of the endoderm with the mesenchyme during development. The media was supplemented with oncostatin M, ITS, and dexamethasone. The resulting hepatocyte like cells expressed hepatospecific genes albumin, alpha-1-antitrypsin (AAT), CK-8, CK-18, TTR, and CYP2A13 and displayed morphology similar to that of primary rat hepatocytes. Immunostaining demonstrated the presence of albumin and CK-18 while functional analysis showed the cells could synthesize urea. This study showed the generation of a homogeneous population of hepatocyte-like cells from ES cells[51]. However, the drawback of this method is that two separate co-cultures are required to direct differentiation, with one feeder cell being the scarce cell type that we are trying to generate.

2.2.3 Metabolic engineering

A distinguishing feature of adult hepatocytes is the high content of mitochondria and high level of oxidative metabolism. On the contrary, ES cells contain a much smaller amount of mitochondria and produce energy mainly through the glycolytic pathway. Recent studies show that metabolic additives that promote carbon backbone oxidation can be used to help direct differentiation towards the hepatocyte lineage. One such method utilizes sodium butyrate treatment to generate an enriched population of hepatocyte-like cells from embryonic stem cell [52]. ES cells were plated on gelatin and the media was supplemented with DMSO for the first 5 days of culture. Sodium butyrate replaced DMSO for the next 6 days, and cells were replated onto collagen coated or non-coated polystyrene at various time points in order to perform metabolic analysis. Significantly higher levels of urea secretion and albumin positive cells were observed in a 2.5 mM sodium butyrate condition on both substrates. It was also shown that mitochondrial mass increased from days 5-8 in culture, which is characteristic of hepatic differentiation. However, the percentage of albumin positive and high mitochondrial activity cells was still less than mouse hepatoma cells. These results imply that these cells represent an immature hepatocyte phenotype. A subsequent study was conducted in order to further differentiate the cells into mature hepatocyte-like cells [53]. The immature cells were treated with S-NitrosoAcetylPenicillamine (SNAP), a nitric oxide donor. Nitric oxide is known to induce the synthesis of mitochondria, thus possibly facilitating a further increase of mitochondrial mass to levels seen in mature liver cells. After the 11 days of culture conditions that were found to induce partial differentiation using sodium butyrate, cells were replated on day 12 and supplemented with various dilutions of SNAP in DMSO for the next 3 days. A 500 μM concentration of SNAP significantly increased glucose consumption, lactate production, and the percentage of albumin positive cells. From a functional perspective, SNAP treatment also increased urea and albumin secretion as well as cytochrome P4507a1 activity relative to the other culture conditions. These studies demonstrate that simply altering the ES cell's metabolic activity to more closely resemble those of mature hepatocytes is an alternative strategy to developing hepatocyte-like cells. This novel method circumvents the need for media supplementation with expensive cocktails of growth factors or co-culture with another cell type.

3. Utilizing hepatocyte-like cells

Techniques aimed at obtaining a homogeneous population of hepatocyte-like cells with functional characteristics similar to native hepatocytes from ES cells are rapidly improving. As these methods progress, applications taking advantage of a constant supply of hepatocytes are being developed in parallel. One application is the use of hepatocytes for the treatment of liver failure. With the gap between those on the waiting list for a liver transplant and the organs available for transplantation growing every year, a renewable source of hepatocyte-like cells could potentially alleviate this problem. Bioartificial livers containing functional hepatocyte-like cells could be used to keep patients alive while waiting for a transplant. In addition, decellularizing livers unsuitable for transplant and reseeding them with functional cells could increase the donor pool. In conjunction, these two cutting-edge methods could reduce the number of patients who die on the waiting list. Finally, the important role the liver plays in the metabolic clearance of drugs makes hepatocytes an important research tool for the pharmaceutical industry. By including microfluidic technology, the number heaptocytes needed per assay can be greatly reduced, facilitating high-throughput screening of new chemical entities. This next section will discuss the current state of these applications of hepatocyte-like cells derived from ES cells.

3.1 Decellularized liver scaffolds for implantation

Using hepatocyte-like cells for transplantation is a potentially very exciting application. As mentioned earlier, a large gap exists between the number of patients waiting for a liver transplant and the number of available liver grafts. With this gap growing each year, an alternative source of transplantable livers is greatly needed. Although the differentiation of hepatocyte-like cells from embryonic stem cells has been accomplished through a variety of methods, creating a three-dimensional organ structure is challenging due to the nutrient and oxygen limitations that occur in the engineered tissue. The liver consists of a complex network of extracellular matrix proteins as well as microvasculature critical to organ function. One approach to provide the complex 3D environment of the liver is not to try to recreate it from scratch, but rather to use natural decellularized liver scaffolds. Data show that the native 3D matrix can promote cell engraftment, survival, and sustained hepatic function over time. In addition, by preserving the native microvasculature structure, the risk of ischemic damage or lack of perfusion is minimized. This approach has the potential of utilizing livers unsuitable for transplantation as a source of scaffolds to seed hepatocyte-like cells derived from ES cells, thereby increasing the number of livers available for transplantation.

Using the liver as a scaffold requires that the organ be decellularized while leaving the 3D architecture intact. Following decellularization, the scaffold must be reseeded with the proper cell types engrafting to their appropriate locations within the tissue to promote function. This has been accomplished by perfusing sodium dodecyl sulfate (SDS) solutions through the portal vein of a rat liver for 72 hours [54]. The result was a translucent structure free of cells which preserved the 3D architecture of the liver, Figure 4a. Most notably, the microvascular tree was preserved, as shown in Figure 4b. Using the scaffold, cells were seeded by injecting 12.5 million cells in 4 doses at 10-minute intervals. This approach resulted in a grafting efficiency greater than 90%, and perfusion of the recellularized scaffold showed 80% viability over 2 days. Since a liver consists of non-parenchymal cells as well as hepatocytes, epithelial cells were also seeded and engrafted in the lining of the vessel. Moreover, epithelial cell seeding did not affect hepatocyte viability, providing proof of concept that other cell types could also be successfully seeded. The scalability of the system was also tested, injecting a total of 200 million cells using the 4-dose approach. This cell total represents 20% of the adult rat liver mass, double the amount required to provide therapeutic benefit.

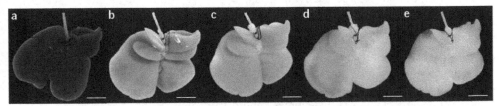

Fig. 4a. Rat liver during the decellularization process. SDS was perfused through the portal vein, leaving a translucent, cell free structure which maintained native liver architecture. From left to right, the images show the liver at 0, 18, 48, 52, and 72 hours of the SDS perfusion, respectively. (Figure taken from [54], Figure 1)

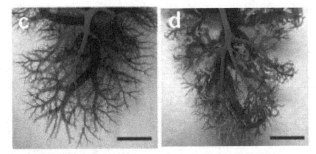

Fig. 4b. Portal (red) and venous (blue) corrosion cast of normal (left) and decellularized liver (right). Comparison of the two shows that the decellularization process preserves the native liver microvasculature. (Figure taken from [54], Figure 2)

Analysis of the reseeded hepatocytes showed gene expression similar to that of long-term stable cultures (e.g. collagen sandwich) of hepatocytes. Immunohistochemical analysis of UGT1a, G6pc, and albumin showed staining at levels comparable to adult livers. Functional analysis showed urea synthesis significantly higher that hepatocyte sandwich and similar albumin secretion rates. However, albumin production was much lower than that of adult rat livers. The recellularized liver was then transplanted into a rat for 8 hours to investigate the effect of shear stress due to blood flow. Transplantation did not affect hepatic function, viability, or morphology in any significant way. Other investigators successfully decellularized a liver and seeded the matrix with both hepatocytes and other epithelial cells

[55]. These studies demonstrate the feasibility of using a decellularized liver matrix as a scaffold for hepatocytes. The inclusion of other non-parenchymal cells and evaluation of the transplant after long periods in vivo still needs to be performed prior to bringing this approach to the bedside. This may further require the development of techniques to derive hepatic nonparenchymal cells from ES cells.

3.2 Bioartificial liver devices

The shortage of donor livers has also prompted researchers to develop bioartificial liver (BAL) devices, **Figure 5**. These devices aim to provide temporary assistance to patients with liver failure while waiting for a donor organ. Early BAL concepts were modified dialysis systems which did not incorporate living cells, [56] and were found to be limited in efficacy. Since the liver provides a host of biochemical processing and detoxification functions that are essential to life, it was thought that an effective device should contain liver parenchymal cells (e.g. hepatocytes). Cells were added to the dialysis systems, and again poor results were obtained, in this case because the bioreactor design itself did not allow for sufficient metabolite transport (especially oxygen), and as a result the cells did not function properly or even survive. Next, a support structure was built that allows for the convective and diffusive transport of plasma metabolites to and from the cells in the device [57]. Many creative operational strategies and designs exist [58]; [59]; [60], ranging from packed bed bioreactors [61, 62], to flat plate bioreactors [63]. It was found that hepatocytes can only

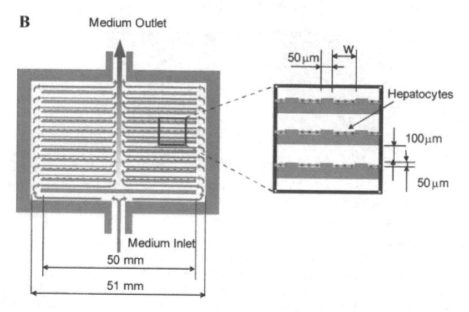

Fig. 5. **Schematic of a radial flow Bioartifical Liver Device.** Red arrows show the direction of medium flow and in blue is the location of the seeded hepatocytes. The design includes patterned microgrooves to decrease shear stress on the seeded hepatocytes. (Figure taken from [67], Figure 1)

withstand low levels of fluid shear stress, therefore in a recent modification of the flat plate geometry, cells were seeded at the bottom of grooves to allow for higher flow rates, thus increasing mass transport within the device, while keeping shear stress at the cell surface to a low level [64, 65].

The high metabolic activity of hepatocytes makes the transport of oxygen a significant technical concern in BAL devices. In fact, transport limitations have led to the loss of hepatic function over time and the failure of many BAL devices based on hollow fiber technology that have undergone clinical trials. To alleviate this issue, semi-permeable membranes have been introduced into devices to increase the oxygen tension within the device. However, a device would require a surface area of approximately 10 m^2 to provide therapeutic benefit [66]. Therefore, the incorporation of an internal membrane oxygenator would create scale up issues. To address these problems, a radial stacked plate bioreactor was developed to increase the surface area to volume ratio of the device. The design was devoid of a semi-permeable membrane and therefore required perfusion at high volumetric flow rates in order to create the necessary oxygen tension to maintain hepatocyte function. Nevertheless, hepatocytes will also lose function above a critical shear stress. Therefore, photolithographically patterned microgrooves were incorporated to shield the cells from the resulting high shear rates required for sufficient convective oxygen transport.

The requirement of high-flow rates and low shear stress is a non-trivial engineering problem. In order to examine the effect of microgrooves, computation fluid dynamics (CFD) was employed to characterize the device. CFD analysis showed that varying width of the microgrooves with the distance from the center of the bioreactor results shear stresses well below detrimental levels throughout the device. Incorporating an oxygenator within the perfusion circuit, design and operating parameters were optimized that provided sufficient convective oxygen delivery and acceptable shear stresses. These critical parameters resulted in 95% viability of hepatocytes under perfusion after 36 hours within the device. In addition, urea and albumin secretion levels were significantly higher than a flat plate bioreactor and comparable to hepatocytes co-cultures with fibroblasts. The device produced 2,100 μg of albumin per day, as compared to 19×10^5 μg/day required for a therapeutic effect. To be clinical useful, this device would need to be scaled by a factor of 905, which would allow the device to be operated without exceeding the recommended clinical priming volume[67].

As opposed to *ex vivo* bioartificial liver devices, an implantable liver assist device (LAD) has been developed by engineering a hepatic organoid. The implantable construct comprised of a PAU-coated PTFE non-woven fabric covered with a polyethylene-vinyl alcohol membrane layered with a polyester supporting fabric. Based on the method described in Section 2.2.2, human cholangiocytes, liver endothelial cells, and hepatic stellate cells were injected into an LAD coated with FGF-2 to facilitate angiogenesis. The LAD performance was evaluated through implantation into mice after a 50% hepatectomy for 7 days. While LAD with only hepatocytes did not survive, devices with non-parenchymal cells exhibited the formation of organotypic structures in the LAD similar to the liver acinus. Additionally, in vitro analysis showed that the organoid significantly improved ammonia and lidociane clearance as well as albumin secretion relative to device with seeded with hepatocytes alone. This study showed that the inclusion of non-parenchymal cells in liver assist devices has the potential of improving *in vivo* performance.

3.3 In vitro drug screening systems

According to the Pharmaceutical Research and Manufacturers of America (PhRMA) U.S. drug companies spent $62.4 billion on research and development in 2009. Studies indicate that it can cost more than $800 million, of which 80% is spent on clinical trials and development, and will take between 8 and 10 years of development to bring a new drug to market. Among candidate drugs that make it past Phase I clinical trials, 50% fail due to human toxicity and bioavailability issues. Moreover, of all candidate drugs, 90% do not make it through final stages of development. This tremendous attrition rate has not improved in recent years. To curb such costly failures, a significant amount of research has been dedicated to identifying in vitro screening systems; i.e., approaches that can be utilized in preclinical phases of discovery and development that offer greater utility in predicting in vivo subcellular and cellular physiological responses.

Currently, a majority of hepatic in vitro screening assays employed within the field of drug metabolism and pharmacokinetics (DPMK) utilize hepatocytes cultured under fully static conditions. In such assays, hepatocytes are either adhered to the bottom of a microtiter well-plate to which culture medium containing candidate drug(s) is subsequently added; or else the hepatocytes are maintained inside the microtiter well in suspension in the media. The microtiter plate is shaken to facilitate mixing and transport, but there is no means for providing a continuous flow of culture media over the cells.

The lack of continuous flow produces functional limitations in these conventional static systems when compared to microfluidic systems. The presence of flow helps regulate the concentrations of both metabolites and cellular by-products in the immediate vicinity of the hepatocytes; whereas in a static system these concentrations are ever-changing until a saturation/depletion condition is attained through accumulation, uptake, and reaction. In a flow system it is possible to maintain a pseudo steady state (equilibrium) which results in optimal working characteristics. Furthermore, in a static well the system is usually mass transport limited; flow can remedy this by the addition of convective mode of mass transport.

A variety of devices have been developed for this purpose [68-70], and in particular to determine parameters for multi-compartmental physiologically-based pharmacokinetic (PBPK) models, Figure 6. For example, a multi-tissue compartmental device has been developed that incorporates a large liver compartment for the assessment of drug absorption both in the liver as well as in other metabolizing tissue types [71-73]. More specifically, the Hµrel® Corporation has developed a liver-specific microfluidic chip that focuses on liver metabolism, with the possible application to liver toxicity assessment, Figure 7. The Hµrel® device allows for the seeding of various cell types to emulate the *in vivo* components affecting pharmacokinetics. The device consists of separate chambers, each seeded with a specific cell type. Device testing demonstrated that the flow co-culture format in the device resulted in better predictions of *in vivo* clearance rates compared to static cultures and flow-based monoculture models, across a wide range of cytochrome P450s. The reason for increased hepatocyte function when flow is incorporated is not yet known for certain. One possibility is that increased mass transport in the system leads to a thinner boundary layer in addition to faster removal of unwanted by-products, together resulting in an observed increased clearance. Regardless of the mechanism, the Hµrel® device yields an in vitro analogue to PBPK models utilizing minimal amounts of cells and drug, thus facilitating high-throughput screening of new chemical entities.

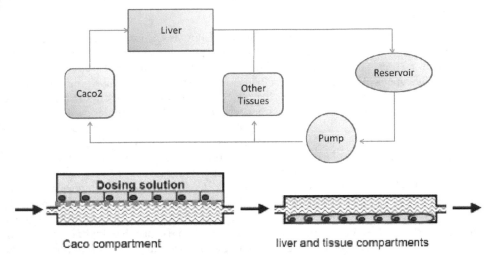

Fig. 6. **Example of multi-compartmental MEMs model utilized to determine PBPK values for use in in silico simulations.** The new chemical entity is dosed on one side of the Caco-2 cells, where it must be absorbed prior to reaching the microchannels. The absorbed drug then passes into the liver for metabolic clearance prior to being re-circulated and reaching the target tissue.

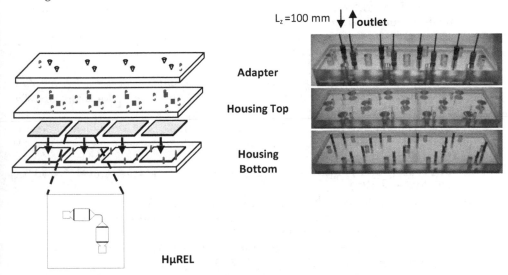

Fig. 7. **Geometry of the static and flow configurations in the HµREL® system.** The assembly of a HµREL® housing set with four biochips. The components of the chip housing and interface are, from the top – adapter, housing top, HµREL® biochips, housing bottom. The complete setup of the HµREL® prototype instrument then involves connecting inlet and outlet tubing to the adapter. The inlet tubing is then fed through a peristaltic pump, and connected to a reservoir that contains the media with the test compound of interest. The outlet tubing is also inserted into the reservoir to complete the recirculation loop. (Figure taken from [75], Figure 1)

4. Future directions

Considerable progress has been made in differentiating ESCs into liver cells; however, current protocols have not yet produced cells that express a completely adult-like mature hepatocyte. In fact, criteria that define what is an acceptable functional human stem cell-derived hepatocyte will need to be established and standardized. ESC differentiation protocols typically do not yield a pure hepatocyte population, and often times sorting protocols are needed. Methods to scale-up such protocols to the therapeutic scale of a human patient will need to be developed. There remains safety concerns (e.g. tumoregenicity) when using ESCs and iPSC for cell transplantation which cannot easily investigated in rodent models and will require further analysis in more "human-like" systems, such as nonhuman primates. On a short-term basis, human hepatocytes derived from ESCs or iPSCs may be effectively used for toxicology studies on xenobiotics as well as drug safety screening. The development of devices that contain such cells for high throughput testing is an important avenue for the future in this area, and special consideration should be taken to make such systems easy to use at the point of care or in the field. The ability to derive cells that are patient-specific provides a unique opportunity to better understand patient variability in their sensitivity to drugs as well as potentially develop individualized patient-specific drug regimens.

5. References

[1] Cho, C.H., et al., *A new technique for primary hepatocyte expansion in vitro.* Biotechnology and Bioengineering, 2008. 101(2): p. 345-356.

[2] Yagi, H., et al., *Long-Term Superior Performance of a Stem Cell/Hepatocyte Device for the Treatment of Acute Liver Failure.* Tissue Engineering Part A, 2009. 15(11): p. 3377-3388.

[3] Maguire, T.J., et al., *Design and Application of Microfluidic Systems for In Vitro Pharmacokinetic Evaluation of Drug Candidates.* Current Drug Metabolism, 2009. 10(10): p. 1192-1199.

[4] Arias, I.M., et al., *The Liver: Biology and Pathobiology.* 1 ed1988, New York: Raven PRess.

[5] Cho, C.H., et al., *Layered patterning of hepatocytes in co-culture systems using microfabricated stencils.* BioTechniques, 2010. 48(1): p. 47-52.

[6] Susick, R., et al., *Hepatic progenitors and strategies for liver cell therapies.* Ann N Y Acad Sci, 2001. 944: p. 398-419.

[7] Forbes, S., et al., *Hepatic stem cells.* J Pathol, 2002. 197(4): p. 510-8.

[8] Wang, X., et al., *The origin and liver repopulating capacity of murine oval cells.* Proc Natl Acad Sci U S A, 2003. 100 Suppl 1: p. 11881-8.

[9] Fausto, N. and J.S. Campbell, *The role of hepatocytes and oval cells in liver regeneration and repopulation.* Mech Dev, 2003. 120(1): p. 117-30.

[10] Zhang, Y., X.F. Bai, and C.X. Huang, *Hepatic stem cells: existence and origin.* World J Gastroenterol, 2003. 9(2): p. 201-4.

[11] Nagy, P., et al., *In vivo infusion of growth factors enhances the mitogenic response of rat hepatic ductal (oval) cells after administration of 2-acetylaminofluorene.* Hepatology, 1996. 23(1): p. 71-9.

[12] LeGasse, E., H. Connors, and M. Al-Dhalimym, *Purified hematopoietic sten cells can differentiate into mature hepatocytes in vivo.* Nature Medicine, 2000. 6(11): p. 1229-1234.

[13] Tan, J., et al., *Immunohistochemical Evidence for Hepatic Progenitor Cells in Liver Diseases.* Liver, 2002. 22: p. 365.

[14] Evans, M.J. and M.H. Kaufman, *Establishment in culture of pluripotential cells from mouse embryos.* Nature, 1981. 292(5819): p. 154-6.

[15] Smith, A.G., et al., *Inhibition of pluripotential embryonic stem cell differentiation by purified polypeptides.* Nature, 1988. 336(6200): p. 688-90.

[16] Takahashi, K. and S. Yamanaka, *Induction of pluripotent stem cells from mouse embryonic and adult fibroblast cultures by defined factors.* Cell, 2006. 126(4): p. 663-76.

[17] Lister, R., et al., *Hotspots of aberrant epigenomic reprogramming in human induced pluripotent stem cells.* Nature, 2011. 471(7336): p. 68-73.

[18] Takahashi, K., et al., *Induction of pluripotent stem cells from adult human fibroblasts by defined factors.* Cell, 2007. 131(5): p. 861-72.

[19] Yamanaka, S., *Strategies and New Developments in the Generation of Patient-Specific Pluripotent Stem Cells.* Cell Stem Cell, 2007. 1(1): p. 39-49.

[20] Yamanaka, S., *A Fresh Look at iPS Cells.* Cell, 2009. 137(1): p. 13-17.

[21] Yu, J., et al., *Human Induced Pluripotent Stem Cells Free of Vector and Transgene Sequences.* Science, 2009. 324(5928): p. 797-801.

[22] Feng, B., et al., *Molecules that Promote or Enhance Reprogramming of Somatic Cells to Induced Pluripotent Stem Cells.* Cell Stem Cell, 2009. 4(4): p. 301-312.

[23] McLin, V.A., S.A. Rankin, and A.M. Zorn, *Repression of Wnt/β-catenin signaling in the anterior endoderm is essential for liver and pancreas development.* Development, 2007. 134(12): p. 2207-2217.

[24] Zorn, A.M. and J.M. Wells, *Vertebrate Endoderm Development and Organ Formation.* Annual Review of Cell and Developmental Biology, 2009. 25(1): p. 221-251.

[25] Bossard, P. and K.S. Zaret, *GATA transcription factors as potentiators of gut endoderm differentiation.* Development, 1998. 125(24): p. 4909-4917.

[26] Liu, J.K., C.M. DiPersio, and K.S. Zaret, *Extracellular signals that regulate liver transcription factors during hepatic differentiation in vitro.* Mol. Cell. Biol., 1991. 11(2): p. 773-784.

[27] Kamiya, A., T. Kinoshita, and A. Miyajima, *Oncostatin M and hepatocyte growth factor induce hepatic maturation via distinct signaling pathways.* FEBS Letters, 2001. 492(1-2): p. 90-94.

[28] Kamiya, A., et al., *Fetal liver development requires a paracrine action of oncostatin M through the gp130 signal transducer.* Embo J, 1999. 18(8): p. 2127-36.

[29] Kinoshita, T. and A. Miyajima, *Cytokine regulation of liver development.* Biochimica et Biophysica Acta (BBA) - Molecular Cell Research, 2002. 1592(3): p. 303-312.

[30] Lemaigre, F. and K.S. Zaret, *Liver development update: new embryo models, cell lineage control, and morphogenesis.* Current Opinion in Genetics & Development, 2004. 14(5): p. 582-590.

[31] Snykers, S., et al., *In Vitro Differentiation of Embryonic and Adult Stem Cells into Hepatocytes: State of the Art.* STEM CELLS, 2009. 27(3): p. 577-605.

[32] Zhao, R. and S.A. Duncan, *Embryonic development of the liver.* Hepatology, 2005. 41(5): p. 956-967.

[33] Sosa-Pineda, B., J.T. Wigle, and G. Oliver, *Hepatocyte migration during liver development requires Prox1.* Nature genetics, 2000. 25(3): p. 254-5.

[34] Battle, M.A., et al., *Hepatocyte nuclear factor 4a orchestrates expression of cell adhesion proteins during the epithelial transformation of the developing liver.* Proceedings of the National Academy of Sciences, 2006. 103(22): p. 8419-8424.

[35] Odom, D.T., et al., *Control of Pancreas and Liver Gene Expression by HNF Transcription Factors.* Science, 2004. 303(5662): p. 1378-1381.

[36] Si-Tayeb, K., et al., *Highly efficient generation of human hepatocyte–like cells from induced pluripotent stem cells.* Hepatology, 2010. 51(1): p. 297-305.

[37] Agarwal, S., K.L. Holton, and R. Lanza, *Efficient Differentiation of Functional Hepatocytes from Human Embryonic Stem Cells.* STEM CELLS, 2008. 26(5): p. 1117-1127.

[38] Song, Z., et al., *Efficient generation of hepatocyte-like cells from human induced pluripotent stem cells.* Cell Res, 2009. 19(11): p. 1233-1242.

[39] Schwartz, R.E., et al., *Defined Conditions for Development of Functional Hepatic Cells from Human Embryonic Stem Cells.* Stem Cells and Development, 2005. 14(6): p. 643-655.

[40] Imamura, T., et al., *Embryonic Stem Cell-Derived Embryoid Bodies in Three-Dimensional Culture System Form Hepatocyte-Like Cells in Vitro and in Vivo.* Tissue Engineering, 2004. 10(11-12): p. 1716-1724.

[41] Matsumoto, K., et al., *Hepatic differentiation of mouse embryonic stem cells in a three-dimensional culture system using polyurethane foam.* Journal of Bioscience and Bioengineering, 2008. 105(4): p. 350-354.

[42] Liu, T., et al., *Hepatic Differentiation of Mouse Embryonic Stem Cells in Three-Dimensional Polymer Scaffolds.* Tissue Engineering Part A, 2010. 16(4): p. 1115-1122.

[43] Maguire, T., et al., *Control of hepatic differentiation via cellular aggregation in an alginate microenvironment.* Biotechnol Bioeng, 2007. 98(3): p. 631-44.

[44] Maguire, T., et al., *Alginate-PLL microencapsulation: effect on the differentiation of embryonic stem cells into hepatocytes.* Biotechnol Bioeng, 2006. 93(3): p. 581-91.

[45] Ishii, T., et al., *Effects of extracellular matrixes and growth factors on the hepatic differentiation of human embryonic stem cells.* American Journal of Physiology - Gastrointestinal and Liver Physiology, 2008. 295(2): p. G313-G321.

[46] Fukumitsu, K., et al., *Establishment of a Cell Line Derived from a Mouse Fetal Liver That Has the Characteristic to Promote the Hepatic Maturation of Mouse Embryonic Stem Cells by a Coculture Method.* Tissue Engineering Part A, 2009. 15(12): p. 3847-3856.

[47] Ishii, T., et al., *In vitro hepatic maturation of human embryonic stem cells by using a mesenchymal cell line derived from murine fetal livers.* Cell and Tissue Research, 2010. 339(3): p. 505-512.

[48] Soto-Gutierrez, A., et al., *Reversal of mouse hepatic failure using an implanted liver-assist device containing ES cell-derived hepatocytes.* Nat Biotech, 2006. 24(11): p. 1412-1419.

[49] Saito, K., et al., *Promoted differentiation of cynomolgus monkey ES cells into hepatocyte-like cells by co-culture with mouse fetal liver-derived cells.* World Journal of Gastroenterology, 2006. 12(42): p. 6818-6827.

[50] Moore, R.N., et al., *Enhanced differentiation of embryonic stem cells using co-cultivation with hepatocytes.* Biotechnology and Bioengineering, 2008. 101(6): p. 1332-1343.

[51] Cho, C.H., et al., *Homogeneous differentiation of hepatocyte-like cells from embryonic stem cells: applications for the treatment of liver failure.* The FASEB Journal, 2008. 22(3): p. 898-909.

[52] Sharma, N.S., et al., *Sodium butyrate-treated embryonic stem cells yield hepatocyte-like cells expressing a glycolytic phenotype*. Biotechnology and Bioengineering, 2006. 94(6): p. 1053-1063.

[53] Sharma, N.S., et al., *Enrichment of Hepatocyte-like Cells with Upregulated Metabolic and Differentiated Function Derived from Embryonic Stem Cells Using S-NitrosoAcetylPenicillamine*. Tissue Engineering Part C: Methods, 2009. 15(2): p. 297-306.

[54] Uygun, B.E., et al., *Organ reengineering through development of a transplantable recellularized liver graft using decellularized liver matrix*. Nat Med, 2010. 16(7): p. 814-820.

[55] Baptista, P.M., et al., *The use of whole organ decellularization for the generation of a vascularized liver organoid*. Hepatology, 2011. 53(2): p. 604-617.

[56] Yarmush, M.L., J.C. Dunn, and R.G. Tompkins, *Assessment of artificial liver support technology*. Cell Transplant, 1992. 1(5): p. 323-41.

[57] Jauregui, H.O., C.J. Mullon, and B.A. Solomon, *Extracorporeal Artificial Liver Support*, in *Principles of Tissue Engineering* 1997, R.G. Landes: Boulder CO.

[58] Nyberg, S.L., et al., *Evaluation of a hepatocyte entrapment hollow fiber bioreactor: a potential bioartificial liver*. Biotechnol Bioeng, 1993. 41(194-203).

[59] Kelly, J.H. and N.L. Sussman, *The hepatix extracorporeal liver assist device in the treatment of fulminant hepatic failure*. Asaio J, 1994. 40(1): p. 83-5.

[60] Roy, P., et al., *Analysis of oxygen transport to hepatocytes in a flat-plate microchannel bioreactor*. Ann Biomed Eng, 2001. 29(11): p. 947-55.

[61] Ohshima, N., K. Yanagi, and H. Miyoshi, *Development of a packed-bed type bioartificial liver: tissue engineering approach*. Transplant Proc, 1999. 31(5): p. 2016-7.

[62] Dixit, V. and G. Gitnick, *The bioartificial liver: state-of-the-art*. Eur J Surg Suppl, 1998(582): p. 71-6.

[63] Roy, P., et al., *Effect of flow on the detoxification function of rat hepatocytes in a bioartificial liver reactor*. Cell Transplant, 2001. 10(7): p. 609-14.

[64] McClelland, R.E., J.M. MacDonald, and R.N. Coger, *Modeling O2 transport within engineered hepatic devices*. Biotechnol Bioeng, 2003. 82(1): p. 12-27.

[65] Park, J., et al., *Microfabricated grooved substrates as platforms for bioartificial liver reactors*. Biotechnol Bioeng, 2005. 90(5): p. 632-44.

[66] Park, J., et al., *Microfabricated grooved substrates as platforms for bioartificial liver reactors*. Biotechnology and Bioengineering, 2005. 90(5): p. 632-644.

[67] Park, J., et al., *Radial flow hepatocyte bioreactor using stacked microfabricated grooved substrates*. Biotechnology and Bioengineering, 2008. 99(2): p. 455-467.

[68] Maguire, T.J., et al., *Design and application of microfluidic systems for in vitro pharmacokinetic evaluation of drug candidates*. Current drug metabolism, 2009. 10(10): p. 1192-9.

[69] Novik, E., et al., *A microfluidic hepatic coculture platform for cell-based drug metabolism studies*. Biochem Pharmacol, 2010. 79(7): p. 1036-44.

[70] Chao, P., et al., *Evaluation of a microfluidic based cell culture platform with primary human hepatocytes for the prediction of hepatic clearance in human*. Biochem Pharmacol, 2009. 78(6): p. 625-32.

[71] Park, T.H. and M.L. Shuler, *Integration of cell culture and microfabrication technology*. Biotechnology progress, 2003. 19(2): p. 243-53.

[72] Ghanem, A. and M.L. Shuler, *Combining cell culture analogue reactor designs and PBPK models to probe mechanisms of naphthalene toxicity.* Biotechnology progress, 2000. 16(3): p. 334-45.

[73] Sweeney, L.M., et al., *A cell culture analogue of rodent physiology: Application to naphthalene toxicology.* Toxicology in vitro : an international journal published in association with BIBRA, 1995. 9(3): p. 307-16.

[74] Zorn, A.M., *StemBook. The Stem Cell Research Community,* in *Liver development,* L. Girard, Editor 2008.

[75] Chao, P., et al., *Evaluation of a microfluidic based cell culture platform with primary human hepatocytes for the prediction of hepatic clearance in human.* Biochemical Pharmacology, 2009. 78(6): p. 625-632.

Part 3

Osteogenic Differentiation

5

Osteogenesis from Pluripotent Stem Cells: Neural Crest or Mesodermal Origin?

Kevin C. Keller and Nicole I. zur Nieden
Department of Cell Biology & Neuroscience and Stem Cell Center, College of Natural and Agricultural Sciences, University of California Riverside
United States of America

1. Introduction

Research in stem cell biology has the potential to dramatically alter the way we understand the vast complexity and coordination that is required for an organism to develop and function. The creation of therapeutic tools that will inevitably accompany these discoveries in this field of research may completely revolutionize our approach to medicine in the 21st century.

In this chapter we will examine one facet of stem cell research that holds great potential to improve the quality of life for millions of individuals; the study of osteogenesis from pluripotent stem cells. Despite its overt rigid structure, which provides mechanical support and protective functions, bone is a highly dynamic tissue that is tightly regulated to serve multiple roles in the body. Bone tissue is constantly being remodeled by the actions of the osteoblasts, the bone forming cells, and the osteoclasts, the bone resorbing cells. The improper balance of these cells can result in a number of bone-related and osteodegenerative diseases. Osteoporosis, for example, is estimated to effect 75 million individuals in Europe, Japan and the US alone, and thus the potential benefits of understanding the processes regulating osteogenesis may be quite far reaching.

Despite the similarity of the bone tissues found in the adult mammalian skeleton, there are three different sources from which bone is derived in the developing embryo (Fig. 1). Two of these bone origins are from mesodermal progenitors, where cells from either the lateral plate or paraxial mesoderm contribute to the appendicular or axial skeleton, respectively. The third origin of bone tissue can be traced back to ectodermal cells where neural crest progenitors differentiate into many of the bones within the craniofacial region. Differences in the origin in bone are also paralleled in differences seen in the bone formation process. Most bones of mesodermal origin develop via the process of endochondral bone formation, whereas the bones of ectodermal origin form by a process called intramembranous bone formation. These processes differ most generally in the series of cell differentiations that lead to the mature tissue. In endochondral bone formation the mesenchymal progenitors differentiate into chondrocytes, which lay down the cartilaginous framework that is eventually replaced by the mineralized matrix of invading osteoblasts, while the chondrocytes undergo apoptosis. In intramembranous bone formation, the progenitors differentiate directly into osteoblasts. In addition, mature bone tissues house adult stem cell niches, such as those composed of mesenchymal or hematopoietic stem cells. These cells are the source for diverse cell types throughout the life of the organism and are critical for normal maintenance and overall physiology.

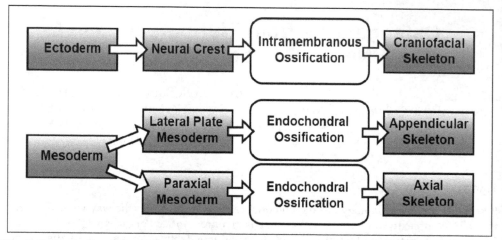

Fig. 1. Embryonic origins of bone tissue

While it is widely accepted that pluripotent stem cells have the capability to give rise to osteoblasts, it has only recently been examined whether they do so through a mesodermal route or through progenitors with neural crest characteristics. This chapter will provide a review of the current understanding of the different progenitors that contribute to the aforementioned bone formation processes and regulatory networks known to play critical roles in these cells. It will further examine the experimental manipulations in stem cell culture systems that have allowed us to derive neural crest and mesodermal type osteoprogenitors *in vitro*. However, it remains elusive whether a neural crest type progenitor and a mesodermal progenitor will have the same capacity to repair bone when transplanted or whether one will be superior to the other in a certain transplantation site. In order to systematically assess the influence of the type of progenitor and the transplantation site as well as the process of bone formation that is typically used as repair mechanism in a particular transplantation site, this chapter therefore also summarizes bone tissue engineering studies that have been undertaken using these diverse progenitors and that will bring us closer to eventual clinical applications that this exciting field of research will provide.

2. Pluripotent stem cells to bone

Both *in vitro* and *in vivo* studies continue to elucidate the developmental program that pluripotent stem cells take to their eventual differentiated states. One such program is the development of bone tissue; and research in this field has already made a positive impact on the lives of individuals in various clinical trials (Giordano et al., 2007). However, before these applications become commonplace in the medical field, further study is required to improve both our understanding and methodologies. This chapter seeks to give a broad overview of a diverse range of topics, from differentiation of pluripotent stem cells along osteogenic lineages, some current approaches in applying stem cell based bone engineering for potential clinical applications, and concluding with a discussion of different bone origins and their respective developmental pathways.

2.1 Embryonic stem cells

Pluripotent stem cells can be distinguished from adult stem cells based on their nature of origin, but first and foremost based on their more versatile differentiation capability. This unsurpassed differentiation capability is known as pluripotency, the potential to generate cell types from the three embryonic germ layers: the mesoderm, the ectoderm and the endoderm. One class of pluripotent stem cells, the embryonic stem cells (ESCs) have been under fervent ethical debate since their initial derivation. The crux of this debate can be attributed to their source being a cluster of cells found in the blastocyst, an early pre-implantation embryonic stage. This cluster of cells, the inner cell mass (ICM), is established directly after the developing embryo has gone through the first fate decision, in which the trophoectoderm secedes from the ICM. While this outer trophoectodermal layer of the blastocyst eventually gives rise to the placenta, the *in vivo* fate of the ICM is to develop into the embryo proper, which contains cell types of the three germ layers. Mirroring this capability of the ICM, isolated ESCs also have the capacity to give rise to cell types of all three germ layers when differentiated *in vitro* (Itskovitz-Eldor et al., 2000).

ESCs were first derived from mouse blastocysts (Evans and Kaufman, 1981; Martin, 1981) and since then their derivation has been reported from a number of mammals including: hamster, rabbit and rat (Doetschman et al., 1988; Giles et al., 1993; Iannaccone et al., 1994). Although these alternative rodent ESC lines have never gained recognition as model systems, their utilization continues to provide insights into stem cell biology. As for primate ESC derivation, the initial challenges that plagued the field for years were finally overcome by Thomson et al. (1995), and this study laid the ground for the establishment of human ESCs by the same team just shortly before the turn of the century (Thomson et al., 1998).

In addition to the pluripotent nature, it is their second characteristic of being capable of unlimited proliferation that ESCs first became an attractive cell source for regenerative therapies. This propagation in the undifferentiated state can be supported in culture with the addition of leukemia inhibitory factor (LIF) (Williams et al., 1988). Since LIF is inefficient in maintaining the undifferentiated state in human ESCs, the molecular cues needed maybe released by murine embryonic fibroblast feeder layers, which both human ESCs and murine ESCs can be grown on (Evans and Kaufman, 1981; Martin, 1981; Thomson et al., 1998). In feeder-independent conditions, basic fibroblast growth factor (bFGF) is able to maintain the pluripotent state of human ESCs (Amit et al., 2003).

2.2 Differentiation of ESCs into bone cells

Historically the developmental program that pluripotent stem cells take to form bone tissue was first elucidated using murine ESCs. Buttery and coworkers were the first to show that mESCs maintained in medium supplemented with beta-glycerophosphate and ascorbic acid had mineralized in culture, a hallmark feature of bone tissue formation (Buttery et al., 2001). In the past decade, numerous protocols have then been established that allow ESC differentiation into bone and cartilage and their characteristic cell types, the osteoblasts and osteoclasts as well as the chondrocytes. The studies that describe formation of osteoblasts typically all assess the ability of the cells to secrete an organic matrix composed of collagen type I (COL I) and proteoglycans, the deposition of inorganic hydroxyapatite and the expression of osteoblast-specific genes (Davis et al., 2011; Handschel et al., 2008; Shimko et al., 2004).

One difference between these protocols however, is the choice of additional osteogenic inducers. While beta-glycerophosphate and ascorbic acid are absolutely necessary for the cells to calcify, the additional supplementation of either dexamethasone, retinoic acid or 1,25alpha (OH)$_2$ vitamin D$_3$ (VD$_3$) each can significantly increase the amount of bone nodules and expression of osteogenic markers in both mouse and human ESC cultures (Buttery et al., 2001; Phillips et al., 2001; Sottile et al., 2003; zur Nieden et al., 2003).

Similar to endochondral bone formation in the embryo, osteogenesis from ESCs *in vitro* can be direct or the future bone can at first undergo a chondrocyte phase. Both processes have been described for ESCs. For example, during ESC *in vitro* intramembranous ossification, osteoblasts would be specified through a mesenchymal precursor and then directly into the osteoblastic fate. In this case, markers for hypertrophic chondrocytes should be absent or should only be minimally expressed. In turn, ESC differentiation would model embryonal endochondral ossification when ESCs would first differentiate into chondrocytes, then undergo hypertrophy and give way to osteoprogenitors that calcify. Hegert and colleagues, supported by data from our group, have shown that chondrogenic ESC cultures indeed can be manipulated to calcify, whereby such ossification results in a lower calcium content of the matrix then the direct (non chondrocyte-mediated) differentiation (Hegert et al., 2002; zur Nieden et al., 2005). This direct chondrocytic differentiation is mediated by growth factors of the transforming growth factor family, including bone morphogenic proteins and TGFβ1 (Kramer et al., 2000; Hegert et al., 2002; zur Nieden et al., 2005; Toh et al., 2007). Under such treatment the cartilage-specific transcription factors Sox9 and scleraxis are up-regulated at early stages of differentiation (Kramer et al., 2002, 2005; zur Nieden et al., 2005). The addition of BMP also increased the formation of cartilaginous matrix, comprised of collagen, proteoglycans and ECM proteins and expression of collagen mRNAs found in cartilage, such as collagen type II and collagen type X, the latter being indicative of chondrocytes undergoing hypertrophy (Kielty et al., 1985). ESC cultures containing such hypertrophic chondrocytes also initiate expression of osteoblast-specific mRNAs. This overlap of the chondrocyte-specific and the osteoblast- specific differentiation program suggest that ESCs may be undergoing the endochondral bone formation process.

In addition to growth factors and chemicals that direct differentiation through the endochondral or intramembranous route, different physical means have also been utilized to induce ESC differentiation into bone. While murine ESCs are typically grown into small (i.e. approximately 300-400 μm) agglomerates of differentiating cells called embryoid bodies (EBs) (Trettner et al., 2011), as the first stage of differentiation, human ESCs can alternatively be induced to differentiate by overgrowing colonies on a plate (Karp et al., 2006). Further osteogenic differentiation can be observed when intact EBs or dissociated EB cells are cultured in the presence of osteogenic supplements (Buttery et al., 2001; Cao et al., 2005; Chaudhry et al., 2004; zur Nieden et al., 2003). Woll and coworkers trypsinized mouse EBs into single cell suspensions and plated those at very low clonal density (Woll et al., 2006). They reported that approximately 60-80% of single-cell derived colony formation exhibited matrix mineralization as determined by von Kossa staining. Further qPCR analysis of osteoblast markers supported the potential of these cells to undergo osteogenesis, although there was heterogeneity between colonies in expression of these specific markers. Despite this heterogeneity between these individual colonies, the clonal expansion from a single cell offers an easy approach to dissect the differentiation pathway leading to bone cell formation.

This seems to be of particular importance as ESCs can be lead to differentiate from pluripotency into mesenchyme and subsequently bone, whereby mesenchyme may be specified either from a mesodermal or neural crest derived origin. More recent studies have indeed reported the generation of mesenchymal stem cell like cells from ESCs as well as the isolation of progenitors with osteogenic properties that were mesoderm or neural crest derived (Aihara et al., 2010; Olivier et al., 2006; Sakurai et al., 2006; Trivedi and Hematti, 2007).

A few days into the differentiation, ESCs will express T-Brachyury, a gene that is typically transcribed in the primitive streak when the early embryo undergoes gastrulation to establish the three germ layers (Beddington et al., 1992). The primitive streak contains cells with mesendodermal character, a subpopulation of cells that can later become osteoblasts. T-Brachyury expression is often used to characterize the output of differentiating mesendoderm (Gadue et al., 2006; Nakanishi et al., 2009) and is thus also informative to the very early differentiation events of osteogenesis. Similarly, modeled after the early lineage decisions *in vivo*, activin and nodal induction may be used to enhance the percentage of mesendodermal cells positive for Goosecoid (Gsc), E-cadherin, and platelet-derived growth factor receptor alpha (PDGFRα) (Tada et al., 2005), which are a combination of markers expressed by organizer cells in the primitive streak region. During subsequent development, this triple-positive cell population diverges to Gsc+ and either E-cadherin or PDGFRα positive intermediates that later differentiate into definitive endoderm and mesodermal lineages, including calcified osteopontin expressing osteoblasts (Tada et al., 2005).

While the mesendodermal progenitors are being established in the process of gastrulation *in vivo*, neurulation has already initiated in the anterior part of the embryo. Therefore, specification of neural crest populations may occur *in vitro* during ESC differentiation at around the same time or slightly after T-Brachyury+ or Gsc+ populations are found. In the embryo, neural crest cells emerge from the dorsal epithelium of the neural tube after it has formed, undergo epithelial-to-mesenchymal transitions and become highly migratory. These cells later disperse to and incorporate within skin tissue (i.e. melanocytes) as well as neurons and glia in the peripheral nervous system (Chung et al., 2009; Dupin et al., 2007; Weston, 1991). Due to the multitude of cell types that arise from the highly specific population of neural crest cells, it is sometimes regarded as the fourth germ layer. In addition, the neural crest is generally considered to be the source of a population of cells deemed the ectomesenchyme, which produces a variety of mesenchymal tissues including craniofacial cartilage and bone (Morrisskay et al., 1993; Smith and Hall, 1990). More recently however, the view that mesenchymal cell types are established from progenitor populations of neural crest origin was challenged by Weston and colleagues, who suggest that neural crest and ectomesenchyme are developmentally distinct progenitor populations, possibly distinguishable by the expression of E-cadherin and PDGFRα (Weston et al., 2004).

While it seems widely established that ESCs have the capacity to differentiate into osteoblasts from these various origins, other questions related to the feasibility of their clinical use are still under investigation. As pluripotent cells, ESCs are particularly attractive for the treatment of critical size bone defects that require large numbers of cells as an illimitable source of progenitors, be it mesoderm or neural crest derived MSCs or even more committed osteoprogenitors. More recently, a new less ethically controversial source of pluripotent cells has been discovered in the artificial creation of induced pluripotent stem cells (iPSCs). In this method mature, fully differentiated cells are reprogrammed to a pluripotent state. Explicitly, pluripotency-associated genes are shuttled into somatic cells, e.g. fibroblasts or keratinocytes (Aasen et al., 2008; Okita et al., 2007; Takahashi and Yamanaka, 2006), and brought to expression before they are silenced, which is just enough to turn the differentiated cells into ESC-like cells with a pluripotent pheno- and genotype. Only five years after their discovery, iPSCs have been recently exploited to study osteogenesis and have already been shown to possess comparable differentiation capacity (Bilousova et al., 2011).

3. Bone tissue engineering

The current gold standard for bone tissue replacement is the autologous graft, which utilizes bone tissue that has been extracted from another site within the patient's own body. However, there is only a limited amount of bone tissue that can feasibly be harvested without inducing considerable donor site morbidity (Rose and Oreffo, 2002). On the other hand, surgical procedures using an allograft, where the bone is harvested from a cadaver, can provide enough material to correct large-scale bone defects. However, this approach carries its own disadvantages including potential immunorejection and pathogen transmission. Techniques involving synthetic materials such as metals and ceramics are continually being used and explored as alternatives to these approaches, but these substitutes continually fall short of bone grafts in areas such as host site integration and tensile strength (Rezwan et al., 2006; Yaszemski et al., 1996). Thus, the attractive features and potential versatility of stem cells offers the investigator an exciting source to improve and develop new technologies that may significantly enhance the efficacy of these procedures.

Currently a popular approach in applying stem cells to *de novo* bone synthesis is the *in vitro* culturing or 'seeding' of cells onto scaffolding materials that can be used for subsequent implantation. In order for this approach to be successful there are a number of essential properties that a researcher must keep in mind when designing the appropriate scaffolding material. These properties will have a direct effect on both the colonization of the scaffold and its successful incorporation into host bone tissue. To achieve an optimal scaffold design a number of considerations such as biocompatibility, porosity, pore size, osteoinductivity and conductivity (including biomolecule incorporation), biodegradability, and mechanical properties must be accounted for (Salgado et al., 2004). Thus, reaching this goal will be a challenge that requires the coordinated efforts of researches across the diverse disciplines of material and biological sciences.

3.1 Mesenchymal stem cells in bone tissue engineering

Beyond the type of scaffold used in a particular study, the choice of seeded cell type will also play a critical role in the creation of *de novo* bone tissue. Starting with the most differentiated cell type, seeding a scaffold with harvested autologous osteoblasts superficially seems attractive because of their inherent cellular program to develop new bone. However, using this cell type is problematic because of low initial concentrations following harvest and relatively poor proliferation capacity *in vitro*. Also, if these treatments are designed to not only amend bone defects, but also to alleviate bone disorders, it is unlikely that harvested osteoblasts will have the suitable characteristics to be effective. Another possible cell type is the multipotent adult mesenchymal stem cell.

Mesenchymal stem cells (MSCs) are unspecialized adult stem cells that reside in mature somatic tissues, predominantly the bone marrow in the long bones. There they share the niche with hematopoietic stem cells, but differ from them in the array of specialized daughter cells that they can generate. MSCs were first described forty five years ago by

Friedenstein and colleagues, when they first found this heterogeneity in differentiation capacity between cells isolated from bone marrow. While they described the cells as ossific progenitor cells of stromal origin in rats in this first study, subsequent studies proved the multilineage differentiation potential of these cells into fibroblasts, chondrocytes and other cells of connective tissue coining the term mesenchymal stem cell (Friedenstein et al., 1966, 1976, 1987; Tondreau et al., 2004a, b; Johnstone et al., 1998; Young et al., 1998; Niemeyer et al., 2004).

Despite the fact that the scientific community has long exploited MSCs to understand the processes of osteogenic and chondrogenic differentiation as well as for the study of adult stem cell maintenance (Bruder et al., 1990; Gazit et al., 1993; Grayson et al., 2006; Hong and Yaffe, 2006), the isolation of the non-hematopoietic mesenchymal stem cell from bone marrow or other tissue sources remains complex. Initially, Friedenstein isolated the MSCs by their tight adherence to plastic (Friedenstein et al. 1976). Yet, newer studies suggest that by isolating MSCs based on their plastic adherence, a portion of mesenchymal stem cells are lost (Zhang et al. 2009). Unfortunately, the fibroblast-like MSCs show a variable profile of surface marker expression (Simmons und Torok-Storb, 1991; Jiang et al. 2002; Vogel et al. 2003), which makes it difficult to isolate them based on a specific marker set. A few years ago, a group of investigators with extensive track records in MSC research has agreed on specific characteristics that need to be met by a cell in order to be called an MSC (Dominici et al., 2006, the International Society for Cellular Therapy position statement). For example, CD14, CD34 or CD45 mark hematopoietic cells and are therefore considered negative markers for MSCs. The most commonly used markers for the detection and purification of MSCs are CD90 (Thy-1 cell surface antigen), CD105 (endoglin) and CD73 (ecto-5'-nucleotidase) (Pittenger et al., 1999; Dominici et al., 2006). Both CD105 and CD73 are constitutively expressed by MSCs, however are also expressed by endothelial cells (Gougos und Letarte, 1988; Airas et al., 1995). Therefore, a combinatorial approach using CD106 (vascular cell adhesion molecule 1) is also recommended in the literature to identify MSCs, as CD106 is only expressed on the MSC surface, but not on endothelial cells (Pittenger et al., 1999; Osborn et al., 1989). Stro1 (Stenderup et al., 2001), glycophorin A (Pittenger et al., 1999; Reyes et al., 2001; Jones et al., 2006), D7-fib (Jones et al., 2002) and p75 (Quirici et al., 2002) have also been associated with MSCs recently, but are not contained in the International Society for Cellular Therapy position statement.

Currently, the use of bone marrow derived mesenchymal stem cells (BDMSCs) to study bone tissue generation is popular because these can be harvested from the patient's own body, thereby removing concerns of immunorejection and disease transmission. Because the transition of BDMSC studies to clinical applications is currently more direct, and not enveloped in ethical considerations, there have been many studies looking at the differentiation capacity of BDMSCs *in vivo* (Arinzeh et al., 2003; Bruder et al., 1998; Gao et al., 2001; Kotobuki et al., 2008). BDMSCs are already used in preclinical trials for treatment of osteogenesis imperfecta and non-union bone fractures (Le Blanc et al., 2005; Tuch, 2006).

However, this does not exclude the necessity to examine ESCs as a potential source of bone engineered cells. In fact, improvements in the techniques of somatic nuclear transfer (Byrne et al., 2007) and creating iPSCs (Nakagawa et al., 2008; Yu et al., 2007), make it quite plausible that the protocols derived from the study of ESCs may someday become more applicable to the future of regenerative medicine than their adult stem cell counterparts. In addition, there are drawbacks from using BDMSCs, including the limited number that can be obtained, more restricted proliferation and differentiation capacities when compared to

ESCs, and they may also harbor undesirable characteristics when harvested from unhealthy bone. So although the use of MSCs has progressed further in clinical applications of bone tissue engineering, the examination of ESCs as a potential source for repairing bone defects and disorders still merits a great deal of attention.

3.2 Embryonic stem cells for bone tissue engineering

Since Levenberg and colleagues (2003) demonstrated the potential to create complex tissue structures on 3D scaffolds using differentiating human ESCs, a number of investigations sought to refine and optimize the conditions required to engineer specific tissue types within 3D scaffolds. In 2004, Chaudhry and colleagues (2004) were the first to demonstrate the feasibility of inducing mineralization of murine ESC derived cells within 3D poly L-lactic acid (PLLA) scaffolds. To accomplish this goal the team initially differentiated murine ESCs into osteoblast progenitor cells in 2D culture. EBs were initially formed, which were then subsequently transferred into suspension dishes for 3 days in the presence of retinoic acid, and then were grown in the presence of β-glycerophosphate and ascorbic acid. EBs were trypsinized and seeded onto PLLA scaffolds. After four weeks of subsequent culture in osteogenic media, the scaffolds showed extensive bone nodule formation on the surface of the scaffold and evidence of cell invasion/mineralization with the interior, as demonstrated by electron microscopy and von Kossa staining. Molecular characterization of the cells that had colonized the scaffold also revealed expression of the osteoblast specific markers osteocalcin, osteopontin and alkaline phosphatase (Alk Phos).

When discussing synthetic scaffolds for tissue engineering it is important to realize that not only the composition of the material itself is important, but that the nano-scale architecture can also play a critical role in the successful colonization of the material. Smith and colleagues (2009) developed a fabrication method of producing a nanofibrous PLLA scaffold in an attempt to mimic a collagen matrix. These were compared to traditional 'solid-walled' PLLA scaffolds in both 2D and 3D osteogenic culture systems. It was found that the 3D nanofibrous matrices expedited differentiation of mouse ESCs as revealed by markers runx2, an osteoblast-specific transcription factor (5 times greater), bone sialoprotein (8.5 times greater) and osteocalcin (2.9 times greater). These scaffolds were also found to contain greater amounts of COL I (5.5 times) and calcium (3 times) when cultured for 28 days. Another point of interest from this study showed that the nanofibrous scaffold, unlike all the other materials tested, was also able to support osteogenesis without the addition of osteogenic supplements. Although, the osteogenic output was not as robust as when cultured with media supplemented with ascorbic acid, β-glycerophosphate, and dexamethasone. Thus, it appears that the nano-scaled architecture of these scaffolds mimics the endogenous ECM.

These differences in geometry presumably create a more appropriate spatial context to facilitate cell-cell interactions and communication for bone tissue development. In addition, it was previously found that this nanofibrous scaffold absorbed four times the amount of serum proteins than their traditional solid walled counterparts (Woo et al., 2003). Thus, the ability of this nano-scaled architecture to both improve the spatial arrangement of cells and to absorb more growth factors, demonstrates how attention to microscopic manufacturing of materials can greatly enhance the potential and success of these scaffolds.

The availability of a blood supply, especially to large bone grafts, is critical for engineered tissue transplant efficacy. The creation of a flap for transplantation is one surgical approach to address this issue. A flap is tissue that already has a vasculature system in place to support nutrient and gas exchange. Although not explored in ESC-derived grafts, studies performed with BDMSCs demonstrate the feasibility of this approach. Warnke and colleagues performed an interesting clinical demonstration of this technique in 2004. Here, a seeded scaffold intended to repair a large resection of the patient's mandible was first implanted within the patient's latissimus dorsi muscle. This *in vivo* incubation period allowed time for the graft, a titanium mesh cage filled with hydroxyapatite blocks coated with recombinant human BMP7, to develop vasculature. The graft was initially seeded with solution containing autologous bone and natural bovine bone-mineral extract. After seven weeks the implant was removed along with the muscle tissue containing the thoracodorsal artery and vein, which had provided the circulation to the implant, and was transplanted into the patient's jaw. Bone mineral density was measured using non-invasive 3D chromatography and revealed continuous improvement for the duration of 38 weeks (Warnke et al., 2004). Due to ethical considerations, a biopsy of the implant was not undertaken. However, mineralized scar tissue in areas of implant overgrowth was histologically examined and showed young cancellous bone formation containing viable osteoblasts and osteocytes. The patient's continual smoking and alcohol abuse compromised the initial favorable prognosis of the treatment, and unfortunately the patient had passed away 15 months following the operation (Warnke et al., 2006). Also due to the nature of the procedure, which precluded the use of control implants, statistical analyses were not performed. However this study provides at least an initial demonstration of principle within a human subject, and may eventually serve as a model to vascularize engineered bone tissue *in vivo*.

To examine the differences in the *in vivo* osteogenic capacity of between BDMSCs and ESCs, Tremoleda and colleagues (2008) implanted chambers that were cell-impermeable. These chambers contained either BDMSCs or ESCs that had been cultured *in vitro* for 4 days in standard osteogenic media. Since the pore size of these chambers precluded the passage of cells but allowed the diffusion of growth factors and other macromolecules, comparison of the intrinsic capacity for differentiation of these cell types became more straightforward. After 79 days post-implantation within nude mice, the authors reported no qualitative differences between the bone tissue formation between the BDMSCs, H7, and H9 embryonic stem cells. Although an interesting finding revealed that the ESC lines used did not require the *in vitro* osteogenic culture prior to implantation to form de novo bone tissue, which was unlike the BDMSCs, which required this pretreatment. Thus, although a significant difference between these cell types with the same osteogenic treatment was not uncovered in this study, the fact that ESCs required less coaxing and were more primed to respond to the bone tissue environment may be capitalized upon in future studies.

However, one of the major concerns when using ESCs for reparative medicine is the potential for residual undifferentiated cells to form teratomas following *in vivo* introduction. As such, undifferentiated murine ESCs form teratomas when injected into a healthy knee joint (Wakitani et al., 2003). The rate at which the teratomas grew in the knee joint however was slower than upon subcutaneous injection, suggesting that the microenvironment in the knee joint is not as favorable for ESC proliferation as for example a subcutaneous injection site. Surprisingly, if cells were injected into an inflammatory environment caused by a full-thickness osteochondral defect, the cells integrated and repaired the defect even in an allogenic setting (Wakitani et al., 2004).

Also, our group was recently able to show that ESCs lose their teratoma formation capacity with progressing osteogenic differentiation and maturation *in vitro*, whereby the *in vitro* microenvironment used to steer differentiation influences their teratoma formation capacity *in vivo*. Whereas spontaneously differentiated cells formed teratomas in 16% of the cases when taken from day 10 old cultures, 30-day osteogenic cultures did not show any sign of teratoma formation upon subcutaneous injection (Taiani et al., 2009).

Highlighting the concern of teratoma formation further, Nakajima and colleagues (2008) seeded mouse ESCs embedded in a collagen matrix into osteochondral defects within the knee joints of mice. Their investigation focused on the differentiation potential of these cells when the joint was either free to move or physically immobilized. They revealed that the mechanical environment appears to have a dramatic effect on the differentiation outcome of these implanted cells. Three weeks post operation, the defects were examined and the free-moving joints were shown to contain cartilaginous tissue formation with favorable histological characteristics. Surprisingly, when the joint was immobilized a teratoma formed in every instance of study. Thus, considering the close link between chondrogenesis and osteogenesis (to be discussed further in next section), it is important to note the results here and recognize that the mechanical environment into which undifferentiated stem cells are placed can have important consequences.

3.3 ESC-derived MSCs

Another cell type that has been recently gained attention as a possible therapeutic source is the embryonic stem cell-derived mesenchymal stem cell (ESC-MSC) in which ESCs are induced along the mesenchymal stem cell lineage. For a more detailed overview of the markers and techniques used to isolate such mesenchymal stem cell like cells from ESCs, the reader is referred to two recent reviews by Hematti (2011) and zur Nieden (2011). In one study of this cell type Barberi and colleagues (2005) demonstrated that cells initially differentiated along a paraxial mesoderm lineage were able to undergo osteogenesis *in vitro*. They found that this induced and sorted cell type (i.e. using the mesenchymal stem cell marker CD73) was able to undergo osteogenesis, by various staining assays and expression of bone specific markers. Similarly, Hu and colleagues derived human ESC-MSCs, and examined their capacity to differentiate into bone forming cells (Hu et al., 2010). When these cells were cultured in the presence of dexamethasone and BMP-7, they found that both Alk Phos levels and calcium deposition was statistically higher in dishes containing both supplements. This improvement found with both supplements was a synergistic one, as revealed through the modest effect when BMP-7 was used independently. When these cells were grown on 3D PLLA nanofibrous scaffolds, similar to that of Smith and colleagues (2009) discussed earlier, they exhibited growth throughout the scaffold and demonstrated extensive mineralization.

The *in vitro* osteogenic capacity between isolated human MSCs and derived human ESC-MSCs, was directly compared by de Peppo and others (2010). In this study they designated human ESC-MSCs as human embryonic stem cell-derived mesodermal progenitors hES-MPs and used a similar approach to that of Hu et al. (2010) to derive this cell type (Karlsson et al., 2009). Here they demonstrated that *in vitro* culture of hES-MPs resulted in faster ECM mineralization as compared to human MSCs. These results were contrary to their Alk Phos assays, which showed significantly greater activity of Alk Phos in human MSCs at every point during the first five weeks of differentiation. This apparent discrepancy may reflect a differential dependence of Alk Phos to mineralize the ECM between these cell types. In addition, this study examined the osteogenic capacity of cells in relation to their passage number. In every assay performed the osteogenic capacity decreased as passage number increased for all cell types examined. Although they reported that the hES-MPs were more buffered against this diminishing capacity, it brings attention to the problem with serial passages, which are inexorably tied to the requirements of tissue engineering, and their resulting potential to undergo osteogenesis.

The apparent discrepancy in relative Alk Phos activity was also found by Bigdeli and others (2010) when they compared the osteogenic capacity of human MSCs and a derived human ESC line (Bigdeli et al., 2008), which could be expanded on culture plastic without the support of feeder layers or other dish coatings such as Matrigel. Utilizing this cell line allowed the investigators to perform more direct comparison of the two cell types, since the typical differences between culture conditions were eliminated. Like the aforementioned study (de Peppo et al., 2010), they found that although Alk Phos expression was significantly lower at each time point examined, the derived human ESC line was better able to mineralize the extracellular matrix when compared to human MSCs. These results were further supported by ion mass spectrometry of the mineralized ECM, which demonstrated the signature of natural hydroxyapatite.

A study comparing osteogenesis of murine MSCs and murine ESCs derived from the same mouse strain (Shimko et al., 2004) also revealed this pattern where the mineral content was not directly correlated to Alk Phos activity. Thus, although Alk Phos activity is used frequently in studies of osteogenic differentiation, the level of enzyme activity may not directly correspond to the potential of the cells to mineralize the extracellular matrix. In addition, diverse Alk Phos levels may not necessarily suggest that more or less osteoblasts were formed, but may simply reflect different maturation kinetics of the different cell types.

Shimko et. al, (2004) went further in characterizing the mineralized matrix between murine MSCs and murine ESCs derived from the same mouse strain and cultured in the same conditions. As compared to natural hydroxyapatite found in bone, where the ratio of calcium to phosphorous is: 1.67:1; murine ESCs exhibited a ratio far closer (1.26:1) than murine MSCs (0.29:1). Mouse ESC cultures also contained, on average, a mineral content 50 times greater than mouse MSCs. However, once again reflecting distinct differentiation kinetics, pathways, or inherent differences in mineralization capacity, Alk Phos activity was significantly higher in MSCs throughout the course of the experiment. In addition, expression of osteocalcin and COL I in mouse ESCs was delayed relative to mouse MSCs. Thus, murine MSC differentiation appeared to be more reflective of natural osteogenesis, when examining organic matrix components and gene expression. On the other hand, the quantity and quality of the mineralization found in murine ESCs significantly surpassed what was exhibited by murine MSCs.

Although transferring the techniques of osteogenic induction of ESCs from flat culture dishes towards 3D scaffolds have demonstrated initial success, there continues to be the need for method refinement in order for these approaches to bone engineering become widely accepted. One such area of study where current knowledge is lacking is an understanding of the possible differentiation pathways that are normally found in vertebrate development these cells take in attempts at bone tissue engineering.

4. Different embryonic bone origins

Both *in vitro* and *in vivo* studies continue to elucidate the developmental program that pluripotent stem cells take to their eventual differentiated states, among them the osteoblast. Because of their capacity to differentiate into any cell type of the body, pluripotent stem cells may differentiate through the neural crest route or the mesodermal route, followed by mesenchymal specification. Similarly, ossification from pluripotent stem cells may occur through intramembranous bone formation or endochondral bone formation. In regard to the *in vivo* source of mesenchymal cells, which differentiate into bone in the appropriate developmental context, there also appears to be multiple developmental origins. The earliest MSCs appear to arise from Sox1+ neuroepithelium through a neural crest intermediate stage (Takashima et al., 2007) and not from mesoderm progenitors as previously believed.

The process of fracture healing also occurs through both intramembranous and endochondral means, which is dependent on the mechanical conditions at the fractured site (Claes et al., 1998). When dissecting the steps of bone development, far more is known about the endochondral pathway than the intramembranous process. The most overt difference between these two pathways is that either chondrocytes will arise from mesenchymal condensations, which subsequently apoptose and are replaced by invading osteoblasts, or there is a direct differentiation into osteoblasts themselves. Thus the differential influence and the necessity of chondrocytes highlight the most apparent differences between these bone-forming pathways. Thus, in order to optimize bone tissue-engineering procedures there is a need to understand the molecular basis underlying different bone formation processes. However, a current review of the literature demonstrates large holes in our understanding of these multiple routes in which bone naturally forms and how they are recapitulated in experimental systems. The remaining part of this chapter will be devoted towards our preliminary understanding of these processes with particular emphasis to their roles in bone tissue engineering.

4.1 Endochondral ossification

In the endochondral process mesenchymal cells condense and differentiate into proliferating chondrocytes, which take on the general shape of the future bone. These chondrocytes eventually fall out of the cell cycle and these post-mitotic chondrocytes undergo hypertrophy. In this stage of development the mature hypertrophic chondrocytes lay down cartilage-specific proteins into the surrounding matrix. This cartilaginous framework provides molecular cues, which attracts invading vasculature along with osteoblasts, which will replace the cartilage intermediate. Osteogenesis occurs directly adjacent to hypertrophic chondrocytes. It appears that both the parathyroid hormone (PTH)-related peptide (PTHrP) and its receptor PPR are critical in the process osteogenesis via the endochondral pathway. In mice, upon disruption of the either PTHrP or PPR, the formation of ectopic hypertrophic chondrocytes is accompanied by ectopic bone collar formation (Karaplis et al., 1994). To determine if the hypertrophic chondrocytes induce osteogenesis in adjacent cells and is not a spatial/temporal coincidence, Chung and colleagues (2001) studied transgenic mice that express constitutively active PPR under the control of a chondrocyte specific promoter. This constitutive action resulted in suppression of hypertrophic chondrocyte formation and concurrent suppression of bone collar and primary spongiosa development. In addition, when these transgenic mice were mated to PTHrP-/- mice the resulting rescue of the ectopic bone formation, supported the conclusion that hypertrophic chondrocytes are responsible for the induction of osteogenesis in adjacent tissue.

Regulation of the PTHrP/PPR signal appears to be controlled by one of the members of the hedgehog family of paracrine factors, Indian hedgehog (Ihh). Members of this signaling family are found throughout the animal kingdom and take on a number of critical roles in the developing organism. Here, Ihh is expressed by both prehypertrophic and hypertrophic chondrocytes. This signal mediates the expression of PTHrP by cells of the perichondrium, which in turn binds to PPR on chondrocytes. Ihh and PTHrP signaling thereby creates a negative feedback loop which suppresses differentiation of the proliferating chondrocytes into hypertrophic ones (Lanske et al., 1996; Vortkamp et al., 1996). Thus, this balance of signals dictates the spatial positioning of the hypertrophic chondrocytes. However, the role of Ihh appears to have a broader impact on osteogenesis than its PTHrP-dependent regulation of chondrocyte maturation.

St-Jacques and colleagues (1999) demonstrated that Ihh also plays a role in chondrocyte proliferation and the direct development of osteoblasts in endochondral bones. Previous studies have demonstrated a critical role of Wnt signaling and β-catenin localization as well (Gong et al., 2001; Kato et al., 2002). Hu and others (2005) found nuclear β-catenin localization within the cells of perichondrium indicating an upstream role of Ihh signaling to facilitate proper Wnt signaling. Furthermore, Ihh null mice do not exhibit osteocalcin expression within endochondral bones, whereas this expression is readily detected within the intramembranous bones of the skull and clavicle. This differential dependence of Ihh signaling underscores one of the differences between endochondral and intramembranous bone formation.

When assessing the role of local synthesis of VD_3 in transgenic mice that exhibited a chondrocyte-specific loss-of-function Cyp27b1, the enzyme that converts 25-hydroxyvitamin D_3 into the active form VD_3, it was found that the hypertrophic zone was expanded (Naja et al., 2009), thereby increasing both bone mass and trabecular size and number. The classical view that VD_3 synthesis (active form) was restricted to the kidneys and that this hormone's influence on bone tissue regulation was an indirect consequence of altering calcium and phosphate homeostasis had to be reevaluated. The authors suggest their results can be explained by a reduced osteoclast recruitment, which follows from a reported delay of vascularization that may be attributed to a reduction of VEGF found. Conversely, overexpression of Cyp27b1 under a chondrocyte-specific promoter resulted in the opposite expression profile and phenotype. These results are in accordance with chondrocyte specific VD_3 receptor ablation experiments, which showed impaired vascularization and osteoclast number in endochondral bone (Masuyama et al., 2006). As opposed to the traditional view of the role of VD_3 in bone biology as an indirect mediator of mineral uptake, these experiments demonstrate a functional role of this metabolite in regulating endochondral bone formation.

Some investigators have explored an approach to bone tissue-engineering by mimicking the development of mammalian long bones, where the creation of cartilage scaffolds *in vitro* are implanted *in vivo*. This approach hinges on the idea that the body will recognize this cartilage scaffold as an intermediate step in the endochondral bone formation process and will then proceed to ossify this construct. In the formation of endochondral bone, chondrocytes are exposed to very low oxygen levels and their survival is dependent on the expression of the transcription factor hypoxia-inducible factor-1 (For review see: Pfander and Gelse, 2007). Thus, the natural ability of chondrocytes to withstand the low oxygen supply can provide the time needed for new vasculature to develop and reach the core of the implant before widespread cell necrosis.

Jukes et al. (2008) tested whether *in vitro* differentiation of ESCs along chondrocyte lineages on scaffolds could improve *in vivo* osteogenesis following implantation. ESCs were initially induced along a chondrogenic pathway for 21 days on ceramic scaffolds. These chondrogenically-primed scaffolds were then subsequently implanted in immunodeficient mice and were found to exhibit nascent bone tissue formation when examined 21 days post-operatively. For comparison, primary chondrocytes and adult MSCs of human, goat, and bovine origin were used in lieu of the chondrocyte-induced ESCs. It was found that each cell type demonstrated differential abilities to form bone tissue *in vivo*. Interestingly, the goat MSCs resulted in the highest degree of bone tissue formation, and it appeared that this formation occurred via an intramembranous pathway.

Farrell et al. (2009) further examined the *in vitro* chondrogenic-priming of scaffolds using human MSCs and reported limited success. After the cells were cultured on collagen–GAG scaffolds for three weeks in chondrogenic media, the scaffolds were implanted subcutaneously in nude mice. Although cell survival and angiogenesis was found higher in the chondrogenically-primed scaffolds, as opposed to scaffolds that were osteogenically-primed, there appeared to be no *de novo* osteogenesis. The authors reported the chondrogenically-primed scaffolds showed evidence of the initial progression of endochondral ossification, yet were unable to proceed through the later stages of osteoblast-induced mineralization. When mineralization was induced *in vitro* prior to implantation, the nascent angiogenesis that was previously obtained was compromised. Thus, it appears that for this approach to be successful, the timed release of additional factors *in vivo* is needed to promote the osteogenic replacement of the cartilaginous scaffold.

When examining the developmental pathway of bone-tissue engineered constructs, by either endochondral or intramembranous routes, it makes sense that different cell types will mature along different pathways even when presented to the same conditions. Tortelli and others (2010) revealed how the differentiated state of implanted cells affects subsequent ossification and host cell recruitment to the graft site. They seeded hydroxyapatite scaffolds with either human MSCs or osteoblasts. When differentiated osteoblasts were used to seed the scaffolds, ossification occurred through an intramembranous pathway, as revealed by the lack of cartilage markers by immunohistological examination. This intramembranous ossification appeared to be more rapid and thus accounted for more bone deposition within the same time period when compared to the MSC-seeded scaffolds. However, MSC scaffolds, which ossified in an endochondral fashion, were able to facilitate nascent vascularization of the graft. This highlights the fact that engineered bone grafts may one day be tailored to a patient's need depending on factors such as speed of graft ossification and site incorporation. In addition this study shows that implanted MSCs can progress through the endochondral pathway, but as the aforementioned study by Farrell et al. (2009) demonstrates this process currently cannot be split into an early *in vitro* stage that can be 'picked up' later *in vivo*. However, if the process of endochondral bone formation is elucidated further and applied to tissue engineering, then it is feasible that this approach may one day become a viable avenue to repair large bone defects.

Although mimicking the development of long bone through endochondral ossification of scaffolds maybe appropriate in some contexts, intramembranous ossification may be suitable for other applications in regenerative medicine. The body utilizes both of these systems in different contexts depending on certain conditions whose reasons remain to be fully characterized. Nonetheless, it appears quite probable that bone tissue engineering need not only be tailored to the individual but also the specific bone defect or disease in order to be completely effective.

4.2 Intramembranous ossification

As for intramembranous bone formation, not only is little known about the process itself, but the developmental pathway of the cells leading to the formation of the tissues within the cranial skeleton is still not well understood.

4.2.1 Neural crest cells

As incipiently indicated, the migrating cranial neural crest cells form bone mostly through intramembranous ossification. Initially neural crest cells become committed to either an ectomesenchymal (i.e. producing tissues such as cartilage, bone and connective tissue) or a non-ectomesenchymal (i.e. producing neurons, glia and pigment cells) lineage. The ectomesenchymal tissue is also referred to in the literature as mesectoderm. Blentic and others (2008) describe how migrating neural crest cells in chick and zebrafish embryos commit to either fate. Cells that migrate into the pharyngeal arches are induced to respond to FGF signaling within these embryonic structures, resulting in the expression of the homeobox gene Dlx2. Concurrently, early neural crest markers Sox10 and FoxD2 are downregulated, which are still expressed in the neural crest cells that have not invaded the pharyngeal arches and thus are fated to become non-ectomesenchyme. Whether or not neural cells migrate into the pharyngeal arches appears to be determined by the timing of their emergence from the neural tube. Although not fully understood, it appears that early migrating cells 'fill up' the pharyngeal arches and the cells that migrate later are thus more likely to find residence outside of the arches and become non-ectomesenchyme (Blentic et al., 2008).

4.2.2 Neural crest and mesodermal progenitors in intramembranous bone formation

The parietal bone, which is of paraxial mesoderm origin and the frontal bone, which is of neural crest origin, both form via intramembranous ossification, thus making the study of calvarial bones an attractive platform to study the possible differences in bones of different embryonic origins. Quarto et al. (2010) examined the osteogenic capacity of first passage osteoblasts that were obtained from these respective bones in mice. Frontal bone-derived osteoblasts from post-natal day 7 and day 60 mice were found to exhibit greater mineralization capacity, as revealed by Alk Phos activity, von Kossa and Alizarin Red S staining. This was also supported by expression data of the bone-specific markers osteocalcin and runx2. These *in vitro* observations were reinforced by the relative healing capacity of these two bones. The successful healing of 2mm defects was found within the frontal bone in the majority of mice at 8 weeks post-injury, whereas complete healing was not typically found in same sized injuries of the parietal bones within the same time period.

The investigators uncovered a higher level of endogenous canonical Wnt signaling in frontal bone osteoblasts as compared to parietal bone osteoblasts that may be responsible for this differential regenerative propensity. By modulating Wnt signaling through exogenous addition of Wnt3a or transfecting osteoblasts with constructs that increase β-catenin signaling in parietal bones to frontal bone levels, and vice versa, the authors showed a reversal of osteogenic potential of these cells. Thus, providing strong evidence that that the enhanced osteogenic potential of frontal bone osteoblasts can be at least be partially attributed to these differences in endogenous Wnt signaling.

Xu and colleagues (2007) found that osteoblasts derived from the frontal bone proliferated faster and attached to culture dishes better than osteoblasts that were harvested from parietal bone. This may be linked to the fourfold greater expression of osteoblast-specific cadherin that they found within frontal bone osteoblasts. The parietal bone osteoblasts did however show double the Alk Phos activity at the time points examined. When cultured in the presence of osteogenic inducing factors, such as VD_3, the frontal bone osteoblasts showed a much more robust bone nodule formation. However, expression of osteogenic differentiation markers, such as osteopontin, Col1, and Wnt5a was significantly greater in the parietal bone derived cells. Members of the FGF signaling cascade were also differentially expressed between these two cell types. Thus, the frontal and parietal bones appear superficially similar yet exhibit an number of different characteristics such as growth kinetics, regulation by signaling cascades and varying marker expression, all of which demonstrate that these bones are not as similar as they initially appear to be.

To further examine the regenerative osteogenic capacity of cells from different embryonic origins Leucht and others (2008) engineered mice in which developing cells of neural crest origin would irreversibly express GFP. Tissues from mesodermal origin were also induced to express β-galactosidase. Following skeletal injury in either the mandible or the tibia resulted in natural bone regeneration where the progenitor pool which became new bone tissue was derived from the same embryonic origin of the injured bone itself (i.e. cells from neural crest origin repaired mandible defects, and cells of mesodermal origin repaired tibia defects). The investigators then performed a number of transplant experiments where skeletal progenitor cells were implanted into bone of different embryonic origin. Interestingly neural crest derived progenitors were able to form more new bone when implanted ectopically into tibia injury sites, than if they were implanted back into their endogenous environment within mandible injuries. Conversely, when mesoderm derived progenitors were implanted into mandible injuries, an abundance of cartilage formed, which over time ossified via an endochondral pathway.

These results suggest a difference in the underlying reparative plasticity of cells from different origins. *In vitro* analysis demonstrated that mesoderm osteoprogenitors proliferated faster than the corresponding neural crest osteoprogenitors. However, the cells of neural crest origin were able to differentiate faster based on Alizarin Red S staining and qPCR of osteogenic markers. The authors went further to try to understand the possible molecular mechanisms underlying this difference (Leucht et al., 2008). They found that in the adult mice Hoxa11 expression was maintained in the tibia and was absent in the mandible. For neural crest osteoprogenitors, which originally lack Hoxa11 expression, they began to express Hoxa11 when ectopically placed in the tibia. This switch in expression was not found in the mesodermal osteoprogenitors, which continued to express Hoxa11 even when placed in the Hoxa11-negative environment of the mandible. This study once again reiterates how the molecular identity of cells used for transplantations can be a crucial factor in determining the success of a stem cell based bone graft. In addition, it may be true that osteoprogenitors of neural crest origin may be best suited as the stem cell source of bone grafts because of their greater plasticity to adapt to local environments.

4.2.3 ESC-derived neural crest stem cells

When ESC cultures are osteogenically induced following standard differentiation procedures, it is seldom examined which developmental progenitors are responsible for the terminally differentiated osteoblasts. Although some studies have differentiated ESCs along defined lineages and then determined their osteogenic capacity, Lee et al. (2008) reported the isolation and propagation of human neural crest cells from human ESCs. Initially they cultured human ESCs in neural induction media and then mechanically removed and replated the resulting neural rosettes. Cells that were doubly positive for the neural crest markers p75 and HNK-1 were further cultured and revealed a CD73 positive population. This marker expression indicates the presence of neural crest-derived mesenchymal stem cells. This CD73+ population could be osteogenically induced as revealed by Alizarin Red S, and Alk Phos staining, and bone sialoprotein expression.

In a similar study Jiang and colleagues (2008) also used a FACS enrichment strategy for p75 and HNK-1 positive neural crest cells after co-culture of human ESCs with PA6 stromal cells, although the osteogenic differentiation potential of such isolated neural crest cells was not determined. In another study cranial neural crest-like cells were derived from human ESCs, not by co-culture but instead though EB formation (Zhou and Snead, 2008). Here, FACS purification of neural crest cells was performed based on the expression of Frizzled3, a Wnt receptor, and cadherin11, a cadherin specifically expressed in the gastrulating embryo and migrating neural crest cells (Kimura et al., 1995). Only about 1% of cells were double positive for these selected markers and were able to self-renew and maintain multipotent differentiation potential, including runx2 positive osteoblasts with the capability to calcify. Although not definitive demonstrations of the isolation of osteoprogenitor stem cells from different germ layer-derived populations, these studies offer compelling evidence that cells existing in *in vitro* culture conditions can recapitulate the neural crest osteogenic pathways found in the developing embryo.

5. Conclusion

In summation, pluripotent stem cells are a particularly attractive source to develop new technologies and techniques to address many debilitating bone disorders and defects, and we have come far in the understanding and characterization of osteogenesis. Although more investigations and innovations are needed before regenerative bone biology becomes commonplace, the future holds great promise in this field of research.

6. Acknowledgment

N.zN. acknowledges support from the German Federal Ministry of Education and Research (BEO31/0312314 and 0315121A), the Tobacco-Related Disease Research Program (19KT-0017) and the Alberta Heritage Foundation for Medical Research. The authors offer sincere apologies to the many colleagues whose work could not be cited because of space limitations.

7. References

Aasen, T.; Raya, A.; Barrero, M. J.; Garreta, E.; Consiglio, A.; Gonzalez, F.; Vassena, R.; Bilic, J.; Pekarik, V.; Tiscornia, G.; Edel, M.; Boué, S. & Izpisúa Belmonte, J.C. (2008). Efficient and rapid generation of induced pluripotent stem cells from human keratinocytes. *Nat Biotechnol* 26, 1276-1284.

Aihara, Y.; Hayashi, Y.; Hirata, M.; Ariki, N.; Shibata, S.; Nagoshi, N.; Nakanishi, M.; Ohnuma, K.; Warashina, M.; Michiue, T.; Uchiyama, H.; Okano, H.; Asashima, M. & Furue, M.K. (2010). Induction of neural crest cells from mouse embryonic stem cells in a serum-free monolayer culture. *Int J Dev Biol* 54, 1287-1294.

Airas, L.; Hellman, J.; Salmi, M.; Bono, P.; Puurunen, T.; Smith, D.J. & Jalkanen, S. (1995). CD73 is involved in lymphocyte binding to the endothelium: characterization of lymphocyte-vascular adhesion protein 2 identifies it as CD73. *J Exp Med* 182(5), 1603-1608.

Amit, M. , Shariki, C. , Margulets, V. & Itskovitz-Eldor, J. (2004) Feeder layer- and serum-free culture of human embryonic stem cells. *Biol Reprod* 70(3), 837-345.

Arinzeh, T. L.; Peter, S. J.; Archambault, M. P.; van den Bos, C.; Gordon, S.; Kraus, K.; Smith, A. & Kadiyala, S. (2003). Allogeneic mesenchymal stem cells regenerate bone in a critical-sized canine segmental defect. *J Bone Joint Surg Am* 85-A, 1927-1935.

Barberi, T.; Willis, L. M.; Socci, N. D. & Studer, L. (2005). Derivation of multipotent mesenchymal precursors from human embryonic stem cells. *Plos Med* 2, 554-560.

Beddington, R. S. P.; Rashbass, P. & Wilson, V. (1992). Brachyury - a Gene Affecting Mouse Gastrulation and Early Organogenesis. *Dev Suppl*, 157-165.

Bigdeli, N.; Andersson, M.; Strehl, R.; Emanuelsson, K.; Kilmare, E.; Hyllner, J. & Lindahl, A. (2008). Adaptation of human embryonic stem cells to feeder-free and matrix-free culture conditions directly on plastic surfaces. *J Biotechnol* 133, 146-153.

Bigdeli, N.; de Peppo, G. M.; Lenneras, M.; Sjovall, P.; Lindahl, A.; Hyllner, J. & Karlsson, C. (2010). Superior osteogenic capacity of human embryonic stem cells adapted to matrix-free growth compared to human mesenchymal stem cells. *Tissue Eng Part A* 16, 3427-3440.

Bilousova, G.; Jun, D. H.; King, K. B.; De Langhe, S.; Chick, W. S.; Torchia, E. C.; Chow, K. S.; Klemm, D. J.; Roop, D. R. & Majka, S. M. (2011). Osteoblasts Derived from Induced Pluripotent Stem Cells Form Calcified Structures in Scaffolds Both in Vitro and in Vivo. *Stem Cells* 29, 206-216.

Blentic, A.; Tandon, P.; Payton, S.; Walshe, J.; Carney, T.; Kelsh, R. N.; Mason, I. & Graham, A. (2008). The emergence of ectomesenchyme. *Dev Dynam* 237, 592-601.

Bruder, S.P.; Gazit, D.; Passi-Even, L.; Bab, I. & Caplan, A.I. (1990). Osteochondral differentiation and the emergence of stage-specific osteogenic cell-surface molecules by bone marrow cells in diffusion chambers. *Bone Miner* 11(2), 141-151.

Bruder, S. P.; Kurth, A. A.; Shea, M.; Hayes, W. C.; Jaiswal, N. & Kadiyala, S. (1998). Bone regeneration by implantation of purified, culture-expanded human mesenchymal stem cells. *J Orthop Res* 16, 155-162.

Buttery, L. D. K.; Bourne, S.; Xynos, J. D.; Wood, H.; Hughes, F. J.; Hughes, S. P. F.; Episkopou, V. & Polak, J. M. (2001). Differentiation of osteoblasts and in vitro bone formation from murine embryonic stem cells. *Tissue Eng* 7, 89-99.

Byrne, J. A.; Pedersen, D. A.; Clepper, L. L.; Nelson, M.; Sanger, W. G.; Gokhale, S.; Wolf, D. P. & Mitalipov, S. M. (2007). Producing primate embryonic stem cells by somatic cell nuclear transfer. *Nature* 450, 497-502.

Cao, T.; Heng, B. C.; Ye, C. P.; Liu, H.; Toh, W. S.; Robson, P.; Li, P.; Hong, Y. H. & Stanton, L. W. (2005). Osteogenic differentiation within intact human embryoid bodies result in a marked increase in osteocalcin secretion after 12 days of in vitro culture, and formation of morphologically distinct nodule-like structures. *Tissue Cell* 37, 325-334.

Chaudhry, G. R.; Yao, D.; Smith, A. & Hussain, A. (2004). Osteogenic cells derived from embryonic stem cells produced bone nodules in three-dimensional scaffolds. *J Biomed Biotechnol*, 203-210.

Chung, I. H.; Yamaza, T.; Zhao, H.; Choung, P. H.; Shi, S. & Chai, Y. (2009). Stem Cell Property of Postmigratory Cranial Neural Crest Cells and Their Utility in Alveolar Bone Regeneration and Tooth Development. *Stem Cells* 27, 866-877.

Chung, U. I.; Schipani, E.; McMahon, A. P. & Kronenberg, H. M. (2001). Indian hedgehog couples chondrogenesis to osteogenesis in endochondral bone development. *J Clin Invest* 107, 295-304.

Claes, L. E.; Heigele, C. A.; Neidlinger-Wilke, C.; Kaspar, D.; Seidl, W.; Margevicius, K. J. & Augat, P. (1998). Effects of mechanical factors on the fracture healing process. *Clin Orthop Relat R*, S132-S147.

Davis, L. A.; Dienelt, A. & zur Nieden, N. I. (2011). Absorption-based assays for the analysis of osteogenic and chondrogenic yield. *Methods Mol Biol* 690, 255-272.

Dominici, M.; Le Blanc, K.; Mueller, I.; Slaper-Cortenbach, I.; Marini, F.; Krause, D.; Deans, R.; Keating, A.; Prockop, D.j. & Horwitz, E. (2006). Minimal criteria for defining multipotent mesenchymal stromal cells. The International Society for Cellular Therapy position statement. *Cytotherapy* 8(4), 315-317.

de Peppo, G. M.; Sjovall, P.; Lenneras, M.; Strehl, R.; Hyllner, J.; Thomsen, P. & Karlsson, C. (2010). Osteogenic potential of human mesenchymal stem cells and human embryonic stem cell-derived mesodermal progenitors: a tissue engineering perspective. *Tissue Eng Part A* 16, 3413-3426.

Doetschman, T.; Williams, P. & Maeda, N. (1988). Establishment of Hamster Blastocyst-Derived Embryonic Stem (ES) Cells. *Dev Biol* 127, 224-227.

Dupin, E.; Calloni, G.; Real, C.; Gongalves-Trentin, A. & Le Douarin, N. M. (2007). Neural crest progenitors and stem cells. *Cr Biol* 330, 521-529.

Evans, M. J. & Kaufman, M. H. (1981). Establishment in Culture of Pluripotential Cells from Mouse Embryos. *Nature* 292, 154-156.

Farrell, E.; van der Jagt, O. P.; Koevoet, W.; Kops, N.; van Manen, C. J.; Hellingman, C. A.; Jahr, H.; O'Brien, F. J.; Verhaar, J. A. N.; Weinans, H. & van Osch, G. J. V. M. (2009). Chondrogenic Priming of Human Bone Marrow Stromal Cells: A Better Route to Bone Repair? *Tissue Eng Part C-Meth* 15, 285-295.

Friedenstein, A.J.; Piatetzky-Shapiro, I.I. & Petrakova, K.V. (1966). Osteogenesis in transplants of bone marrow cells. *J Embryol Exp Morphol* 16(3), 381-390.

Friedenstein, A.J.; Gorskaja, J.F. & Kulagina, N.N. (1976). Fibroblast precursors in normal and irradiated mouse hematopoietic organs. *Exp Hematol* 4(5), 267-274.

Friedenstein, A.J.; Chailakhyan, R.K. & Gerasimov, U.V. (1987). Bone marrow osteogenic stem cells: in vitro cultivation and transplantation in diffusion chambers. *Cell Tissue Kinet* 20(3), 263-272.

Gadue, P.; Huber, T. L.; Paddison, P. J. & Keller, G. M. (2006). Wnt and TGF-beta signaling are required for the induction of an in vitro model of primitive streak formation using embryonic stem cells. *P Natl Acad Sci USA* 103, 16806-16811.

Gao, J. Z.; Dennis, J. E.; Solchaga, L. A.; Awadallah, A. S.; Goldberg, V. M. & Caplan, A. I. (2001). Tissue-engineered fabrication of an osteochondral composite graft using rat bone marrow-derived mesenchymal stem cells. *Tissue Eng* 7, 363-371.

Gazit, D.; Ebner, R.; Kahn, A.J. & Derynck, R. (1993). Modulation of expression and cell surface binding of members of the transforming growth factor-beta superfamily during retinoic acid-induced osteoblastic differentiation of multipotential mesenchymal cells. *Mol Endocrinol* 7(2), 189-198.

Giles, J. R.; Yang, X.; Mark, W. & Foote, R. H. (1993). Pluripotency of cultured rabbit inner cell mass cells detected by isozyme analysis and eye pigmentation of fetuses following injection into blastocysts or morulae. *Mol Reprod Dev* 36, 130-138.

Giordano, A., Galderisi, U., Marino, I.R. (2007). From the laboratory bench to the patient's bedside: an update on clinical trials with mesenchymal stem cells. *J Cell Physiol* 211(1), 27-35.

Gong, Y.; Slee, R. B.; Fukai, N.; Rawadi, G.; Roman-Roman, S.; Reginato, A. M.; et al. Osteoporosis-Pseudoglioma Syndrome Collaborative Group (2001). LDL receptor-related protein 5 (LRP5) affects bone accrual and eye development. *Cell* 107, 513-523.

Gougos, A. & Letarte, M. (1988). Identification of a human endothelial cell antigen with monoclonal antibody 44G4 produced against a pre-B leukemic cell line. *J Immunol* 141(6), 1925-1933.

Grayson, W.L.; Zhao, F.; Izadpanah, R.; Bunnell, B. & Ma, T. (2006). Effects of hypoxia on human mesenchymal stem cell expansion and plasticity in 3D constructs. *J Cell Physiol* 207(2), 331-339.

Handschel, J.; Berr, K.; Depprich, R. A.; Kubler, N. R.; Naujoks, C.; Wiesmann, H. P.; Ommerborn, M. A. & Meyer, U. (2008). Induction of osteogenic markers in differentially treated cultures of embryonic stem cells. *Head Face Med* 4, 10.

Hegert, C.; Kramer, J.; Hargus, G.; Muller, J.; Guan, K.; Wobus, A.M.; Müller, P.K. & Rohwedel, J. (2002). Differentiation plasticity of chondrocytes derived from mouse embryonic stem cells. *J Cell Sci* 115(Pt 23), 4617-4628.

Hematti, P. (2011). Human embryonic stem cell-derived mesenchymal progenitors: an overview. *Methods Mol Biol* 690, 163-174.

Hong, J.H. & Yaffe, M.B. (2006). TAZ: a beta-catenin-like molecule that regulates mesenchymal stem cell differentiation. *Cell Cycle* 5(2), 176-179.

Hu, H.; Hilton, M. J.; Tu, X.; Yu, K.; Ornitz, D. M. & Long, F. (2005). Sequential roles of Hedgehog and Wnt signaling in osteoblast development. *Development* 132, 49-60.

Hu, J.; Smith, L. A.; Feng, K.; Liu, X.; Sun, H. & Ma, P. X. (2010). Response of human embryonic stem cell-derived mesenchymal stem cells to osteogenic factors and architectures of materials during in vitro osteogenesis. *Tissue Eng Part A* 16, 3507-3514.

Iannaccone, P. M.; Taborn, G. U.; Garton, R. L.; Caplice, M. D. & Brenin, D. R. (1994). Pluripotent Embryonic Stem-Cells from the Rat Are Capable of Producing Chimeras. *Dev Biol* 163, 288-292.

Itskovitz-Eldor, J.; Schuldiner, M.; Karsenti, D.; Eden, A.; Yanuka, O.; Amit, M.; Soreq, H. & Benvenisty, N. (2000). Differentiation of human embryonic stem cells into embryoid bodies comprising the three embryonic germ layers. *Mol Med* 6, 88-95.

Jiang, Y.; Jahagirdar, B.N.; Reinhardt, R.L.; Schwartz, R.E.; Keene, C.D.; Ortiz-Gonzalez, X.R.; Reyes, M.; Lenvik, T.; Lund, T.; Blackstad, M.; Du, J.; Aldrich, S.; Lisberg, A.; Low, W.C.; Largaespada, D.A. & Verfaillie, C.M. (2002). Pluripotency of mesenchymal stem cells derived from adult marrow. *Nature* 418(6893), 41-49.

Jiang, X.; Gwye, Y.; McKeown, S.J.; Bronner-Fraser, M.; Lutzko, C. & Lawlor, E.R. (2009). Isolation and characterization of neural crest stem cells derived from in vitro-differentiated human embryonic stem cells. *Stem Cells Dev* 18(7), 1059-1070.

Johnstone, B.; Hering, T.M.; Caplan, A.I.; Goldberg, V.M. & Yoo, J.U. (1998). In vitro chondrogenesis of bone marrow-derived mesenchymal progenitor cells. *Exp Cell Res* 238(1), 265-272.

Jukes, J. M.; Both, S. K.; Leusink, A.; Sterk, L. M. T.; Van Blitterswijk, C. A. & De Boer, J. (2008). Endochondral bone tissue engineering using embryonic stem cells. *P Natl Acad Sci USA* 105, 6840-6845.

Jones, E.A.; Kinsey, S.E.; English, A.; Jones, R.A.; Straszynski, L.; Meredith, D.M.; Markham, A.F.; Jack, A.; Emery, P. & McGonagle D. (2002). Isolation and characterization of bone marrow multipotential mesenchymal progenitor cells. *Arthritis Rheum* 46(12), 3349-3360.

Jones, E.A.; English, A.; Kinsey, S.E.; Straszynski, L.; Emery, P.; Ponchel, F. & McGonagle, D. (2006). Optimization of a flow cytometry-based protocol for detection and phenotypic characterization of multipotent mesenchymal stromal cells from human bone marrow. *Cytometry B Clin Cytom* 70(6), 391-399.

Karaplis, A. C.; Luz, A.; Glowacki, J.; Bronson, R. T.; Tybulewicz, V. L. J.; Kronenberg, H. M. & Mulligan, R. C. (1994). Lethal Skeletal Dysplasia from Targeted Disruption of the Parathyroid Hormone-Related Peptide Gene. *Genes Dev* 8, 277-289.

Karlsson, C.; Emanuelsson, K.; Wessberg, F.; Kajic, K.; Axell, M. Z.; Eriksson, P. S.; Lindahl, A.; Hyllner, J. & Strehl, R. (2009). Human embryonic stem cell-derived mesenchymal progenitors-Potential in regenerative medicine. *Stem Cell Res* 3, 39-50.

Karp, J. M.; Ferreira, L. S.; Khademhosseini, A.; Kwon, A. H.; Yeh, J. & Langer, R. S. (2006). Cultivation of human embryonic stem cells without the embryoid body step enhances osteogenesis in vitro. *Stem Cells* 24, 835-843.

Kato, M.; Patel, M. S.; Levasseur, R.; Lobov, I.; Chang, B. H.; Glass, D. A., 2nd; Hartmann, C.; Li, L.; Hwang, T. H.; Brayton, C. F., Lang, R.A.; Karsenty, G. & Chan, L. (2002). Cbfa1-independent decrease in osteoblast proliferation, osteopenia, and persistent embryonic eye vascularization in mice deficient in Lrp5, a Wnt coreceptor. *J Cell Biol* 157, 303-314.

Kielty, C.M.; Kwan, A.P.; Holmes, D.F.; Schor, S.L. & Grant, M.E. (1985). Type X collagen, a product of hypertrophic chondrocytes. *Biochem J* 227(2), 545-554.

Kimura, Y.; Matsunami, H.; Inoue, T.; Shimamura, K.; Uchida, N.; Ueno, T.; Miyazaki, T. & Takeichi, M. (1995). Cadherin-11 expressed in association with mesenchymal morphogenesis in the head, somite, and limb bud of early mouse embryos. *Dev Biol* 169, 347–358.

Kotobuki, N.; Katsube, Y.; Katou, Y.; Tadokoro, M.; Hirose, M. & Ohgushi, H. (2008). In vivo survival and osteogenic differentiation of allogeneic rat bone marrow mesenchymal stem cells (MSCs). *Cell Transplant* 17, 705-712.

Kramer, J; Hegert, C.; Guan, K.; Wobus, A.M.; Müller, P.K. & Rohwedel, J. (2000). Embryonic stem cell-derived chondrogenic differentiation in vitro: activation by BMP-2 and BMP-4. *Mech Dev* 92(2), 193-205.

Kramer, J.; Hegert, C.; Hargus, G. & Rohwedel, J. (2005). Mouse ES cell lines show a variable degree of chondrogenic differentiation in vitro. *Cell Biol Int* 29(2), 139-146.

Lanske, B.; Karaplis, A. C.; Lee, K.; Luz, A.; Vortkamp, A.; Pirro, A.; Karperien, M.; Defize, L. H. K.; Ho, C.; Mulligan, R. C.; Abou-Samra, A.B.; Jüppner, H.; Segre, G.V. & Kronenberg HM. (1996). PTH/PTHrP receptor in early development and Indian hedgehog-regulated bone growth. *Science* 273, 663-666.

Le Blanc, K.; Gotherstrom, C.; Ringden, O.; Hassan, M.; McMahon, R.; Horwitz, E.; Anneren, G.; Axelsson, O.; Nunn, J.; Ewald, U.; Nordén-Lindeberg, S.; Jansson, M.; Dalton, A.; Aström, E. & Westgren, M. (2005). Fetal mesenchymal stem-cell engraftment in bone after in utero transplantation in a patient with severe osteogenesis imperfecta. *Transplantation* 79(11), 1607-1614.

Lee, G.; Kim, H.; Elkabetz, Y.; Al Shamy, G.; Panagiotakos, G.; Barberi, T.; Tabar, V. & Studer, L. (2008). Corrigendum: Isolation and directed differentiation of neural crest stem cells derived from human embryonic stem cells (vol 25, pg 1468, 2007). *Nat Biotechnol* 26, 831-831.

Leucht, P.; Kim, J. B.; Amasha, R.; James, A. W.; Girod, S. & Helms, J. A. (2008). Embryonic origin and Hox status determine progenitor cell fate during adult bone regeneration. *Development* 135, 2845-2854.

Levenberg, S.; Huang, N. F.; Lavik, E.; Rogers, A. B.; Itskovitz-Eldor, J. & Langer, R. (2003). Differentiation of human embryonic stem cells on three-dimensional polymer scaffolds. *Proc Natl Acad Sci U S A* 100, 12741-12746.

Martin, G. R. (1981). Isolation of a Pluripotent Cell-Line from Early Mouse Embryos Cultured in Medium Conditioned by Teratocarcinoma Stem-Cells. *P Natl Acad Sci USA* 78, 7634-7638.

Masuyama, R.; Stockmans, I.; Torrekens, S.; Van Looveren, R.; Maes, C.; Carmeliet, P.; Bouillon, R. & Carmeliet, G. (2006). Vitamin D receptor in chondrocytes promotes osteoclastogenesis and regulates FGF23 production in osteoblasts. *J Clin Invest* 116, 3150-3159.

Morrisskay, G.; Ruberte, E. & Fukiishi, Y. (1993). Mammalian Neural Crest and Neural Crest Derivatives. *Ann Anat* 175, 501-507.

Naja, R. P.; Dardenne, O.; Arabian, A. & St Arnaud, R. (2009). Chondrocyte-specific modulation of Cyp27b1 expression supports a role for local synthesis of 1,25-dihydroxyvitamin D3 in growth plate development. *Endocrinology* 150, 4024-4032.

Nakagawa, M.; Koyanagi, M.; Tanabe, K.; Takahashi, K.; Ichisaka, T.; Aoi, T.; Okita, K.; Mochiduki, Y.; Takizawa, N. & Yamanaka, S. (2008). Generation of induced pluripotent stem cells without Myc from mouse and human fibroblasts. *Nat Biotechnol* 26, 101-106.

Nakajima, M.; Wakitani, S.; Harada, Y.; Tanigami, A. & Tomita, N. (2008). In vivo mechanical condition plays an important role for appearance of cartilage tissue in ES cell transplanted joint. *J Orthopaed Res* 26, 10-17.

Nakanishi, M.; Kurisaki, A.; Hayashi, Y.; Warashina, M.; Ishiura, S.; Kusuda-Furue, M. & Asashima, M. (2009). Directed induction of anterior and posterior primitive streak by Wnt from embryonic stem cells cultured in a chemically defined serum-free medium. *Faseb J* 23, 114-122.

Niemeyer, P.; Mehlhorn, A.; Jaeger, M.; Kasten, P.; Simank, H.G.; Krause, U. & Südkamp, N.P. (2004). Adult mesenchymal stem cells for the regeneration of musculoskeletal tissue. *MMW Fortschr Med* 146(51-52), 45.

Okita, K.; Ichisaka, T. & Yamanaka, S. (2007). Generation of germline-competent induced pluripotent stem cells. *Nature* 448, 313-U311.

Olivier, E. N.; Rybicki, A. C. & Bouhassira, E. E. (2006). Differentiation of human embryonic stem cells into bipotent mesenchymal stem cells. *Stem Cells* 24, 1914-1922.

Osborn, L.; Hession, C.; Tizard, R.; Vassallo, C.; Luhowskyj, S.; Chi-Rosso, G. & Lobb, R. (1989). Direct expression cloning of vascular cell adhesion molecule 1, a cytokine-induced endothelial protein that binds to lymphocytes. *Cell* 59(6), 1203-1211.

Pfander, D. & Gelse, K. (2007). Hypoxia and osteoarthritis: how chondrocytes survive hypoxic environments. *Curr Opin Rheumatol* 19, 457-462.

Phillips, B. W.; Belmonte, N.; Vernochet, C.; Ailhaud, G. & Dani, C. (2001). Compactin enhances osteogenesis in murine embryonic stem cells. *Biochem Biophys Res Commun* 284, 478-484.

Pittenger, M.F.; Mackay, A.M.; Beck, S.C.; Jaiswal, R.K.; Douglas, R.; Mosca, J.D.; Moorman, M.A.; Simonetti, D.W.; Craig, S. & Marshak, D.R. (1999). Multilineage potential of adult human mesenchymal stem cells. *Science* 284(5411), 143-147.

Quarto, N.; Wan, D. C.; Kwan, M. D.; Panetta, N. J.; Li, S. & Longaker, M. T. (2010). Origin matters: differences in embryonic tissue origin and Wnt signaling determine the osteogenic potential and healing capacity of frontal and parietal calvarial bones. *J Bone Miner Res* 25, 1680-1694.

Quirici, N.; Soligo, D.; Bossolasco, P.; Servida, F.; Lumini, C. & Deliliers, G.L. (2002). Isolation of bone marrow mesenchymal stem cells by anti-nerve growth factor receptor antibodies. *Exp Hematol* 30(7), 783-791.

Reyes, M.; Lund, T.; Lenvik, T.; Aguiar, D.; Koodie, L. & Verfaillie, C.M. (2001). Purification and ex vivo expansion of postnatal human marrow mesodermal progenitor cells. *Blood* 98(9), 2615-2625.

Rezwan, K.; Chen, Q. Z.; Blaker, J. J. & Boccaccini, A. R. (2006). Biodegradable and bioactive porous polymer/inorganic composite scaffolds for bone tissue engineering. *Biomaterials* 27, 3413-3431.

Rose, F. R. & Oreffo, R. O. (2002). Bone tissue engineering: hope vs hype. *Biochem Biophys Res Commun* 292, 1-7.

Sakurai, H.; Era, T.; Jakt, L. M.; Okada, M.; Naki, S.; Nishikawa, S. & Nishikawa, S. I. (2006). In vitro Modeling of paraxial and lateral mesoderm differentiation reveals early reversibility. *Stem Cells* 24, 575-586.

Salgado, A. J.; Coutinho, O. P. & Reis, R. L. (2004). Bone tissue engineering: state of the art and future trends. *Macromol Biosci* 4, 743-765.

Shimko, D. A.; Burks, C. A.; Dee, K. C. & Nauman, E. A. (2004). Comparison of in vitro mineralization by murine embryonic and adult stem cells cultured in an osteogenic medium. *Tissue Eng* 10, 1386-1398.

Simmons, P.J. & Torok-Storb, B. (1991). CD34 expression by stromal precursors in normal human adult bone marrow. *Blood* 78(11), 2848-2853.

Smith, L. A.; Liu, X. H.; Hu, J. & Ma, P. X. (2009). The influence of three-dimensional nanofibrous scaffolds on the osteogenic differentiation of embryonic stem cells. *Biomaterials* 30, 2516-2522.

Smith, M. M. & Hall, B. K. (1990). Development and Evolutionary Origins of Vertebrate Skeletogenic and Odontogenic Tissues. *Biol Rev* 65, 277-373.

Sottile, V.; Thomson, A. & McWhir, J. (2003). In vitro osteogenic differentiation of human ES cells. *Cloning Stem Cells* 5, 149-155.

Stenderup, K.; Justesen, J.; Eriksen, E.F.; Rattan, S.I. & Kassem, M. (2001). Number and proliferative capacity of osteogenic stem cells are maintained during aging and in patients with osteoporosis. *J Bone Miner Res* 16(6), 1120-1129.

St-Jacques, B.; Hammerschmidt, M.; & McMahon, A. P. (1999). Indian hedgehog signaling regulates proliferation and differentiation of chondrocytes and is essential for bone formation. *Genes Dev* 13, 2617-2617.

Tada, S.; Era, T.; Furusawa, C.; Sakurai, H.; Nishikawa, S.; Kinoshita, M.; Nakao, K.; Chiba, T. & Nishikawa, S. I. (2005). Characterization of mesendoderm: a diverging point of the definitive endoderm and mesoderm in embryonic stem cell differentiation culture. *Development* 132, 4363-4374.

Taiani, J.; Krawetz, R.J.; zur Nieden, N.I.; Wu, E.Y.; Kallos, M.S.; Matyas, J.R. & Rancourt, D.E. (2010). Reduced differentiation efficiency of murine embryonic stem cells in stirred suspension bioreactors. *Stem Cells Dev* 19(7), 989-998.

Takahashi, K. & Yamanaka, S. (2006). Induction of pluripotent stem cells from mouse embryonic and adult fibroblast cultures by defined factors. *Cell* 126, 663-676.

Takashima, Y.; Era, T.; Nakao, K.; Kondo, S.; Kasuga, M.; Smith, A. G. & Nishikawa, S. I. (2007). Neuroepithelial cells supply an initial transient wave of MSC differentiation. *Cell* 129, 1377-1388.

Thomson, J. A.; Itskovitz-Eldor, J.; Shapiro, S. S.; Waknitz, M. A.; Swiergiel, J. J.; Marshall, V. S. & Jones, J. M. (1998). Embryonic stem cell lines derived from human blastocysts. *Science* 282, 1145-1147.

Thomson, J. A.; Kalishman, J.; Golos, T. G.; Durning, M.; Harris, C. P.; Becker, R. A. & Hearn, J. P. (1995). Isolation of a primate embryonic stem cell line. *Proc Natl Acad Sci U S A* 92, 7844-7848.

Toh, W.S.; Yang, Z.; Liu, H.; Heng, B.C.; Lee, E.H. & Cao, T. (2007). Effects of culture conditions and bone morphogenetic protein 2 on extent of chondrogenesis from human embryonic stem cells. *Stem Cells* 25(4), 950-960.

Tondreau, T.; Lagneaux, L.; Dejeneffe, M.; Delforge, A.; Massy, M.; Mortier, C. & Bron, D. (2004a). Isolation of BM mesenchymal stem cells by plastic adhesion or negative selection: phenotype, proliferation kinetics and differentiation potential. *Cytotherapy* 6(4), 372-379.

Tondreau, T.; Lagneaux, L.; Dejeneffe, M.; Massy, M.; Mortier, C.; Delforge, A. & Bron, D. (2004b). Bone marrow-derived mesenchymal stem cells already express specific neural proteins before any differentiation. *Differentiation* 72(7), 319-312.

Tortelli, F.; Tasso, R.; Loiacono, F. & Cancedda, R. (2010). The development of tissue-engineered bone of different origin through endochondral and intramembranous ossification following the implantation of mesenchymal stem cells and osteoblasts in a murine model. *Biomaterials* 31, 242-249.

Tremoleda, J. L.; Forsyth, N. R.; Khan, N. S.; Wojtacha, D.; Christodoulou, I.; Tye, B. J.; Racey, S. N.; Collishaw, S.; Sottile, V.; Thomson, A. J.; Simpson, A.H.; Noble, B.S. & McWhir, J. (2008). Bone tissue formation from human embryonic stem cells in vivo. *Cloning Stem Cells* 10, 119-132.

Trettner, S.; Seeliger, A. & zur Nieden, N. I. (2011). Embryoid body formation: recent advances in automated bioreactor technology. *Methods Mol Biol* 690, 135-149.

Trivedi, P. & Hematti, P. (2007). Simultaneous generation of CD34(+) primitive hematopoietic cells and CD73(+) mesenchymal stem cells from human embryonic stem cells cocultured with murine OP9 stromal cells. *Exp Hematol* 35, 146-154.

Tuch, B.E. (2006) Stem cells--a clinical update. *Aust Fam Physician* 35(9), 719-721.

Vogel, W.; Grünebach, F.; Messam, C.A.; Kanz, L.; Brugger, W. & Bühring, H.J. (2003). Heterogeneity among human bone marrow-derived mesenchymal stem cells and neural progenitor cells. *Haematologica* 88(2), 126-133.

Vortkamp, A.; Lee, K.; Lanske, B.; Segre, G. V.; Kronenberg, H. M. & Tabin, C. J. (1996). Regulation of rate of cartilage differentiation by Indian hedgehog and PTH-related protein. *Science* 273, 613-622.

Wakitani, S.; Takaoka, K.; Hattori, T.; Miyazawa, N.; Iwanaga, T.; Takeda, S.; Watanabe, T.K. & Tanigami, A. (2003). Embryonic stem cells injected into the mouse knee joint form teratomas and subsequently destroy the joint. *Rheumatology* 42(1), 162-165.

Wakitani, S.; Aoki, H.; Harada, Y.; Sonobe, M.; Morita, Y.; Mu, Y.; Tomita, N.; Nakamura, Y.; Takeda, S.; Watanabe, T.K. & Tanigami, A. (2004). Embryonic stem cells form articular cartilage, not teratomas, in osteochondral defects of rat joints. *Cell Transplant* 13(4), 331-336.

Warnke, P. H.; Springer, I. N. G.; Wiltfang, J.; Acil, Y.; Eufinger, H.; Wehmoller, M.; Russo, P. A. J.; Bolte, H.; Sherry, E.; Behrens, E. & Terheyden, H. (2004). Growth and transplantation of a custom vascularised bone graft in a man. *Lancet* 364, 766-770.

Warnke, P. H.; Wiltfang, J.; Springer, I.; Acil, Y.; Bolte, H.; Kosmahl, M.; Russo, P. A. J.; Sherry, E.; Lutzen, U.; Wolfart, S. & Terheyden, H. (2006). Man as living bioreactor: Fate of an exogenously prepared customized tissue-engineered mandible. *Biomaterials* 27, 3163-3167.

Weston, J. A. (1991). Sequential Segregation and Fate of Developmentally Restricted Intermediate Cell-Populations in the Neural Crest Lineage. *Curr Top Dev Biol* 25, 133-153.

Weston, J. A.; Yoshida, H.; Robinson, V.; Nishikawa, S.; Fraser, S. T. & Nishikawa, S. (2004). Neural crest and the origin of ectomesenchyme: Neural fold heterogeneity suggests an alternative hypothesis. *Dev Dynam* 229, 118-130.

Williams, R. L.; Hilton, D. J.; Pease, S.; Willson, T. A.; Stewart, C. L.; Gearing, D. P.; Wagner, E. F.; Metcalf, D.; Nicola, N. A. & Gough, N. M. (1988). Myeloid-Leukemia Inhibitory Factor Maintains the Developmental Potential of Embryonic Stem-Cells. *Nature* 336, 684-687.

Woll, N. L.; Heaney, J. D. & Bronson, S. K. (2006). Osteogenic nodule formation from single embryonic stem cell-derived progenitors. *Stem Cells Dev* 15, 865-879.

Woo, K. M.; Chen, V. J. & Ma, P. X. (2003). Nano-fibrous scaffolding architecture selectively enhances protein adsorption contributing to cell attachment. *J Biomed Mater Res A* 67A, 531-537.

Xu, Y.; Malladi, P.; Zhou, D. & Longaker, M. T. (2007). Molecular and cellular characterization of mouse calvarial osteoblasts derived from neural crest and paraxial mesoderm. *Plast Reconstr Surg* 120, 1783-1795.

Yaszemski, M. J.; Payne, R. G.; Hayes, W. C.; Langer, R. & Mikos, A. G. (1996). Evolution of bone transplantation: molecular, cellular and tissue strategies to engineer human bone. *Biomaterials* 17, 175-185.

Yu, J.; Vodyanik, M. A.; Smuga-Otto, K.; Antosiewicz-Bourget, J.; Frane, J. L.; Tian, S.; Nie, J.; Jonsdottir, G. A.; Ruotti, V.; Stewart, R.; Slukvin, I.I. & Thomson, J.A. (2007). Induced pluripotent stem cell lines derived from human somatic cells. *Science* 318, 1917-1920.

Young, R.G.; Butler, D,L.; Weber, W.; Caplan, A.I.; Gordon, S.L. & Fink, D.J. (1998). Use of mesenchymal stem cells in a collagen matrix for Achilles tendon repair. *J Orthop Res* 16(4), 406-413.

Zhang, Z.L.; Tong, J.; Lu, R.N.; Scutt, A.M.; Goltzman, D. & Miao, D.S. (2009). Therapeutic potential of non-adherent BM-derived mesenchymal stem cells in tissue regeneration. *Bone Marrow Transplant* 43(1), 69-81.

Zhou, Y. & Snead, M.L. (2008). Derivation of cranial neural crest-like cells from human embryonic stem cells. *Biochem Biophys Res Commun* 376(3), 542-547.

zur Nieden, N. I. (2011). Embryonic stem cells for osteo-degenerative diseases. *Methods Mol Biol* 690, 1-30.

zur Nieden, N. I.; Kempka, G. & Ahr, H. J. (2003). In vitro differentiation of embryonic stem cells into mineralized osteoblasts. *Differentiation* 71, 18-27.

zur Nieden, N.I.; Kempka, G.; Rancourt, D.E. & Ahr, H.J. (2005). Induction of chondro-, osteo- and adipogenesis in embryonic stem cells by bone morphogenetic protein-2: effect of cofactors on differentiating lineages. *BMC Dev Biol* 5(1), 1.

Part 4

Pluripotent Alternatives –
Induced Pluripotent Stem Cells (iPSCs)

6

New Techniques in the Generation of Induced Pluripotent Stem Cells

Raymond C.B. Wong[1,3], Ellen L. Smith[1,3] and Peter J. Donovan[1,2,3]
[1]*Department of Biological Chemistry,*
[2]*Department of Developmental and Cell Biology,*
[3]*Sue and Bill Gross Stem Cell Research Center, University of California at Irvine, Irvine,*
USA

1. Introduction

Pluripotent stem cells have the ability to differentiate into cells of the three primary germ layer lineages, ectoderm, mesoderm and endoderm. The most studied type of pluripotent stem cells are embryonic stem cells (ESC), cells derived from the inner cell mass of embryos at the blastocyst stage of development (Evans and Kaufman, 1981; Martin, 1981; Thomson et al., 1998). The pluripotent property of human embryonic stem cells (hESC) makes them useful for the development of cellular therapies to replace diseased or degenerated cells in the body. Moreover, hESC also possess the ability to propagate indefinitely *in vitro* while maintaining a normal karyotype, and thus can provide an unlimited source of cells for the development of cell replacement therapies (Pera et al., 2000). However, one of the major hurdles in hESC research has been the ethical implications of using stem cells derived from embryos. Furthermore, generation of patient-specific stem cell lines may overcome some of the issues associated with immuno-compatibility in cell replacement therapy.

The breakthrough studies conducted by Shinya Yamanaka's group demonstrated direct reprogramming of mouse or human fibroblasts back to pluripotent cells, creating so-called induced pluripotent stem cells (iPSC) (Takahashi et al., 2007; Takahashi and Yamanaka, 2006). Studies of iPSC revolutionized stem cell research by creating a more reproducible method to generate sufficient amounts of patient-specific pluripotent cells and bypassing the ethical implications surrounding research utilizing human embryos. iPSC also provide an alternative approach to generate disease-specific lines for mechanistic studies in disease modeling, as well as high throughput screening for drug discovery or toxicology studies (Amabile and Meissner, 2009). As the area of iPSC research is rapidly evolving, this review aims to summarize and discuss the current techniques used for the generation of iPSC.

2. Reprogramming factors used in generation of induced pluripotent stem cells (iPSC)

The initial derivation of iPSC by Shinya Yamanaka's group was achieved by overexpressing four transcription factors first in mouse and then human fibroblasts, namely Octamer-binding transcription factor 4 (Oct4), Sex-determining region Y HMG box 2 (Sox2), Krüppel-like factor 4 (Klf4) and v-myc myelocytomatosis viral oncogene homolog (c-Myc), often referred to as the 'Yamanaka factors' (Takahashi et al., 2007; Takahashi and Yamanaka, 2006). Alternatively, a study from James Thomson's lab identified a different combination of factors for the generation of human iPSC, using Oct4, Sox2, Nanog and Lin28 (Yu et al., 2007). Subsequent reports from many labs have contributed to a growing list of reprogramming factors used for iPSC generation, including Estrogen-related receptor beta (Esrrb), Sal-like 4 (Sall4), microRNAs (miRNA), simian virus 40 large-T (SV40LT) antigen and human telomerase reverse transcriptase (hTERT). This section will provide a background of our understanding of these reprogramming factors in regulating the cell fate of pluripotent stem cells and discuss their role during direct somatic cell reprogramming. Other strategies to enhance reprogramming efficiency will also be discussed, such as supplementation with small molecules as well as knockdown of p53, p21 and p16.

2.1 Oct4

Oct4 was one of the first transcription factors identified to be a master regulator of cellular pluripotency (Okamoto et al., 1990; Rosner et al., 1990; Scholer et al., 1989). During mouse development *in vivo*, Oct4 expression is restricted to the inner cell mass, primitive ectoderm and primordial germ cells (Pesce and Scholer, 2001). Similarly *in vitro*, ESC and embryonal carcinoma cells (ECC) have high expression of Oct4, which is reduced upon their differentiation (Assou et al., 2007; Rosner et al., 1990).

Although expression of Oct4 is fundamental for the maintenance of pluripotency and development of the inner cell mass in mice (Nichols et al., 1998), complex regulation of its precise level is required to prevent cells from differentiating into other lineages. A transient increase in endogenous Oct4 levels has been observed upon mesodermal differentiation of mouse embryonic stem cells (mESC) (Zeineddine et al., 2006). Furthermore in various over-expression studies, an increase in Oct4 expression can cause mESC to differentiate into endoderm, mesoderm and neuroectoderm lineages (Niwa et al., 2000; Shimozaki et al., 2003; Zeineddine et al., 2006). On the other hand, repression of Oct4 levels results in a loss of pluripotency and promotes trophectodermal differentiation in mESC and hESC (Matin et al., 2004; Niwa et al., 2000). Consistent with these studies, Oct4 has been shown to directly inhibit the expression of major trophectoderm differentiation regulators such as caudal type homeobox 2 (Cdx2) and Eomesdermin (Eomes) (Liu et al., 1997; Liu and Roberts, 1996; Niwa et al., 2005). Together these studies highlight the significance of the critical range of Oct4 level required to maintain ESC pluripotency (Niwa et al., 2000).

As a master regulator of pluripotency, Oct4 was one of the original four factors utilized by Yamanaka and colleagues in the generation of iPSC in both mouse and human (Takahashi et al., 2007; Takahashi and Yamanaka, 2006). As seen in Oct4 over-expression and down-regulation experiments in ESC, the precise level of Oct4 in combination with other reprogramming factors is also essential for efficient generation of iPSC (Papapetrou et al., 2009). Using bicistronic vectors, Papapetrou *et al.* (2009) showed that a 3-fold higher expression of Oct4 compared to Sox2, Klf4 and c-Myc enhanced iPSC generation (Papapetrou et al., 2009). Interestingly, overexpression of Oct4 alone was sufficient to induce reprogramming in neural stem cells that already express high endogenous level of Sox2, c-Myc and Klf4 (Kim et al., 2009b; Kim et al., 2009c). To date, most protocols for generation of iPSC require ectopic expression of Oct4, underlying the important role of Oct4 during direct somatic cell reprogramming (Feng et al., 2009b). Recently, Heng *et al.* (2010) demonstrated that an orphan nuclear receptor Nr5a2 can functionally replace Oct4 in the generation of mouse iPSC (Heng et al., 2010). However, the precise role of Nr5a2 in regulating cell fate in pluripotent stem cells remains unclear. Further research is also needed to confirm the ability of Nr5a2 to replace Oct4 in human iPSC generation.

2.2 Sox2

Sox2 is an important transcription factor in pluripotent stem cells as well as precursor cells of the neural compartment. It is expressed in the inner cell mass, epiblast and extraembryonic ectodermal cells during mouse embryo development (Avilion et al., 2003; Miyagi et al., 2004). Unlike Oct4, Sox2 expression is maintained in neural stem cells (Ellis et al., 2004; Graham et al., 2003) and over-expression of Sox2 favors neural differentiation in mESC (Kopp et al., 2008; Zhao et al., 2004). Sox2 is known to interact with several binding partners, including Oct4 in the maintenance of pluripotency (Yuan et al., 1995). In a genome-wide chromatin immunoprecipitation study in hESC, Sox2 and Oct4 were found to share many target genes, many of which are transcription factors important in development (Boyer et al., 2005).

Importantly, Sox2 was shown to be indispensable for maintaining pluripotency. Sox2 knockout mouse embryos are unable to form an epiblast and fail to develop past the implantation stage (Avilion et al., 2003). Down-regulation of Sox2 in mESC and hESC results in loss of pluripotency and differentiation towards the trophectoderm cell lineage (Adachi et al., 2010; Fong et al., 2008; Li et al., 2007; Masui et al., 2007). Somewhat surprising was the finding that expression of many Sox2 target genes were not affected by the loss of Sox2 (Masui et al., 2007). The authors in this study suggested potential compensation of Sox2 function by other members of the Sox family. Consistent with this idea, Nakagawa *et al.* (2008) demonstrated that Sox1, Sox3, Sox15 and Sox18 have the ability to replace Sox2 to some extent in iPSC generation (Nakagawa et al., 2008). To date, Sox2 and Oct4 remain to be the two fundamental reprogramming factors and are widely used in various protocols to generate iPSC. Similar to Oct4, it should be noted that ectopic expression of Sox2 can be omitted in the generation of iPSC, if the starting cell type expresses substantial levels of Sox2 (Utikal et al., 2009a).

2.3 Nanog

Nanog is a homeodomain protein that is widely considered as a master regulator for stem cell pluripotency (Chambers et al., 2003; Mitsui et al., 2003). Nanog expression is restricted to the inner cell mass, epiblast and primordial germ cells in the early embryo, as well as a number of pluripotent cells lines such as ESC, ECC and embryonic germ cells (Chambers et al., 2003). During embryo development, Nanog plays a role in suppressing Cdx2, a master regulator of trophectoderm differentiation, and in turn suppression of Cdx2 specifies the inner cell mass fate (Chen et al., 2009). Moreover, Nanog can also physically interact with Oct4 (Wang et al., 2006) and cooperates extensively with Oct4 and Sox2 to form an autoregulated core-transcriptional network that maintain stem cell pluripotency (Boyer et al., 2005; Chen et al., 2008; Kim et al., 2008).

Unlike Oct4 or Sox2, sustained expression of Nanog renders mESC and hESC resistant to differentiation (Chambers et al., 2003; Darr et al., 2006; Ivanova et al., 2006). However in the absence of Oct4, Nanog alone is not sufficient to maintain mESC self-renewal, suggesting that Nanog plays a subservient role in maintaining self-renewal (Chambers et al., 2003). This is also supported by evidence from Nanog knockdown studies. Although early studies suggested that a reduction of Nanog resulted in differentiation of mESC and hESC (Fong et al., 2008; Hyslop et al., 2005; Ivanova et al., 2006; Mitsui et al., 2003), it was later discovered that transient down-regulation of Nanog can be reversible and does not necessarily mark commitment to differentiation (Chambers et al., 2007). In this respect, mESC can remain undifferentiated in the absence of Nanog, but are more prone to differentiation (Chambers et al., 2007).

Given the important role of Nanog in establishing cell pluripotency, it was somewhat surprising that the initial derivation of iPSC could be achieved without the ectopic expression of Nanog (Takahashi et al., 2007; Takahashi and Yamanaka, 2006). However, Nanog has proved to be a valuable marker for identification of fully reprogrammed iPSC that are germline competent (Maherali et al., 2007; Okita et al., 2007; Wernig et al., 2007). Furthermore, ectopic expression of Nanog in combination with Oct4, Sox2, Klf4 and c-Myc seems to accelerate the reprogramming kinetics of somatic cells to iPSC, but has no effect on the overall reprogramming efficiency (Hanna et al., 2009).

2.4 Klf4

Klf4 and its family members have emerged as important regulators for maintaining pluripotency. Klf4 belongs to the Krüppel-like factor (Klf) family of zinc finger transcription factors. Klf4 can act as an oncogene or a tumor suppressor gene depending on the physiological context (McConnell et al., 2007; Rowland and Peeper, 2006). Klf4 is usually expressed in adult tissues that possess some degree of regenerative capability, including intestine, gut, skin and testis (Nandan and Yang, 2009). Li *et al.* (2005) provided the first evidence that Klf4 plays a role in regulating stem cell pluripotency, by showing that overexpression of Klf4 prevents differentiation of mESC into erythroid progenitors (Li et al., 2005). In conjunction with Oct4, Sox2 and c-Myc, Klf4 was among the first factors to be used to generate iPSC (Takahashi et al., 2007; Takahashi and Yamanaka, 2006). However, the current view is that Klf4 acts only as a secondary factor to enhance somatic cell reprogramming, as iPSC can be generated without Klf4 using a different combination of reprogramming factors (Yu et al., 2007). Klf4 was later discovered to be an important component of the core transcriptional network that regulates expression of Oct4, Sox2, Nanog, Myc and also Klf4 itself (Chen et al., 2008; Kim et al., 2008). Furthermore, Klf4 can directly interact and cooperate with Oct4 and Sox2 to activate a subset of ESC specific genes, including Nanog and Lefty1 (Nakatake et al., 2006; Wei et al., 2009). Klf4 also acts to inhibit apoptosis by suppressing p53 (Rowland et al., 2005), which helps to reprogram somatic cells to a pluripotent state (See discussion below).

Importantly, other Klf family members including Klf1, Klf2 or Klf5, can substitute for Klf4 in iPSC generation (Nakagawa et al., 2008), which suggests that functional redundancies exist among the Klf family members in establishing cell pluripotency. This also explains the observation that Klf4 knockdown in mESC exhibited no obvious phenotype (Jiang et al., 2008; Nakatake et al., 2006), whereas triple knockdown of Klf2, Klf4 and Klf5 resulted in rapid differentiation of mESC (Jiang et al., 2008). However, isoform-specific functions of Klf4 and Klf5 are also observed. Previous studies showed that Klf5 knockout mice result in embryo lethality and defects in implantation (Ema et al., 2008), whereas Klf4 knockout mice are normal during early embryo development but die soon after birth due to loss of skin barrier function (Segre et al., 1999). Furthermore, Ema *et al.* (2008) demonstrated that knocking out Klf5 in mESC results in spontaneous differentiation. Although introduction of

Klf4 can rescue the spontaneous differentiation phenotype, proliferation is significantly decreased (Ema et al., 2008). Further studies are needed to dissect the precise roles of different Klf members in regulating cell pluripotency.

2.5 Lin28

Lin28 encodes for a cytoplasmic RNA binding protein that acts as a translational enhancer (Polesskaya et al., 2007). It was first identified as a heterochronic gene that regulates the developmental timing pathway in *Caenorhabditis elegans* (Moss et al., 1997). A previous transcriptome study has shown that Lin28 is a hESC-specific gene, suggesting that it may play a role in regulating stem cell pluripotency (Richards et al., 2004). However, functional studies of Lin28 in hESC and mESC yielded opposing results. In mESC, Lin28 knockdown resulted in decreased cell proliferation while overexpression of Lin28 enhanced cell proliferation (Xu et al., 2009a). In sharp contrast, Lin28 knockdown in hESC had no obvious phenotype, whereas Lin28 overexpression reduced proliferation and promoted extraembryonic endoderm differentiation (Darr and Benvenisty, 2009). Further studies are clearly needed to elucidate whether Lin28 has a different role in maintenance of pluripotent stem cells in mice and humans.

Lin28 was first used in combination with Nanog, Oct4 and Sox2 to generate human iPSC, acting as an enhancer for somatic cell reprogramming much like Klf4 (Yu et al., 2007). However, it remains unclear how Lin28 contributes to induction of pluripotency. It was demonstrated that Lin28 can block the processing of let7 microRNA family members, a group of pro-differentiation microRNA that also act as tumor suppressors (Melton et al., 2010; Viswanathan et al., 2008). Members of the let7 microRNA family have been shown to repress expression of oncogenes such as c-Myc and Ras. Hence, down-regulation of let7 by Lin28 could increase cell proliferation and drive cellular transformation (Viswanathan et al., 2009). Consistent with this idea, a recent study in mice demonstrated that Lin28 accelerates reprogramming kinetics by enhancing cell proliferation (Hanna et al., 2009). Another proposed mechanism of Lin28 action is that it can selectively regulate gene expression at a post-transcriptional level, enhancing translation of anti-differentiation mRNAs while degrading pro-differentiation mRNAs to maintain pluripotency. A previous study demonstrated that Lin28 can reside in polysomal ribosome fractions, in which mRNAs are translated (Balzer and Moss, 2007). Indeed, Lin28 has been shown to bind directly to Oct4 mRNA in hESC to facilitate translation via interaction with RNA helicase A (Qiu et al., 2010). Lin28 can also reside in P-bodies, in which mRNAs are degraded (Balzer and Moss, 2007). Therefore, it remains speculative that Lin28 may be able to selectively degrade certain pro-differentiation mRNA to support stem cell pluripotency. Further studies are needed to confirm this hypothesis.

2.6 c-Myc

The basic helix–loop–helix/leucine zipper transcription factor c-Myc has a well documented role in cellular transformation and tumor progression, by controlling cell cycle, apoptosis, protein biosynthesis and metabolism (Kendall et al., 2006; Patel et al., 2004). c-Myc has been shown to regulate its target genes through interactions with the transcription machinery, as well as exerting epigenetic regulation via interactions with chromatin remodeling complexes, DNA methyltransferases and histone modifying enzymes (Eilers and Eisenman, 2008). Subsequent studies also identified a critical role of c-Myc in mESC maintenance.

Overexpression of c-Myc enables mESC to be resistant to differentiation, whereas expression of a dominant negative form of c-Myc promotes differentiation (Cartwright et al., 2005). However, a functional study of c-Myc in hESC yielded rather different results. Overexpression of c-Myc drives hESC to apoptosis and differentiation into extraembryonic endoderm and trophectoderm (Sumi et al., 2007).

c-Myc was identified as one of the four 'Yamanaka factors' initially used to generate both mouse and human iPSC (Takahashi et al., 2007; Takahashi and Yamanaka, 2006). Other reports have also shown that c-Myc can be substituted by two other related family members, N-Myc and L-Myc, during somatic cell reprogramming (Blelloch et al., 2007; Nakagawa et al., 2008). Subsequent studies demonstrated that somatic cell reprogramming can be achieved without c-Myc, albeit with significantly reduced efficiency and slower kinetics (Nakagawa et al., 2008; Wernig et al., 2008). Furthermore, reactivation of c-Myc has been observed in iPSC following blastocyst incorporation, resulting in tumor formation in the chimeric mice (Okita et al., 2007). This finding raises concerns about the safety of using iPSC generated with c-Myc for clinical applications. Understanding the molecular mechanism of c-Myc contributions during somatic cell reprogramming may help identify alternative enhancers for iPSC generation that are less tumorigenic.

Recent studies have shed light on the function of c-Myc during somatic cell reprogramming. Genome-wide analysis of promoter binding demonstrated that c-Myc regulates a different set of target genes compared to other pluripotency factors Oct4, Sox2 and Klf4 in mESC and iPSC (Chen et al., 2008; Kim et al., 2008; Sridharan et al., 2009). This suggests that c-Myc may have a very different function than the other transcription factors associated with induction of pluripotency. One proposed function is that c-Myc acts to repress expression of somatic genes during the early reprogramming stage, a process that is necessary before the activation of pluripotency gene networks (Sridharan et al., 2009). Another proposed mechanism of action of c-Myc is that it may induce a cell cycle program that is necessary for self-renewal of stem cells, activating genes which promote proliferation (i.e. cyclin A, cyclin E or E2F) and repressing genes associated with growth arrest (i.e. p21, p27) (Vermeulen et al., 2003). Finally, c-Myc may exert epigenetic control by modifying the chromatin structure to become suitable for activation of the self-renewal gene program, thus allowing somatic cells to revert back to a pluripotent state (Knoepfler et al., 2006).

2.7 Esrrb

Esrrb belongs to a subfamily of orphan nuclear receptors that are closely related to estrogen receptors   (Giguere, 2002). The natural ligands for Esrrb are currently unknown. Nevertheless, Esrrb and its family members can bind to DNA and function as transcriptional activators without exogenous ligands (Giguere, 2002). Most of our knowledge of the role of Esrrb in regulating self-renewal comes from studies in mice. Overexpression of Esrrb is sufficient to maintain self-renewal of mESC in conditions that favour differentiation, possibly by maintaining the level of Oct4 expression (Zhang et al., 2008). Also, knockdown of Esrrb level in mESC induces differentiation (Ivanova et al., 2006; Loh et al., 2006). These results identify Esrrb as a positive regulator of ESC pluripotency.

Indeed, Esrrb has been used as a factor to reprogram somatic cells back to a pluripotent state. In the presence of Oct4 and Sox2, Feng et al. (2009) demonstrated that Esrrb could replace Klf4 as an enhancer to reprogram mouse fibroblasts into iPSC, albeit with lower reprogramming efficiency (Feng et al., 2009a). Furthermore, another family member Esrrg also possesses a similar reprogramming ability when used in conjunction with Oct4 and Sox2 (Feng et al., 2009a). Genome-wide analysis of promoter binding suggested that Essrb shares many target genes with Oct4 and Sox2. Further studies demonstrated that Esrrb is a binding partner for Oct4 and Nanog in mESC (van den Berg et al., 2010; Wang et al., 2006), but whether it physically interacts with Sox2 remains to be determined. In summary, Esrrb was found to have a partially overlapping role with Klf4 in enhancing somatic cell reprogramming in mice, by cooperating with other pluripotency factors Oct4 and Nanog. To date, it has not yet been determined whether Esrrb plays a similar role in human cells.

2.8 Sall4

Sall4 belongs to the family of *Spalt* transcription factors that are characterized by highly conservative C2H2 zinc-finger domains (Sweetman and Munsterberg, 2006). Mutations of Sall4 in humans results in Okihiro syndrome, a disease characterized by limb deformities and eye movement deficits (Kohlhase et al., 2002). Sall4 is highly enriched in ESC, and is one of the 'embryonic cell associated transcripts' identified by Shinya Yamanaka's group. A previous study indicated that knockdown of Sall4 promoted mESC differentiation, most notably into the trophectoderm lineage (Zhang et al., 2006). However, follow-up reports showed that Sall4-null mESC are able to remain pluripotent, albeit with impaired proliferation (Tsubooka et al., 2009; Yuri et al., 2009). A study by Yuri *et al.* (2009) also demonstrated high expression of trophectoderm markers in Sall4-null mESC (Yuri et al., 2009). These results suggest that Sall4 is not essential to maintain pluripotency in mESC, but rather functions to stabilize the stem cell phenotype by promoting proliferation and possibly repressing trophectoderm differentiation. Furthermore, it is becoming clear that Sall4 is an integral part of the autoregulatory transcriptional network of Oct4, Sox2 and Nanog in mESC (Lim et al., 2008; Yang et al., 2008). These results suggest Sall4 is a possible candidate reprogramming factor for induced pluripotency.

Recently, Wong *et al.* (2008) discovered that Sall4 can enhance the efficiency of reprogramming mouse fibroblasts through fusion with mESC (Wong et al., 2008). Sall4 also increases the reprogramming efficiency of mouse fibroblasts when used in combination with Oct4, Sox2 and Klf4 (Tsubooka et al., 2009). However, this enhancing effect of Sall4 in reprogramming is inconsistent in different human fibroblast cell types, possibly due to variations in endogenous levels of Sall4 in different samples (Tsubooka et al., 2009). Further studies of Sall4 in human pluripotent stem cells will clarify whether the role of Sall4 in regulating cell pluripotency is conserved between mouse and human.

2.9 miRNA

miRNA are small RNAs that provide post-transcriptional control of gene regulation. Once transcribed, primary miRNA undergo multiple processing steps to become mature miRNA that promote degradation or repress translation of target mRNA (Siomi and Siomi, 2010). A previous report provided evidence that miRNA play an important role in the inter-connected transcriptional network regulated by pluripotency factors Oct4, Sox2 and Nanog in mESC (Marson et al., 2008). The pluripotency factors Oct4, Sox2 and Nanog are able to bind and regulate expression of specific miRNA, activating ESC specific miRNA while repressing those associated with differentiation (Barroso-delJesus et al., 2008; Marson et al., 2008). It is believed that miRNA serve as a mechanism for Oct4, Sox2 and Nanog to fine-tune the expression level of their target genes.

Recently, Robert Blelloch's group described a subset of miRNA that play an important role in regulating the cell cycle of mESC, termed ESC-specific cell cycle regulatory miRNA (ESCC miRNA) (Wang et al., 2008b). These ESCC miRNA promote G1 to S transition in mESC by repressing expression of various cyclin E-Cdk2 inhibitors (Wang et al., 2008b). In a follow-up study, the same group demonstrated that ESCC miRNA, in particular mir-291-3p, mir-294 and mir-295, are able to enhance reprogramming efficiency when used in combination with Oct4, Sox2 and Klf4. These ESCC miRNA are found to be downstream effectors of c-Myc, and thus are able to act as substitutes for c-Myc albeit to a lesser extent (Judson et al., 2009). Another set of ESCC miRNA, the mir-302 cluster, is able to reprogram human melanoma and prostate cancer cells to ESC-like cells in the absence of any other reprogramming factors (Lin et al., 2008). However, it remains unclear whether miRNA on their own can reprogram normal human primary cells to obtain genuine iPSC, as the effectiveness of miRNA-based reprogramming strategies may be cell-type dependent. Alternatively, others have shown that suppression of pro-differentiation let-7 miRNA can also enhance reprogramming efficiency in mouse fibroblasts when used in combination with the Yamanaka factors (Melton et al., 2010). This result is consistent with the previous identification of Lin28 as a reprogramming factor for iPSC generation, which presumably acts by blocking the processing of the let-7 family of miRNA (see discussion above). Together, these results demonstrate opposing roles played by different miRNA in somatic cell reprogramming and identify miRNA as important regulators of cell pluripotency. Future research to screen for reprogramming effects of other miRNA members will prove helpful in deriving a more efficient somatic cell reprogramming method. For instance, a recent report showed that miRNA-145 can regulate expression of Oct4, Sox2 and Klf4 and represses pluripotency in hESC (Xu et al., 2009b). Therefore, it will be interesting to see whether miRNA-145 can contribute to somatic cell reprogramming.

2.10 SV40 LT antigen and hTERT

The SV40LT antigen and the catalytic subunit of hTERT are well documented for their roles in establishing immortalized cells. Overexpression of SV40LT and hTERT along with another oncogene Ras are sufficient to confer tumorigenic transformation of normal human cells (Hahn et al., 1999). One proposed mechanism by which SV40 functions in tumorigenesis is by perturbing cellular senescence pathways through suppression of p53 activity. As discussed below, reduced p53 activity during reprogramming has been shown to improve the efficiency. On the other hand, reduction in telomere length during the normal aging process results in replicative senescence and limits the cellular lifespan of human cells. Studies have shown that this can be prevented by ectopic expression of hTERT to drive cellular immortalization (Bodnar et al., 1998). High telomerase activity is observed in the vast majority of tumors and is vital for the progression of malignant tumor cells (Kim et al., 1994). Interestingly, a previous study has also shown that c-Myc overexpression can activate hTERT activity (Wu et al., 1999). Therefore, SV40LT and hTERT may be able to contribute to somatic cell reprogramming by activating a cell cycle program that is required for pluripotent cells, much like the role of c-Myc in induced pluripotency.

Two recent studies sought to enhance the efficiency of generating human iPSC by supplementing reprogramming factors with hTERT and/or SV40LT (Mali et al., 2008; Park et al., 2008). In the study by Mali et al. (2008), the reprogramming cocktails were supplemented with the SV40LT transgene and resulted in accelerated reprogramming kinetics and up to a 70-fold increase in reprogramming efficiency, depending on the combination of reprogramming factors used (Mali et al., 2008). Similar results were obtained by Park *et al.* (2008) when hTERT and SV40LT were included in their reprogramming strategy (Park et al., 2008). Interestingly, while the addition of both SV40LT and hTERT was reported to increase cell proliferation, there were no viral integrations of either transgene in the genomes of the iPSC derived by this method (Park et al., 2008). This suggests that SV40LT and hTERT might be acting indirectly on supportive cells to enhance reprogramming. However, concerns remain about the safety of using SV40LT and hTERT in somatic cell reprogramming for clinical purposes. In this regard, future research studying whether iPSC generated using these two factors are more tumorigenic will help address this issue.

2.11 Silencing of the p53/p21/p16 pathway

One of the major roadblocks in iPSC generation is overcoming cellular senescence. p53 is known as the guardian of the genome and deregulation of p53 function promotes cell immortalization and bypasses cell senescence (Bond et al., 1994). Recent discoveries suggested that high-passage somatic cells with short telomeres show a dramatic decrease in the efficiency for iPSC generation (Marion et al., 2009; Utikal et al., 2009b). In this regard, bypassing cellular senescence may help improve the reprogramming efficiency of iPSC generation.

Key studies have shown that knockdown of senescence factors like p53, p21^{CIP1} or p16^{INK4a} enhances the efficiency of generating iPSC (Banito et al., 2009; Hanna et al., 2009; Hong et al., 2009; Kawamura et al., 2009; Marion et al., 2009). Furthermore, p53 knockdown can be used to replace c-Myc and/or Klf4 in the Yamanaka factors (Hong et al., 2009; Kawamura et al., 2009). When used in combination with UTF1, a chromatin bound factor highly expressed in pluripotent stem cells, the addition of p53 further enhanced reprogramming efficiency by 100-fold when used with the Yamanaka factors (Zhao et al., 2008). Together these studies show that the p53 pathway not only acts as a roadblock for cancer but also for iPSC generation. As p53 is a major tumor suppressor, further studies will be required to evaluate the safety of p53 knockdown in iPSC generation before these iPSC can be used in clinical applications.

2.12 Small molecules used to enhance somatic cell reprogramming

It is becoming clear that reversion of somatic cells to a pluripotent state involves epigenetic changes to chromatin that allow different sets of genes to be expressed (Feng et al., 2009b). Several reports have investigated the use of small molecules to enhance current cellular reprogramming methods towards developing a completely transgene-free strategy. Huangfu *et al.* (2008) discovered that the addition of valproic acid (VPA), a histone deacetylase (HDAC) inhibitor, can increase the efficiency and kinetics of reprogramming (Huangfu et al., 2008a). Moreover, two other HDAC inhibitors, suberoylanilide hydroxamic acid (SAHA) and trichostatin A (TSA), can also improve the reprogramming efficiency, albeit to a lesser extent. This provides supporting evidence for the notion that chromatin modifiers can help to overcome the epigenetic barrier to achieving complete reprogramming. Furthermore, addition of VPA was also able to substitute for c-Myc and Klf4 during reprogramming, thus reducing the number of reprogramming factors required to derive iPSC (Huangfu et al., 2008b). Similar effects on enhancing reprogramming efficiency were also observed with DNA methyltransferase inhibitors, including azacytidine

(AZA) (Huangfu et al., 2008a) and RG108 (Shi et al., 2008a), as well as a histone methyltransferase inhibitor, BIX-01294 (Shi et al., 2008b). In addition, a calcium channel agonist, BayK864, was shown to enhance the effect of BIX-01294 and further improve the efficiency of reprogramming (Shi et al., 2008a). However, it remains unclear whether or not the enhancing effect of these small molecules is dependent on the cell type used for iPSC generation. Altogether, it is thought that histone deacetylase inhibitors (VPA, TSA, SAHA), methyltransferase inhibitors (AZA, RG108, BIX-01294) and possibly other, yet to be identified, chromatin modifiers may function by relaxing chromatin to allow ectopically expressed transcription factors to bind.

Other researchers have screened small molecule libraries to identify chemical compounds that can directly substitute for the known reprogramming factors. This led to the discovery of RepSox (replacement of Sox2), a small molecule used to substitute for Sox2 in the reprogramming strategy (Ichida et al., 2009). RepSox acts by inhibiting transforming growth factor-ß (TGF-ß) signaling, in turn increasing Nanog expression that ultimately promotes partially reprogrammed cells to become fully reprogrammed (Ichida et al., 2009). However, future research will need to address the specificity of RepSox in order to fulfill its potential in generating iPSC for clinical purposes.

Finally, an interesting study by Esteban *et al.* (2010) demonstrated that antioxidants, in particular vitamin C, also help to enhance somatic cell reprogramming when used in combination with Oct4, Sox2 and Klf4 (Esteban et al., 2010). During early stages of reprogramming, vitamin C is able to overcome, at least partially, the cellular senescence roadblock by down-regulating p53 to allow the conversion of partially reprogrammed cells into fully reprogrammed iPSC (Esteban et al., 2010). This study provides a natural alternative to synthesized small molecules and may be easier to obtain approval for clinical usage.

3. Techniques for delivery of reprogramming factors

Since the seminal iPSC work by Shinya Yamanaka and colleagues, the field has moved forward at a rapid pace. Significant progress has been made in identifying new strategies to enhance the reprogramming efficiency and new methods to improve clinical safety. In this section, we will discuss the current techniques employed to introduce the reprogramming factors required for iPSC generation. It is important to note that the reprogramming efficiencies discussed in this section are only subject to the context described in the particular studies. Actual efficiency can be highly affected by many factors including the cell type of origin, the reprogramming factors and enhancer molecules used, as well as the methods to calculate reprogramming efficiencies.

3.1 Integrating Viral Vectors
3.1.1 Retroviral vectors
Retroviruses are efficient gene delivery vectors widely used in a broad range of dividing cell types. They can integrate into the host cell genome to produce continuous transgene expression. However, slow dividing or non-dividing cells are extremely resistant to retroviral transduction and the random sites of transgene integration can lead to unpredicatable genetic mutations within the genome and aberrant transgene expression. The initial derivation of iPSC utilized retroviral-mediated introduction of Oct4, Sox2, Klf4 and c-Myc to convert mouse fibroblasts back to a pluripotent state (Takahashi and Yamanaka, 2006), and subsequently human iPSC derived from adult dermal fibroblasts,

fetal and neonatal cells (Lowry et al., 2008; Park et al., 2008; Takahashi et al., 2007). Also, it was observed that retroviral mediated expression of transgenes were silenced during the iPSC reprogramming process (Hotta and Ellis, 2008). Even with a low efficiency (0.001%-0.5%), these pioneering studies revealed a potential alternative to the controversial use of ESC as a cell source for cellular transplantation therapies.

3.1.2 Lentiviral vectors

At the same time Yamanaka and colleagues reported the generation of human iPSC by retroviral transduction, Yu *et al.* (2007) demonstrated successful derivation of human iPSC using lentiviral methods to deliver a different set of factors Oct4, Sox2, Nanog and Lin28 (Yu et al., 2007). Lentiviruses, a subclass of retroviruses, offer the capability of high-efficiency infection in both dividing and non-dividing cells with stable expression of the transgenes and low immunogenicity. These distinguishing characteristics allow lentiviral vectors to be used for reprogramming a broader range of somatic cell types. However, lentiviruses integrate randomly into the host genome, similar to other retroviruses, which may hinder the use of iPSC generated using these methods for clinical applications. Initial derivation of human iPSC using lentiviral transduction yielded reprogramming efficiencies of 0.01%, significantly lower than previous retroviral methods (Yu et al., 2007). Subsequent improvements have been made by using lentiviral vectors to deliver SV40T, UTF1 or p53 shRNA to supplement the reprogramming cocktails, resulting in a 70-100 fold increase in reprogramming efficiency (Mali et al., 2008; Zhao et al., 2008). Moreover, reporter and antibiotic selection casettes have also been incorporated into lentiviral vectors to aid in the isolation of iPSC (Hotta et al., 2009a; Hotta et al., 2009b).

Previous studies indicated that transient expression of reprogramming factors is sufficient to activate the endogenous pluripotent gene program to allow for direct cell reprogramming (Takahashi et al., 2007; Takahashi and Yamanaka, 2006). This led to the development of inducible lentiviral vectors for direct cell reprogramming. Inducible lentiviral methods provide for improved temporal control over the levels of reprogramming factor expression and have been used to study the timing of reprogramming as well as the molecular changes that occur during the process. This system relies on inclusion of an additional vector that constitutively expresses the reverse tetracycline transactivator (rtTA). In the presence of the drug doxycycline, the rtTA functions to drive expression of the reprogramming factors, while in the absence of doxycycline the reprogramming transgenes are not expressed. Utilizing this type of inducible system, it has been established that exogenous transgene expression is necessary for 8-12 days to induce reprogramming of mouse fibroblasts and dispensable thereafter (Brambrink et al., 2008; Maherali et al., 2008; Stadtfeld et al., 2008a). Moreover, when doxycycline was removed eight days after initial transduction, the partially reprogrammed cells were unable to survive in the ESC growth conditions due to incomplete reactivation of their self-renewal programs. This provides a useful system to select for cells that have completely reverted back to a pluripotent stem cell state.

A major obstacle encountered when attempting to transduce cells with multiple viruses is that only a small proportion of the total cells will become infected with all the viruses. During reprogramming of somatic cells, those cells infected with few viruses may fail to become reprogrammed; leading to a low reprogramming efficiency. In this regard, development of a system to express the transgenes from a single vector may substantially improve the efficiency. One method to express the four transgenes from a single promoter is to insert the self-cleaving 2A and 2A-like sequences between each cDNA sequence

(Donnelly et al., 1997). These 2A sequences act by triggering ribosomal skipping that result in expression of each sequence in a stoichiometric fashion. Importantly, efficient polycistronic expression by 2A-mediated separation of transgenes was achieved in hESC (Hasegawa et al., 2007). This strategy was recently applied to derive mouse and human iPSC using a single lentiviral vector expressing Oct4, Sox2, Klf4, and c-Myc (Carey et al., 2009; Shao et al., 2009; Sommer et al., 2009). One of the advantages of using polycistronic vectors is that it reduces the difficulty of handling multiple lentiviral vectors for different reprogramming factors. Moreover, the mouse and human iPSC generated using this method had less viral integration sites compared to those developed using lentiviral delivery with individual gene. Indeed, the results showed as few as a single viral integration was sufficient for reprogramming (Carey et al., 2009; Shao et al., 2009). Minimizing the number of viral integrations reduces the risk of tumorigenesis and genomic instability. Also, the use of polycistronic vectors ensures expression of all four factors in the transduced cells. However, reprogramming efficiencies using this method were significantly lower (0.05%) than previous methods and reprogramming kinetics were also notably slower. One possible explanation for this low reprogramming efficiency is that the reprogramming factors are required to be expressed at an optimal stoichiometry in order to achieve efficient direct cell reprogramming (Papapetrou et al., 2009). Further studies are needed to clarify if the use of polycistronic vectors is an ideal technique to generate iPSC.

3.2 Non-integrating and excisable approaches

A major concern with employing retroviral or lentiviral-based methods to derive iPSC is random, uncontrollable integrations of the foreign transgenes into the host chromosomes. While many of these integrations prove harmless to the cells, residual viral portions have been shown to contribute to tumor formation. Moreover, it has been suggested that viral integrations may be a possible cause for some of the gene expression and differentiation potential differences observed between blastocyst-derived ESC and iPSC. These differences could affect the interpretation of results during mechanistic studies and, due to the safety concerns, severely limit the clinical applicability of these genetically modified cells. The previous approaches were extremely inefficient processes and most required multiple integration sites to induce reprogramming. Therefore, many groups have focused on developing novel, non-integrating methods for deriving iPSC. Some of these methods include the use of non-integrating vectors, excisable vectors, as well as RNA- or protein-based reprogramming.

3.2.1 Adenoviral vectors

The use of adenoviral vectors is advantageous for somatic cell reprogramming as they lack the machinery to integrate into the host's genome. This allows for high-level expression of exogenous genes with a low risk of integration of viral transgenes into the host genome. The viral titer becomes diluted after every cell division, which allows transient expression of the transgenes. On the other hand, multiple rounds of infections can achieve prolonged expression of transgenes, but it can be difficult to control gene expression levels. Reprogramming somatic cells with adenoviral vectors was first reported by Stadtfeld et al (Stadtfeld et al., 2008b). Using adenoviral vectors, mouse and human iPSC were generated using the Yamanaka factors in various donor cell types, albeit with a low reprogramming efficiency as compared to integrating viral vectors (0.0001%-0.001%) (Stadtfeld et al., 2008b;

Zhou and Freed, 2009). Similarly, a low reprogramming efficiency was also observed using polycistronic adenoviral vectors (Okita et al., 2008). One explanation for this is that it is difficult to maintain high enough transgene levels for multiple days to allow for reprogramming in many of the cells. Also, roughly 20% of the transduced cells were tetraploid, a phenomenon which was not seen in retroviral or lentiviral induced iPSC (Stadtfeld et al., 2008b). The reason for this observed tetraploidy is not clear, but it was suggested that cellular fusion or the presence of a rare aneuploid cell population in the starting culture may account for this result. Therefore, further research is needed to refine the use of adenoviral vectors in reprogramming somatic cells back to pluripotency.

3.2.2 Plasmids

Another non-integrating approach to transiently express reprogramming factors is the use of conventional plasmids. Previous reports have successfully generated integration-free mouse iPSC using polycistronic plasmids to express the Yamanaka factors (Gonzalez et al., 2009; Okita et al., 2008). However, a substantial amount of iPSC colonies contained integration of the transgenes. Therefore, screening of transgene integration sites is still necessary for iPSC generated using this technique to ensure their safety for clinical purposes. Furthermore, multiple rounds of transfection are required to sustain transgene expression at the level required to induce reprogramming and the observed reprogramming efficiency remained significantly lower than seen with the retroviral vectors (Gonzalez et al., 2009; Okita et al., 2008). Improvements to this plasmid-based method were made by the use of a polycistronic nonviral minicircle plasmid to reprogram human adult adipose stem cells (Jia et al., 2010). Minicircle DNA offers a higher transfection rate and is diluted at a slower rate than conventional plasmids when the cells divide. As a result, fewer rounds of transfections are required to generate iPSC. Using this method, Jia *et al.* (2010) generated integration-free human iPSC with a reprogramming efficiency of 0.005%, an efficiency still much lower than the integrating viral methods (Jia et al., 2010).

Episomal plasmids are another non-integrating method used to reprogram somatic cells into iPSC. Unlike conventional plasmids where transient transgene expression is gradually depleted after each cell division, episomal plasmids can be stably established in a number of cell types by drug selection and removed when the drug selection is withdrawn. Using this technique, Yu *et al.* (2009) generated a polycistronic episomal vector to co-express seven transgenes to reprogram human foreskin fibroblasts into iPSC (Yu et al., 2009). It was observed that different positioning of the transgene in the polycistronic vector resulted in varying reprogramming efficiencies, with the highest efficiency achieved being 0.006%. In summary, these studies provide proof-of-principle of the derivation of human iPSC free of genomic integration. However, all plasmid-based methods used to date yield a lower reprogramming efficiency compared to integrative viral methods, possibly due to difficulties in sustaining high transgene expression. Further research combining enhancing factors, such as small molecules, may help improve the reprogramming efficiency of these plasmid-based methods.

3.2.3 Cre recombinase /loxP system

Early non-integrating methods, such as those utilizing adenoviral and plasmid introduction of reprogramming factors, were substantially less efficient than the retroviral methods. Excisable integrating vectors offer a plausible reprogramming strategy to overcome the shortcomings of both the integrating retroviral and the transient expression methods. These excisable systems allow high initial transgene expression followed by subsequent removal of exogenous factors. Soldner *et al.* (2009) used inducible lentiviral vectors to derive human iPSC from fibroblasts collected from Parkinson's disease patients followed by Cre-recombinase mediated excision of the viral transgenes (Soldner et al., 2009). In this study, a constitutively active reverse tetracycline transactivator lentivirus was infected along with doxycycline-inducible lentiviruses for expression of the reprogramming factors, Oct4, Sox2, Klf4 and c-Myc. The inducible lentiviruses were engineered to contain a loxP site in the 3' LTR that becomes duplicated into the 5' LTR during viral replication, producing loxP sites flanking the transgenes. Subsequent expression of Cre-recombinase by electroporation allows the transgenes to be excised. Using this technique, the authors reported successful derivation of integration-free human iPSC (Soldner et al., 2009). Interestingly, the authors also demonstrated that the gene expression profile of these iPSC are more similar to hESC following transgene excision, suggesting that residual integrated reprogramming factors perturb the transcriptional profile of human iPSC (Soldner et al., 2009). Although the Cre-loxP system is the most efficient recombination system known, screening of integration-free iPSC clones is still required, as the authors reported that only sixteen out of 180 clones analyzed were integration-free following excision of transgene. Moreover, Cre-mediated excision of the transgenes does not remove the loxP sites, which raises concern of the possibility of disruption of endogenous gene expression. In this regard, a recent report by Chang *et al.* (2009) demonstrated successful generation of integration-free human iPSC where residual loxP sites did not interrupt expression of any genes or other functional sequences (Chang et al., 2009).

3.2.4 piggyBac transposon-based system

Unlike the Cre-loxP system, the advantage of transposon-based system is that transposases can remove all exogenous transposon elements from the host DNA. In particular, the piggyBac transposons have been demonstrated to be an efficient system for excisable gene delivery, delivering up to 10kb DNA fragments (Ding et al., 2005). Following transfection of the piggyBac transposons, transient expression of the transposase enzyme catalyzes the insertion or the excision event (Fraser et al., 1996). The advantage of the piggyBac transposon system is that it can be completely removed from the host genomes without altering the DNA sequences at the integration sites (Wang et al., 2008a). This led to the development of piggyBac-based reprogramming strategy that allowed generation of mouse and human iPSC using tetracycline-inducible or polycistronic expression of reprogramming factors (Kaji et al., 2009; Woltjen et al., 2009; Yusa et al., 2009). A high reprogramming efficiency of 2.5% was reported in the generation of mouse iPSC using this technique (Kaji et al., 2009). Furthermore, the integration sites were sequenced to confirm that excision of transgenes did not alter the host genome. Therefore, the piggyBac transposon system represents an efficient non-integrative approach to generate iPSC. However, excision of the transgenes by the transposase may still lead to micro-deletions of the genomic DNA (Wang et al., 2008a), which could hinder the clinical application of iPSC generated using this method.

3.2.5 RNA and protein-based reprogramming

Since all of the reprogramming strategies highlighted above create the risk of unexpected genetic modifications, many groups have begun to devise ways to reprogram somatic cells in the absence of genetic modification. Yakubov *et al.* (2010) recently developed a reprogramming technique by transfecting RNA synthesized *in vitro* from cDNA of Oct4, Lin28, Sox2, and Nanog to generate iPSC from human fibroblasts (Yakubov et al., 2010). This method harnesses the power of the endogenous translational machinery for proper protein folding and post-translational modifications. Also, this method of generating iPSC eliminates the risks associated with the use of viruses and DNA transfection methods. However, at least five consecutive transfections were necessary to reprogram these human fibroblasts as the transfected RNAs have a limited half-life. Finally, the reprogramming efficiency (0.05%) remained lower than those observed for integrating viral methods. Further characterization is also needed to confirm the pluripotency of the iPSC-like cells generated using this method and to prove the feasibility of RNA-based reprogramming.

An alternate approach to somatic cell reprogramming without genetic modification is using protein transduction. Importantly, a previous study demonstrated that protein tagged with a C-terminus poly-arginine domain allows efficient protein transduction through the cell membrane (Matsushita et al., 2001). Using direct protein delivery of reprogramming factors, two groups have report successful derivation of iPSC with the Yamanaka factors (Kim et al., 2009a; Zhou et al., 2009). Zhou *et al.* (2009) was the first to use recombinant reprogramming factors tagged with the poly-arginine domain to generate mouse iPSC. This virus-free and DNA-free method yielded a reprogramming efficiency of 0.006% with the use of an enhancer molecule VPA (Zhou et al., 2009). In addition, Kim *et al.* (2009) used whole cell extract from human embryonic kidney cells overexpressing the Yamanaka factors for the generation of human iPSC, yielding a reprogramming efficiency of 0.001% (Kim et al., 2009a). Both studies generated iPSC without any genetic modification, making them suitable for clinical applications. This direct protein transduction method also eradicates the need to screen for integration-free iPSC, thus shortening the time required for generating clinical grade iPSC. However, the reprogramming efficiency achieved with this method is still far lower than those obtained with viral mediated reprogramming. Moreover, multiple rounds of treatment are required during the reprogramming process as the recombinant proteins become degraded overtime. Nevertheless, these studies proved the feasibility of protein-based reprogramming methods and improvements to this technique could be important for final clinical application of iPSC.

4. Conclusions

The clinical potential of hESC for cell replacement therapies and for studying human diseases is undeniable. However, the use of these cells has been constantly burdened by both ethical (destruction of human embryos) and practical concerns (lack of available embryos, difficulties with generation of histo-compatible hESC). The conversion of somatic cells into pluripotent cells may overcome many of these roadblocks. Large numbers of embryos are no longer needed to create banks of patient-matched lines, since cells can now be harvested directly from each patient to create iPSC that are genetically identical and immune-compatible. Since the initial derivation of iPSC using the four Yamanaka factors, a growing list of reprogramming factors have been identified that either permit or enhance the reprogramming process. Moreover, researchers have begun to study other ways to improve the reprogramming efficiency, including the use of miRNA, small molecules, and several different methods to overcome barriers that prevent direct somatic cell reprogramming.

The first generation iPSC methods involved integration of viral transgenes, but the clinical necessity for deriving iPSC without these viral transgenes has pushed many researchers to develop alternative methods. The use of inducible polycistronic lentiviral vectors has already evolved to the utilization of excisable Cre-loxP and piggyBac expression systems, non-integrating plasmids, and recombinant proteins and RNA transfection as tools for generating iPSC. Advances in these non-viral, non-integrating methods will presumably continue until a method is discovered that can, with high efficiency, be used to derive patient-specific iPSC lines in a technically simple manner which can be adopted by many researchers and clinicians. In this regard, pursuing the development of protein-based and small molecule-based reprogramming methods may be most beneficial. However, these methods are still at an early stage and further improvements are needed to achieve high reprogramming efficiencies. Interestingly, a recent report utilized lentiviral vectors to deliver three transgenes and demonstrated direct conversion of mouse fibroblasts into neuronal like cells, bypassing the need of reprogramming back to a pluripotent state (Vierbuchen et al., 2010). Further research is needed to develop similar non-viral methods and to translate these techniques to human cells for clinical applications. Many methodologies used in the derivation of iPSC can be applied to study direct conversion of a somatic cell into another cell type of interest. However, the disadventagous of such direct reprogramming of a somatic cell into another lineage is that the reprogrammed cells are terminally differentiated and are not proliferating. Therefore, this reprogramming strategy is not ideal for large scale production to yield cells for the development of cell replacement therapies. In this regard, direct reprogramming of a somatic cell to a progenitor stage, where the progenitor cells remain proliferative, may prove advantageous. Recent studies also showed that iPSC retain an 'epigenetic memory' of their origins, where differentiation of iPSC to their tissue of origin is more efficient than other lineages (Kim et al., 2010; Polo et al., 2010). This could be used as a strategy to derive efficient protocols for differentiating iPSC to a particular cell type of interest. In summary, the field of stem cell biology was radically altered by the derivation of iPSC. Since their generation, the field has moved forward at a staggering speed, in large part due to the potential of iPSC to transform modern medicine as well as our understanding of human development.

5. Acknowledgements

The authors wish to thank Dr. Gemma Rooney and Dr. Sandy Hung for critical reading of the manuscript. The authors are also grateful for support from the California Institute of Regenerative Medicine to E. L. Smith (TG2-01152), R.C.B. Wong (TG1-00008) and P.J. Donovan (RC1-00110-1).

6. References

Adachi, K., Suemori, H., Yasuda, S.Y., Nakatsuji, N., and Kawase, E. (2010). Role of SOX2 in maintaining pluripotency of human embryonic stem cells. Genes Cells 15, 455-470.

Amabile, G., and Meissner, A. (2009). Induced pluripotent stem cells: current progress and potential for regenerative medicine. Trends Mol Med 15, 59-68.

Assou, S., Le Carrour, T., Tondeur, S., Strom, S., Gabelle, A., Marty, S., Nadal, L., Pantesco, V., Reme, T., Hugnot, J.P., et al. (2007). A meta-analysis of human embryonic stem cells transcriptome integrated into a web-based expression atlas. Stem Cells 25, 961-973.

Avilion, A.A., Nicolis, S.K., Pevny, L.H., Perez, L., Vivian, N., and Lovell-Badge, R. (2003). Multipotent cell lineages in early mouse development depend on SOX2 function. Genes Dev 17, 126-140.

Balzer, E., and Moss, E.G. (2007). Localization of the developmental timing regulator Lin28 to mRNP complexes, P-bodies and stress granules. RNA Biol 4, 16-25.

Banito, A., Rashid, S.T., Acosta, J.C., Li, S., Pereira, C.F., Geti, I., Pinho, S., Silva, J.C., Azuara, V., Walsh, M., et al. (2009). Senescence impairs successful reprogramming to pluripotent stem cells. Genes Dev 23, 2134-2139.

Barroso-delJesus, A., Romero-Lopez, C., Lucena-Aguilar, G., Melen, G.J., Sanchez, L., Ligero, G., Berzal-Herranz, A., and Menendez, P. (2008). Embryonic stem cell-specific miR302-367 cluster: human gene structure and functional characterization of its core promoter. Mol Cell Biol 28, 6609-6619.

Blelloch, R., Venere, M., Yen, J., and Ramalho-Santos, M. (2007). Generation of induced pluripotent stem cells in the absence of drug selection. Cell Stem Cell 1, 245-247.

Bodnar, A.G., Ouellette, M., Frolkis, M., Holt, S.E., Chiu, C.P., Morin, G.B., Harley, C.B., Shay, J.W., Lichtsteiner, S., and Wright, W.E. (1998). Extension of life-span by introduction of telomerase into normal human cells. Science 279, 349-352.

Bond, J.A., Wyllie, F.S., and Wynford-Thomas, D. (1994). Escape from senescence in human diploid fibroblasts induced directly by mutant p53. Oncogene 9, 1885-1889.

Boyer, L.A., Lee, T.I., Cole, M.F., Johnstone, S.E., Levine, S.S., Zucker, J.P., Guenther, M.G., Kumar, R.M., Murray, H.L., Jenner, R.G., et al. (2005). Core transcriptional regulatory circuitry in human embryonic stem cells. Cell 122, 947-956.

Brambrink, T., Foreman, R., Welstead, G.G., Lengner, C.J., Wernig, M., Suh, H., and Jaenisch, R. (2008). Sequential expression of pluripotency markers during direct reprogramming of mouse somatic cells. Cell Stem Cell 2, 151-159.

Carey, B.W., Markoulaki, S., Hanna, J., Saha, K., Gao, Q., Mitalipova, M., and Jaenisch, R. (2009). Reprogramming of murine and human somatic cells using a single polycistronic vector. Proceedings of the National Academy of Sciences of the United States of America 106, 157-162.

Cartwright, P., McLean, C., Sheppard, A., Rivett, D., Jones, K., and Dalton, S. (2005). LIF/STAT3 controls ES cell self-renewal and pluripotency by a Myc-dependent mechanism. Development 132, 885-896.

Chambers, I., Colby, D., Robertson, M., Nichols, J., Lee, S., Tweedie, S., and Smith, A. (2003). Functional expression cloning of Nanog, a pluripotency sustaining factor in embryonic stem cells. Cell 113, 643-655.

Chambers, I., Silva, J., Colby, D., Nichols, J., Nijmeijer, B., Robertson, M., Vrana, J., Jones, K., Grotewold, L., and Smith, A. (2007). Nanog safeguards pluripotency and mediates germline development. Nature 450, 1230-1234.

Chang, C.W., Lai, Y.S., Pawlik, K.M., Liu, K., Sun, C.W., Li, C., Schoeb, T.R., and Townes, T.M. (2009). Polycistronic Lentiviral Vector for "Hit and Run" Reprogramming of Adult Skin Fibroblasts to Induced Pluripotent Stem Cells. Stem Cells 27, 1042-1049.

Chen, L., Yabuuchi, A., Eminli, S., Takeuchi, A., Lu, C.W., Hochedlinger, K., and Daley, G.Q. (2009). Cross-regulation of the Nanog and Cdx2 promoters. Cell Res 19, 1052-1061.

Chen, X., Xu, H., Yuan, P., Fang, F., Huss, M., Vega, V.B., Wong, E., Orlov, Y.L., Zhang, W., Jiang, J., *et al.* (2008). Integration of external signaling pathways with the core transcriptional network in embryonic stem cells. Cell *133*, 1106-1117.

Darr, H., and Benvenisty, N. (2009). Genetic analysis of the role of the reprogramming gene LIN-28 in human embryonic stem cells. Stem Cells *27*, 352-362.

Darr, H., Mayshar, Y., and Benvenisty, N. (2006). Overexpression of NANOG in human ES cells enables feeder-free growth while inducing primitive ectoderm features. Development *133*, 1193-1201.

Ding, S., Wu, X., Li, G., Han, M., Zhuang, Y., and Xu, T. (2005). Efficient transposition of the piggyBac (PB) transposon in mammalian cells and mice. Cell *122*, 473-483.

Donnelly, M.L.L., Gani, D., Flint, M., Monaghan, S., and Ryan, M.D. (1997). The cleavage activities of aphthovirus and cardiovirus 2A proteins. Journal of General Virology *78*, 13-21.

Eilers, M., and Eisenman, R.N. (2008). Myc's broad reach. Genes Dev *22*, 2755-2766.

Ellis, P., Fagan, B.M., Magness, S.T., Hutton, S., Taranova, O., Hayashi, S., McMahon, A., Rao, M., and Pevny, L. (2004). SOX2, a persistent marker for multipotential neural stem cells derived from embryonic stem cells, the embryo or the adult. Dev Neurosci *26*, 148-165.

Ema, M., Mori, D., Niwa, H., Hasegawa, Y., Yamanaka, Y., Hitoshi, S., Mimura, J., Kawabe, Y., Hosoya, T., Morita, M., *et al.* (2008). Kruppel-like factor 5 is essential for blastocyst development and the normal self-renewal of mouse ESCs. Cell Stem Cell *3*, 555-567.

Esteban, M.A., Wang, T., Qin, B.M., Yang, J.Y., Qin, D.J., Cai, J.L., Li, W., Weng, Z.H., Chen, J.K., Ni, S., *et al.* (2010). Vitamin C Enhances the Generation of Mouse and Human Induced Pluripotent Stem Cells. Cell Stem Cell *6*, 71-79.

Evans, M.J., and Kaufman, M.H. (1981). Establishment in culture of pluripotential cells from mouse embryos. Nature *292*, 154-156.

Feng, B., Jiang, J., Kraus, P., Ng, J.H., Heng, J.C., Chan, Y.S., Yaw, L.P., Zhang, W., Loh, Y.H., Han, J., *et al.* (2009a). Reprogramming of fibroblasts into induced pluripotent stem cells with orphan nuclear receptor Esrrb. Nat Cell Biol *11*, 197-203.

Feng, B., Ng, J.H., Heng, J.C., and Ng, H.H. (2009b). Molecules that promote or enhance reprogramming of somatic cells to induced pluripotent stem cells. Cell Stem Cell *4*, 301-312.

Fong, H., Hohenstein, K.A., and Donovan, P.J. (2008). Regulation of self-renewal and pluripotency by Sox2 in human embryonic stem cells. Stem Cells *26*, 1931-1938.

Fraser, M.J., Ciszczon, T., Elick, T., and Bauser, C. (1996). Precise excision of TTAA-specific lepidopteran transposons piggyBac (IFP2) and tagalong (TFP3) from the baculovirus genome in cell lines from two species of Lepidoptera. Insect Mol Biol *5*, 141-151.

Giguere, V. (2002). To ERR in the estrogen pathway. Trends Endocrinol Metab *13*, 220-225.

Gonzalez, F., Monasterio, M.B., Tiscornia, G., Pulido, N.M., Vassena, R., Morera, L.B., Piza, I.R., and Belmonte, J.C.I. (2009). Generation of mouse-induced pluripotent stem cells by transient expression of a single nonviral polycistronic vector. Proceedings of the National Academy of Sciences of the United States of America *106*, 8918-8922.

Graham, V., Khudyakov, J., Ellis, P., and Pevny, L. (2003). SOX2 functions to maintain neural progenitor identity. Neuron 39, 749-765.

Hahn, W.C., Counter, C.M., Lundberg, A.S., Beijersbergen, R.L., Brooks, M.W., and Weinberg, R.A. (1999). Creation of human tumour cells with defined genetic elements. Nature 400, 464-468.

Hanna, J., Saha, K., Pando, B., van Zon, J., Lengner, C.J., Creyghton, M.P., van Oudenaarden, A., and Jaenisch, R. (2009). Direct cell reprogramming is a stochastic process amenable to acceleration. Nature 462, 595-601.

Hasegawa, K., Cowan, A.B., Nakatsuji, N., and Suemori, H. (2007). Efficient multicistronic expression of a transgene in human embryonic stem cells. Stem Cells 25, 1707-1712.

Heng, J.C., Feng, B., Han, J., Jiang, J., Kraus, P., Ng, J.H., Orlov, Y.L., Huss, M., Yang, L., Lufkin, T., et al. (2010). The nuclear receptor Nr5a2 can replace Oct4 in the reprogramming of murine somatic cells to pluripotent cells. Cell Stem Cell 6, 167-174.

Hong, H., Takahashi, K., Ichisaka, T., Aoi, T., Kanagawa, O., Nakagawa, M., Okita, K., and Yamanaka, S. (2009). Suppression of induced pluripotent stem cell generation by the p53-p21 pathway. Nature 460, 1132-1135.

Hotta, A., Cheung, A.Y., Farra, N., Garcha, K., Chang, W.Y., Pasceri, P., Stanford, W.L., and Ellis, J. (2009a). EOS lentiviral vector selection system for human induced pluripotent stem cells. Nat Protoc 4, 1828-1844.

Hotta, A., Cheung, A.Y., Farra, N., Vijayaragavan, K., Seguin, C.A., Draper, J.S., Pasceri, P., Maksakova, I.A., Mager, D.L., Rossant, J., et al. (2009b). Isolation of human iPS cells using EOS lentiviral vectors to select for pluripotency. Nat Methods 6, 370-376.

Hotta, A., and Ellis, J. (2008). Retroviral vector silencing during iPS cell induction: an epigenetic beacon that signals distinct pluripotent states. J Cell Biochem 105, 940-948.

Huangfu, D.W., Maehr, R., Guo, W.J., Eijkelenboom, A., Snitow, M., Chen, A.E., and Melton, D.A. (2008a). Induction of pluripotent stem cells by defined factors is greatly improved by small-molecule compounds. Nature Biotechnology 26, 795-797.

Huangfu, D.W., Osafune, K., Maehr, R., Guo, W., Eijkelenboom, A., Chen, S., Muhlestein, W., and Melton, D.A. (2008b). Induction of pluripotent stem cells from primary human fibroblasts with only Oct4 and Sox2. Nature Biotechnology 26, 1269-1275.

Hyslop, L., Stojkovic, M., Armstrong, L., Walter, T., Stojkovic, P., Przyborski, S., Herbert, M., Murdoch, A., Strachan, T., and Lako, M. (2005). Downregulation of NANOG induces differentiation of human embryonic stem cells to extraembryonic lineages. Stem Cells 23, 1035-1043.

Ichida, J.K., Blanchard, J., Lam, K., Son, E.Y., Chung, J.E., Egli, D., Loh, K.M., Carter, A.C., Di Giorgio, F.P., Koszka, K., et al. (2009). A Small-Molecule Inhibitor of Tgf-beta Signaling Replaces Sox2 in Reprogramming by Inducing Nanog. Cell Stem Cell 5, 491-503.

Ivanova, N., Dobrin, R., Lu, R., Kotenko, I., Levorse, J., DeCoste, C., Schafer, X., Lun, Y., and Lemischka, I.R. (2006). Dissecting self-renewal in stem cells with RNA interference. Nature 442, 533-538.

Jia, F.J., Wilson, K.D., Sun, N., Gupta, D.M., Huang, M., Li, Z.J., Panetta, N.J., Chen, Z.Y., Robbins, R.C., Kay, M.A., et al. (2010). A nonviral minicircle vector for deriving human iPS cells. Nature Methods 7, 197-U146.

Jiang, J., Chan, Y.S., Loh, Y.H., Cai, J., Tong, G.Q., Lim, C.A., Robson, P., Zhong, S., and Ng, H.H. (2008). A core Klf circuitry regulates self-renewal of embryonic stem cells. Nat Cell Biol 10, 353-360.

Judson, R.L., Babiarz, J.E., Venere, M., and Blelloch, R. (2009). Embryonic stem cell-specific microRNAs promote induced pluripotency. Nat Biotechnol 27, 459-461.

Kaji, K., Norrby, K., Paca, A., Mileikovsky, M., Mohseni, P., and Woltjen, K. (2009). Virus-free induction of pluripotency and subsequent excision of reprogramming factors. Nature.

Kawamura, T., Suzuki, J., Wang, Y.V., Menendez, S., Morera, L.B., Raya, A., Wahl, G.M., and Belmonte, J.C. (2009). Linking the p53 tumour suppressor pathway to somatic cell reprogramming. Nature 460, 1140-1144.

Kendall, S.D., Adam, S.J., and Counter, C.M. (2006). Genetically engineered human cancer models utilizing mammalian transgene expression. Cell Cycle 5, 1074-1079.

Kim, D., Kim, C.H., Moon, J.I., Chung, Y.G., Chang, M.Y., Han, B.S., Ko, S., Yang, E., Cha, K.Y., Lanza, R., et al. (2009a). Generation of Human Induced Pluripotent Stem Cells by Direct Delivery of Reprogramming Proteins. Cell Stem Cell 4, 472-476.

Kim, J., Chu, J., Shen, X., Wang, J., and Orkin, S.H. (2008). An extended transcriptional network for pluripotency of embryonic stem cells. Cell 132, 1049-1061.

Kim, J.B., Greber, B., Arauzo-Bravo, M.J., Meyer, J., Park, K.I., Zaehres, H., and Scholer, H.R. (2009b). Direct reprogramming of human neural stem cells by OCT4. Nature 461, 649-643.

Kim, J.B., Sebastiano, V., Wu, G., Arauzo-Bravo, M.J., Sasse, P., Gentile, L., Ko, K., Ruau, D., Ehrich, M., van den Boom, D., et al. (2009c). Oct4-induced pluripotency in adult neural stem cells. Cell 136, 411-419.

Kim, K., Doi, A., Wen, B., Ng, K., Zhao, R., Cahan, P., Kim, J., Aryee, M.J., Ji, H., Ehrlich, L.I., et al. (2010). Epigenetic memory in induced pluripotent stem cells. Nature 467, 285-290.

Kim, N.W., Piatyszek, M.A., Prowse, K.R., Harley, C.B., West, M.D., Ho, P.L.C., Coviello, G.M., Wright, W.E., Weinrich, S.L., and Shay, J.W. (1994). Specific Association of Human Telomerase Activity with Immortal Cells and Cancer. Science 266, 2011-2015.

Knoepfler, P.S., Zhang, X.Y., Cheng, P.F., Gafken, P.R., McMahon, S.B., and Eisenman, R.N. (2006). Myc influences global chromatin structure. EMBO J 25, 2723-2734.

Kohlhase, J., Heinrich, M., Schubert, L., Liebers, M., Kispert, A., Laccone, F., Turnpenny, P., Winter, R.M., and Reardon, W. (2002). Okihiro syndrome is caused by SALL4 mutations. Hum Mol Genet 11, 2979-2987.

Kopp, J.L., Ormsbee, B.D., Desler, M., and Rizzino, A. (2008). Small increases in the level of Sox2 trigger the differentiation of mouse embryonic stem cells. Stem Cells 26, 903-911.

Li, J., Pan, G., Cui, K., Liu, Y., Xu, S., and Pei, D. (2007). A dominant-negative form of mouse SOX2 induces trophectoderm differentiation and progressive polyploidy in mouse embryonic stem cells. J Biol Chem 282, 19481-19492.

Li, Y., McClintick, J., Zhong, L., Edenberg, H.J., Yoder, M.C., and Chan, R.J. (2005). Murine embryonic stem cell differentiation is promoted by SOCS-3 and inhibited by the zinc finger transcription factor Klf4. Blood 105, 635-637.

Lim, C.Y., Tam, W.L., Zhang, J., Ang, H.S., Jia, H., Lipovich, L., Ng, H.H., Wei, C.L., Sung, W.K., Robson, P., et al. (2008). Sall4 regulates distinct transcription circuitries in different blastocyst-derived stem cell lineages. Cell Stem Cell 3, 543-554.

Lin, S.L., Chang, D.C., Chang-Lin, S., Lin, C.H., Wu, D.T., Chen, D.T., and Ying, S.Y. (2008). Mir-302 reprograms human skin cancer cells into a pluripotent ES-cell-like state. RNA 14, 2115-2124.

Liu, L., Leaman, D., Villalta, M., and Roberts, R.M. (1997). Silencing of the gene for the alpha-subunit of human chorionic gonadotropin by the embryonic transcription factor Oct-3/4. Mol Endocrinol 11, 1651-1658.

Liu, L., and Roberts, R.M. (1996). Silencing of the gene for the beta subunit of human chorionic gonadotropin by the embryonic transcription factor Oct-3/4. J Biol Chem 271, 16683-16689.

Loh, Y.H., Wu, Q., Chew, J.L., Vega, V.B., Zhang, W., Chen, X., Bourque, G., George, J., Leong, B., Liu, J., et al. (2006). The Oct4 and Nanog transcription network regulates pluripotency in mouse embryonic stem cells. Nat Genet 38, 431-440.

Lowry, W.E., Richter, L., Yachechko, R., Pyle, A.D., Tchieu, J., Sridharan, R., Clark, A.T., and Plath, K. (2008). Generation of human induced pluripotent stem cells from dermal fibroblasts. Proc Natl Acad Sci U S A 105, 2883-2888.

Maherali, N., Ahfeldt, T., Rigamonti, A., Utikal, J., Cowan, C., and Hochedlinger, K. (2008). A high-efficiency system for the generation and study of human induced pluripotent stem cells. Cell Stem Cell 3, 340-345.

Maherali, N., Sridharan, R., Xie, W., Utikal, J., Eminli, S., Arnold, K., Stadtfeld, M., Yachechko, R., Tchieu, J., Jaenisch, R., et al. (2007). Directly reprogrammed fibroblasts show global epigenetic remodeling and widespread tissue contribution. Cell Stem Cell 1, 55-70.

Mali, P., Ye, Z.H., Hommond, H.H., Yu, X.B., Lin, J., Chen, G.B., Zou, J.Z., and Cheng, L.Z. (2008). Improved efficiency and pace of generating induced pluripotent stem cells from human adult and fetal fibroblasts. Stem Cells 26, 1998-2005.

Marion, R.M., Strati, K., Li, H., Murga, M., Blanco, R., Ortega, S., Fernandez-Capetillo, O., Serrano, M., and Blasco, M.A. (2009). A p53-mediated DNA damage response limits reprogramming to ensure iPS cell genomic integrity. Nature 460, 1149-1153.

Marson, A., Levine, S.S., Cole, M.F., Frampton, G.M., Brambrink, T., Johnstone, S., Guenther, M.G., Johnston, W.K., Wernig, M., Newman, J., et al. (2008). Connecting microRNA genes to the core transcriptional regulatory circuitry of embryonic stem cells. Cell 134, 521-533.

Martin, G.R. (1981). Isolation of a pluripotent cell line from early mouse embryos cultured in medium conditioned by teratocarcinoma stem cells. Proc Natl Acad Sci U S A 78, 7634-7638.

Masui, S., Nakatake, Y., Toyooka, Y., Shimosato, D., Yagi, R., Takahashi, K., Okochi, H., Okuda, A., Matoba, R., Sharov, A.A., et al. (2007). Pluripotency governed by Sox2 via regulation of Oct3/4 expression in mouse embryonic stem cells. Nat Cell Biol 9, 625-635.

Matin, M.M., Walsh, J.R., Gokhale, P.J., Draper, J.S., Bahrami, A.R., Morton, I., Moore, H.D., and Andrews, P.W. (2004). Specific knockdown of Oct4 and beta2-microglobulin expression by RNA interference in human embryonic stem cells and embryonic carcinoma cells. Stem Cells 22, 659-668.

Matsushita, M., Tomizawa, K., Moriwaki, A., Li, S.T., Terada, H., and Matsui, H. (2001). A high-efficiency protein transduction system demonstrating the role of PKA in long-lasting long-term potentiation. J Neurosci 21, 6000-6007.

McConnell, B.B., Ghaleb, A.M., Nandan, M.O., and Yang, V.W. (2007). The diverse functions of Kruppel-like factors 4 and 5 in epithelial biology and pathobiology. Bioessays 29, 549-557.

Melton, C., Judson, R.L., and Blelloch, R. (2010). Opposing microRNA families regulate self-renewal in mouse embryonic stem cells. Nature 463, 621-626.

Mitsui, K., Tokuzawa, Y., Itoh, H., Segawa, K., Murakami, M., Takahashi, K., Maruyama, M., Maeda, M., and Yamanaka, S. (2003). The homeoprotein Nanog is required for maintenance of pluripotency in mouse epiblast and ES cells. Cell 113, 631-642.

Miyagi, S., Saito, T., Mizutani, K., Masuyama, N., Gotoh, Y., Iwama, A., Nakauchi, H., Masui, S., Niwa, H., Nishimoto, M., et al. (2004). The Sox-2 regulatory regions display their activities in two distinct types of multipotent stem cells. Mol Cell Biol 24, 4207-4220.

Moss, E.G., Lee, R.C., and Ambros, V. (1997). The cold shock domain protein LIN-28 controls developmental timing in C. elegans and is regulated by the lin-4 RNA. Cell 88, 637-646.

Nakagawa, M., Koyanagi, M., Tanabe, K., Takahashi, K., Ichisaka, T., Aoi, T., Okita, K., Mochiduki, Y., Takizawa, N., and Yamanaka, S. (2008). Generation of induced pluripotent stem cells without Myc from mouse and human fibroblasts. Nat Biotechnol 26, 101-106.

Nakatake, Y., Fukui, N., Iwamatsu, Y., Masui, S., Takahashi, K., Yagi, R., Yagi, K., Miyazaki, J., Matoba, R., Ko, M.S., et al. (2006). Klf4 cooperates with Oct3/4 and Sox2 to activate the Lefty1 core promoter in embryonic stem cells. Mol Cell Biol 26, 7772-7782.

Nandan, M.O., and Yang, V.W. (2009). The role of Kruppel-like factors in the reprogramming of somatic cells to induced pluripotent stem cells. Histol Histopathol 24, 1343-1355.

Nichols, J., Zevnik, B., Anastassiadis, K., Niwa, H., Klewe-Nebenius, D., Chambers, I., Scholer, H., and Smith, A. (1998). Formation of pluripotent stem cells in the mammalian embryo depends on the POU transcription factor Oct4. Cell 95, 379-391.

Niwa, H., Miyazaki, J., and Smith, A.G. (2000). Quantitative expression of Oct-3/4 defines differentiation, dedifferentiation or self-renewal of ES cells. Nat Genet 24, 372-376.

Niwa, H., Toyooka, Y., Shimosato, D., Strumpf, D., Takahashi, K., Yagi, R., and Rossant, J. (2005). Interaction between Oct3/4 and Cdx2 determines trophectoderm differentiation. Cell 123, 917-929.

Okamoto, K., Okazawa, H., Okuda, A., Sakai, M., Muramatsu, M., and Hamada, H. (1990). A novel octamer binding transcription factor is differentially expressed in mouse embryonic cells. Cell 60, 461-472.

Okita, K., Ichisaka, T., and Yamanaka, S. (2007). Generation of germline-competent induced pluripotent stem cells. Nature 448, 313-317.

Okita, K., Nakagawa, M., Hong, H.J., Ichisaka, T., and Yamanaka, S. (2008). Generation of Mouse Induced Pluripotent Stem Cells Without Viral Vectors. Science 322, 949-953.

Papapetrou, E.P., Tomishima, M.J., Chambers, S.M., Mica, Y., Reed, E., Menon, J., Tabar, V., Mo, Q., Studer, L., and Sadelain, M. (2009). Stoichiometric and temporal requirements of Oct4, Sox2, Klf4, and c-Myc expression for efficient human iPSC induction and differentiation. Proc Natl Acad Sci U S A 106, 12759-12764.

Park, I.H., Zhao, R., West, J.A., Yabuuchi, A., Huo, H.G., Ince, T.A., Lerou, P.H., Lensch, M.W., and Daley, G.Q. (2008). Reprogramming of human somatic cells to pluripotency with defined factors. Nature 451, 141-U141.

Patel, J.H., Loboda, A.P., Showe, M.K., Showe, L.C., and McMahon, S.B. (2004). Analysis of genomic targets reveals complex functions of MYC. Nat Rev Cancer 4, 562-568.

Pera, M.F., Reubinoff, B., and Trounson, A. (2000). Human embryonic stem cells. J Cell Sci 113 (Pt 1), 5-10.

Pesce, M., and Scholer, H.R. (2001). Oct-4: gatekeeper in the beginnings of mammalian development. Stem Cells 19, 271-278.

Polesskaya, A., Cuvellier, S., Naguibneva, I., Duquet, A., Moss, E.G., and Harel-Bellan, A. (2007). Lin-28 binds IGF-2 mRNA and participates in skeletal myogenesis by increasing translation efficiency. Genes Dev 21, 1125-1138.

Polo, J.M., Liu, S., Figueroa, M.E., Kulalert, W., Eminli, S., Tan, K.Y., Apostolou, E., Stadtfeld, M., Li, Y., Shioda, T., et al. (2010). Cell type of origin influences the molecular and functional properties of mouse induced pluripotent stem cells. Nat Biotechnol 28, 848-855.

Qiu, C., Ma, Y., Wang, J., Peng, S., and Huang, Y. (2010). Lin28-mediated post-transcriptional regulation of Oct4 expression in human embryonic stem cells. Nucleic Acids Res 38, 1240-1248.

Richards, M., Tan, S.P., Tan, J.H., Chan, W.K., and Bongso, A. (2004). The transcriptome profile of human embryonic stem cells as defined by SAGE. Stem Cells 22, 51-64.

Rosner, M.H., Vigano, M.A., Ozato, K., Timmons, P.M., Poirier, F., Rigby, P.W., and Staudt, L.M. (1990). A POU-domain transcription factor in early stem cells and germ cells of the mammalian embryo. Nature 345, 686-692.

Rowland, B.D., Bernards, R., and Peeper, D.S. (2005). The KLF4 tumour suppressor is a transcriptional repressor of p53 that acts as a context-dependent oncogene. Nat Cell Biol 7, 1074-1082.

Rowland, B.D., and Peeper, D.S. (2006). KLF4, p21 and context-dependent opposing forces in cancer. Nat Rev Cancer 6, 11-23.

Scholer, H.R., Balling, R., Hatzopoulos, A.K., Suzuki, N., and Gruss, P. (1989). Octamer binding proteins confer transcriptional activity in early mouse embryogenesis. EMBO J 8, 2551-2557.

Segre, J.A., Bauer, C., and Fuchs, E. (1999). Klf4 is a transcription factor required for establishing the barrier function of the skin. Nat Genet 22, 356-360.

Shao, L.J., Feng, W., Sun, Y., Bai, H., Liu, J., Currie, C., Kim, J.J., Gama, R., Wang, Z., Qian, Z.J., et al. (2009). Generation of iPS cells using defined factors linked via the self-cleaving 2A sequences in a single open reading frame. Cell Research 19, 296-306.

Shi, Y., Desponts, C., Do, J.T., Hahm, H.S., Scholer, H.R., and Ding, S. (2008a). Induction of Pluripotent Stem Cells from Mouse Embryonic Fibroblasts by Oct4 and Klf4 with Small-Molecule Compounds. Cell Stem Cell 3, 568-574.

Shi, Y., Do, J.T., Desponts, C., Hahm, H.S., Scholer, H.R., and Ding, S. (2008b). A combined chemical and genetic approach for the generation of induced pluripotent stem cells. Cell Stem Cell 2, 525-528.

Shimozaki, K., Nakashima, K., Niwa, H., and Taga, T. (2003). Involvement of Oct3/4 in the enhancement of neuronal differentiation of ES cells in neurogenesis-inducing cultures. Development 130, 2505-2512.

Siomi, H., and Siomi, M.C. (2010). Posttranscriptional regulation of microRNA biogenesis in animals. Mol Cell 38, 323-332.

Soldner, F., Hockemeyer, D., Beard, C., Gao, Q., Bell, G.W., Cook, E.G., Hargus, G., Blak, A., Cooper, O., Mitalipova, M., et al. (2009). Parkinson's Disease Patient-Derived Induced Pluripotent Stem Cells Free of Viral Reprogramming Factors. Cell 136, 964-977.

Sommer, C.A., Stadtfeld, M., Murphy, G.J., Hochedlinger, K., Kotton, D.N., and Mostoslavsky, G. (2009). Induced Pluripotent Stem Cell Generation Using a Single Lentiviral Stem Cell Cassette. Stem Cells 27, 543-549.

Sridharan, R., Tchieu, J., Mason, M.J., Yachechko, R., Kuoy, E., Horvath, S., Zhou, Q., and Plath, K. (2009). Role of the murine reprogramming factors in the induction of pluripotency. Cell 136, 364-377.

Stadtfeld, M., Maherali, N., Breault, D.T., and Hochedlinger, K. (2008a). Defining molecular cornerstones during fibroblast to iPS cell reprogramming in mouse. Cell Stem Cell 2, 230-240.

Stadtfeld, M., Nagaya, M., Utikal, J., Weir, G., and Hochedlinger, K. (2008b). Induced Pluripotent Stem Cells Generated Without Viral Integration. Science 322, 945-949.

Sumi, T., Tsuneyoshi, N., Nakatsuji, N., and Suemori, H. (2007). Apoptosis and differentiation of human embryonic stem cells induced by sustained activation of c-Myc. Oncogene 26, 5564-5576.

Sweetman, D., and Munsterberg, A. (2006). The vertebrate spalt genes in development and disease. Dev Biol 293, 285-293.

Takahashi, K., Tanabe, K., Ohnuki, M., Narita, M., Ichisaka, T., Tomoda, K., and Yamanaka, S. (2007). Induction of pluripotent stem cells from adult human fibroblasts by defined factors. Cell 131, 861-872.

Takahashi, K., and Yamanaka, S. (2006). Induction of pluripotent stem cells from mouse embryonic and adult fibroblast cultures by defined factors. Cell 126, 663-676.

Thomson, J.A., Itskovitz-Eldor, J., Shapiro, S.S., Waknitz, M.A., Swiergiel, J.J., Marshall, V.S., and Jones, J.M. (1998). Embryonic stem cell lines derived from human blastocysts. Science 282, 1145-1147.

Tsubooka, N., Ichisaka, T., Okita, K., Takahashi, K., Nakagawa, M., and Yamanaka, S. (2009). Roles of Sall4 in the generation of pluripotent stem cells from blastocysts and fibroblasts. Genes Cells.

Utikal, J., Maherali, N., Kulalert, W., and Hochedlinger, K. (2009a). Sox2 is dispensable for the reprogramming of melanocytes and melanoma cells into induced pluripotent stem cells. J Cell Sci 122, 3502-3510.

Utikal, J., Polo, J.M., Stadtfeld, M., Maherali, N., Kulalert, W., Walsh, R.M., Khalil, A., Rheinwald, J.G., and Hochedlinger, K. (2009b). Immortalization eliminates a roadblock during cellular reprogramming into iPS cells. Nature 460, 1145-1148.

van den Berg, D.L., Snoek, T., Mullin, N.P., Yates, A., Bezstarosti, K., Demmers, J., Chambers, I., and Poot, R.A. (2010). An Oct4-centered protein interaction network in embryonic stem cells. Cell Stem Cell 6, 369-381.

Vermeulen, K., Berneman, Z.N., and Van Bockstaele, D.R. (2003). Cell cycle and apoptosis. Cell Prolif 36, 165-175.

Vierbuchen, T., Ostermeier, A., Pang, Z.P., Kokubu, Y., Sudhof, T.C., and Wernig, M. (2010). Direct conversion of fibroblasts to functional neurons by defined factors. Nature 463, 1035-U1050.

Viswanathan, S.R., Daley, G.Q., and Gregory, R.I. (2008). Selective blockade of microRNA processing by Lin28. Science 320, 97-100.

Viswanathan, S.R., Powers, J.T., Einhorn, W., Hoshida, Y., Ng, T.L., Toffanin, S., O'Sullivan, M., Lu, J., Phillips, L.A., Lockhart, V.L., et al. (2009). Lin28 promotes transformation and is associated with advanced human malignancies. Nat Genet 41, 843-848.

Wang, J., Rao, S., Chu, J., Shen, X., Levasseur, D.N., Theunissen, T.W., and Orkin, S.H. (2006). A protein interaction network for pluripotency of embryonic stem cells. Nature 444, 364-368.

Wang, W., Lin, C., Lu, D., Ning, Z., Cox, T., Melvin, D., Wang, X., Bradley, A., and Liu, P. (2008a). Chromosomal transposition of PiggyBac in mouse embryonic stem cells. Proc Natl Acad Sci U S A 105, 9290-9295.

Wang, Y., Baskerville, S., Shenoy, A., Babiarz, J.E., Baehner, L., and Blelloch, R. (2008b). Embryonic stem cell-specific microRNAs regulate the G1-S transition and promote rapid proliferation. Nat Genet 40, 1478-1483.

Wei, Z., Yang, Y., Zhang, P., Andrianakos, R., Hasegawa, K., Lyu, J., Chen, X., Bai, G., Liu, C., Pera, M., et al. (2009). Klf4 interacts directly with Oct4 and Sox2 to promote reprogramming. Stem Cells 27, 2969-2978.

Wernig, M., Meissner, A., Cassady, J.P., and Jaenisch, R. (2008). c-Myc is dispensable for direct reprogramming of mouse fibroblasts. Cell Stem Cell 2, 10-12.

Wernig, M., Meissner, A., Foreman, R., Brambrink, T., Ku, M., Hochedlinger, K., Bernstein, B.E., and Jaenisch, R. (2007). In vitro reprogramming of fibroblasts into a pluripotent ES-cell-like state. Nature 448, 318-324.

Woltjen, K., Michael, I.P., Mohseni, P., Desai, R., Mileikovsky, M., Hamalainen, R., Cowling, R., Wang, W., Liu, P.T., Gertsenstein, M., et al. (2009). piggyBac transposition reprograms fibroblasts to induced pluripotent stem cells. Nature 458, 766-U106.

Wong, C.C., Gaspar-Maia, A., Ramalho-Santos, M., and Reijo Pera, R.A. (2008). High-efficiency stem cell fusion-mediated assay reveals Sall4 as an enhancer of reprogramming. PLoS One 3, e1955.

Wu, K.J., Grandori, C., Amacker, M., Simon-Vermot, N., Polack, A., Lingner, J., and Dalla-Favera, R. (1999). Direct activation of TERT transcription by c-MYC. Nature Genetics 21, 220-224.

Xu, B., Zhang, K., and Huang, Y. (2009a). Lin28 modulates cell growth and associates with a subset of cell cycle regulator mRNAs in mouse embryonic stem cells. RNA 15, 357-361.

Xu, N., Papagiannakopoulos, T., Pan, G., Thomson, J.A., and Kosik, K.S. (2009b). MicroRNA-145 regulates OCT4, SOX2, and KLF4 and represses pluripotency in human embryonic stem cells. Cell 137, 647-658.

Yakubov, E., Rechavi, G., Rozenblatt, S., and Givol, D. (2010). Reprogramming of human fibroblasts to pluripotent stem cells using mRNA of four transcription factors. Biochemical and Biophysical Research Communications 394, 189-193.

Yang, J., Chai, L., Fowles, T.C., Alipio, Z., Xu, D., Fink, L.M., Ward, D.C., and Ma, Y. (2008). Genome-wide analysis reveals Sall4 to be a major regulator of pluripotency in murine-embryonic stem cells. Proc Natl Acad Sci U S A 105, 19756-19761.

Yu, J., Vodyanik, M.A., Smuga-Otto, K., Antosiewicz-Bourget, J., Frane, J.L., Tian, S., Nie, J., Jonsdottir, G.A., Ruotti, V., Stewart, R., et al. (2007). Induced pluripotent stem cell lines derived from human somatic cells. Science 318, 1917-1920.

Yu, J.Y., Hu, K.J., Smuga-Otto, K., Tian, S.L., Stewart, R., Slukvin, I.I., and Thomson, J.A. (2009). Human Induced Pluripotent Stem Cells Free of Vector and Transgene Sequences. Science 324, 797-801.

Yuan, H., Corbi, N., Basilico, C., and Dailey, L. (1995). Developmental-specific activity of the FGF-4 enhancer requires the synergistic action of Sox2 and Oct-3. Genes Dev 9, 2635-2645.

Yuri, S., Fujimura, S., Nimura, K., Takeda, N., Toyooka, Y., Fujimura, Y., Aburatani, H., Ura, K., Koseki, H., Niwa, H., et al. (2009). Sall4 is essential for stabilization, but not for pluripotency, of embryonic stem cells by repressing aberrant trophectoderm gene expression. Stem Cells 27, 796-805.

Yusa, K., Rad, R., Takeda, J., and Bradley, A. (2009). Generation of transgene-free induced pluripotent mouse stem cells by the piggyBac transposon. Nature Methods 6, 363-U369.

Zeineddine, D., Papadimou, E., Chebli, K., Gineste, M., Liu, J., Grey, C., Thurig, S., Behfar, A., Wallace, V.A., Skerjanc, I.S., et al. (2006). Oct-3/4 dose dependently regulates specification of embryonic stem cells toward a cardiac lineage and early heart development. Dev Cell 11, 535-546.

Zhang, J., Tam, W.L., Tong, G.Q., Wu, Q., Chan, H.Y., Soh, B.S., Lou, Y., Yang, J., Ma, Y., Chai, L., et al. (2006). Sall4 modulates embryonic stem cell pluripotency and early embryonic development by the transcriptional regulation of Pou5f1. Nat Cell Biol 8, 1114-1123.

Zhang, X., Zhang, J., Wang, T., Esteban, M.A., and Pei, D. (2008). Esrrb activates Oct4 transcription and sustains self-renewal and pluripotency in embryonic stem cells. J Biol Chem 283, 35825-35833.

Zhao, S., Nichols, J., Smith, A.G., and Li, M. (2004). SoxB transcription factors specify neuroectodermal lineage choice in ES cells. Mol Cell Neurosci 27, 332-342.

Zhao, Y., Yin, X.L., Qin, H., Zhu, F.F., Liu, H.S., Yang, W.F., Zhang, Q., Xiang, C.A., Hou, P.P., Song, Z.H., et al. (2008). Two Supporting Factors Greatly Improve the Efficiency of Human iPSC Generation. Cell Stem Cell 3, 475-479.

Zhou, H.Y., Wu, S.L., Joo, J.Y., Zhu, S.Y., Han, D.W., Lin, T.X., Trauger, S., Bien, G., Yao, S., Zhu, Y., et al. (2009). Generation of Induced Pluripotent Stem Cells Using Recombinant Proteins. Cell Stem Cell 4, 381-384.

Zhou, W.B., and Freed, C.R. (2009). Adenoviral Gene Delivery Can Reprogram Human Fibroblasts to Induced Pluripotent Stem Cells. Stem Cells 27, 2667-2674.

7

The Past, Present and Future of Induced Pluripotent Stem Cells

Koji Tanabe and Kazutoshi Takahashi
Center for iPS Cell Research and Application
Japan

1. Introduction

Our body is derived from only one cell, a fertilized egg. At the birth, the body consists of 220 kinds of somatic cells. The fertilized egg divides many times during development. The resulting cells differentiate into many kinds of somatic cells, and a fertilized egg can differentiate into all of the different types of cells, including intraembryonic and extraembryonic tissues. This ability is called totipotency. Fertilized eggs differentiate into various kinds of somatic cells. However, somatic cells do not divide and differentiate into other types of somatic cells after differentiation in a disorderly manner. There are two possibilities to explain this. First, somatic cells can completely lose their potential to differentiate into other kinds of cells during development, or second, they may retain their potential, but such potential may be suppressed after development. The studies to elucidate how these processes occur were the origin of reprogramming science and regenerative medicine.

In 1938, Spemann was the first person to carry out nuclear transplantation, but the experiment failed (Spemann, 1938). In 1952, Briggs and King transplanted the nucleus of a frog blastula into enucleated unfertilized eggs. The eggs developed into tadpoles. This was the first cloned animal with nuclear transplantation, and the origin of the cloning technique. An interesting discovery was that the later the nucleuses were taken during the developmental stage, the lower the efficiency of generating clone frogs. It was impossible to produce a cloned frog using the nucleus from a stage later than the development of a tailbud. At that time, they thought the information in the nucleus changed during development (Brigge & King, 1952). However, Gurdon arrived at a different conclusion from Briggs and King. He transplanted the nuclei of small intestinal epithelial cells into enucleated unfertilized eggs and obtained tadpoles (Gurdon, 1962). His data suggested that the nucleus of a somatic cell could be reprogrammed, and thereby regain the ability to differentiate into many kinds of cells. In 1997, the cloning of a sheep demonstrated that mammalian somatic cells could also be reprogrammed (Wilmut, 1997). These data suggested that the information in the nucleus did not change irreversibly during development, and indicated that somatic cells have the potentially ability to differentiate into other kinds of cells after development.

2. What are ES cells?

It was necessary for the growth of developmental engineering and reprogramming science to make cells that can easily expand and maintain the ability to differentiate into many kinds of cells in a cell culture system. Embryonic stem (ES) cells fulfilled these characteristics. ES cells have two important abilities, self-renewal and pluripotency. The ability for self-renewal allows these cells to grow semipermanently. Pluripotency, as described above, is the potential for differentiation into many kinds of cells which make up the body, such as muscle cells, neural cells and so on. Mouse ES cells injected into mouse blastocysts contribute to the formation of all tissues in the body. The mice generated from embryos injected with ES cells are called chimeric mice. These abilities of the ES cells made it possible to generate a large number of any type of cells that is desired.

ES cells are established from fertilized eggs. The inner cell mass of blastocyst-stage embryos are transformed into ES cells. The fertilized egg is first cultured on feeder cells, which provide several necessary factors to the egg and ES cells. A few days later, the cells of the inner cell mass start to grow under culture conditions. ES cells are established from these growing cells. In 1981, mouse ES cells were established (Evans & Kaufman, 1981), and human ES cells were established in 1998 (Thomson et al 1998). Interestingly, the characteristics of human ES cells are different from those of mouse ES cells. The morphology of human ES cells was more like that of cynomolgus ES cells, which had been established several years before the mouse ES cells. Moreover, the optimal culture conditions differ between human ES cells and mouse ES cells. For example, leukemia inhibitory factor (LIF) and bone morphogenic protein (BMP) are important for maintaining the abilities of mouse ES cells in vitro. On the other hand, basic fibroblast growth factor (bFGF) and Activin A are required for the maintenance of human ES cells (Boiani & Schöler 2005).

Mouse ES cells are commonly used as a tool to generate transgenic and gene-targeted animals. These animal models have controbuted to the progress made in basic and medical sciences. Human pluripotent stem cells, including ES cells, are expected to be a good source of regenerative medicine, because of their outstanding capacities such as self-renewal and pluripotency.

3. Why generate artificial pluripotent stem cells?

There are several outstanding issues surrounding the use of ES cells for clinical applications. One of them is immunological rejection. ES cells are generated from fertilized eggs, which can have different immunizing antigens from the recipient who received the regenerative medicine developed using these cells. If the somatic cells from ES cells are transplanted into recipients, then the cells are rejected by the patient's own immune system. To overcome this problem, a new technique was developed. In this technique, the nuclei of an individual's somatic cells are transplanted into enucleated unfertilized eggs. The eggs can then be used to make ES cells expressing the individual's own immunizing antigens. These ES cells were called nuclear transfer ES cells (ntES cell), and the somatic cells derived from ntES cells are not rejected by the recipient after transplantation. These ntES cells have been established from not only mouse, but also from monkey cells (Rideout et al., 2000; Byrne et al., 2007). However, there have been no reports of human ntES cells. A likely reason for this is that the efficiency of generating ntES cells is very low, thus requiring a lot of embryos. This is not only a technical challange but also poses ethical problems. Generating human embryos for research is questionable and in case human nuclear transplanted embryos are implanted in a uterus, a cloned human would be generated.

Another ethical problem is the use of ES cells for clinical applications. To generate ES cells, it is necessary to either injure or break up embryos, which are the origin of human life. To avoid these problems, ES cells were generated from embryos which arrested their own development or from poor-quality embryos generated for in vitro fertilization treatments. The embryos which would be discarded as of low quality for fertilization treatment are used to make ES cells. Moreover, ES cells can be generated from single blastomers of embryos, and the biopsied embryos still can grow normally (Chung et al., 2006; Klimanskaya et al., 2006; Chung et al., 2008). That is, ES cells can be generated without embryonic destruction. However, there are still discussions ongoing about how these "origins of human life" are handled by humans, and many countries have legislation preventing the development and use of ES cells. Therefore, it is necessary to be able to make pluripotent stem cells artificially for clinical applications. One of the major goals of nuclear reprogramming research is to generate ES-like cells by the conversion of somatic cells.

4. The search for reprogramming factors

One of the most difficult points for finding ways to convert somatic cells to pluripotent stem cell was to identify reprogramming factors. There had been hints based on the previous research on ES cells. For example, it was known that ES cells could induce pluripotency in somatic cells. When mouse somatic cells were hybridized with mouse ES cells, the nuclei of the somatic cells were reprogrammed. The genes which were normally expressed specifically in ES cells started to be expressed from the genome of somatic cells after hybridization. These hybridized somatic cells could differentiate into all three germ layers. When human ES cells were used for hybridization, the nuclei of human somatic cells were also reprogrammed. These data demonstrated that there were factors (reprogramming factors) which could induce pluripotency in somatic cells that were present not only in oocytes, but also in ES cells.

It was hypothesized that tsuch reprogramming factors would be important factors for maintaining pluripotency in ES cells, and that the identification of the factors required by ES cells would also indicate the factors required for the reprogramming of somatic cells. These factors would be expressed highly and specifically in ES cells. Next, Then gene expression pattern was compared between ES cells and somatic cells to narrow down the candidates of reprogramming factors using a computer database. The selected genes were named ES cell associated transcripts (ECATs). These ECATs were expressed highly and specifically in ES cells. They also were shown to play important roles in maintaining the properties of ES cells. For example, Nanog is one of the ECATs. In the absence of Nanog, mouse ES cells differentiate into visceral or parietal endoderm, and do not maintain the properties of ES cells. An overexpression of Nanog also maintains the self-renewal of ES cells, independent of LIF (Mitsui, et al., 2003; Chambers, et al., 2003).

In the 1990s, the transcription network involved in maintaining the pluripotency and self-renewal of ES cells gradually started to become clearer. Oct3/4 was discovered to be one of key factors that make ES cells unique. Oct3/4 is expressed in ES cells, germ cells and also differentiated cells. However, the expression level of Oct3/4 is strictly regulated strictly by the transcription network in ES cells. A mere 1.5-fold increase in the expression of Oct3/4 induces the differentiation of ES cells to primitive endoderm. A reduction in the expression of Oct3/4 by half leads ES cells to generate trophectoderm (Niwa et al, 2000).

Moreover, several oncogenes were also shown to be important for maintaining ES cells. The Myc family of genes plays an important role in maintaining ES cells. Max is an important partner required for the functions of Myc. If max is knocked out, Myc family genes such as c-Myc, L-Myc and N-Myc cannot exert their effects. Max knockout ES cells cannot survive. Several genes were selected from the ECATs, important transcripts for ES cells and oncogenes as candidates of reprogramming factors. It was necessary to create an assay system which evaluated candidates reprogramming factors for their ability to reprogram somatic cells. Fbx15 is another of the ECATs. That is, Fbx15 is expressed specifically in ES cells, and not in somatic cells. Fibroblasts with a G418 antibiotic resistance gene in the Fbx15 locus were used for the assay system. Normal cells cannot survive in the presence of G418. If the fibroblasts are reprogrammed by the candidates, their Fbx15 locus is activated, the G418 resistance genes are expressed, and the fibroblasts are resistant to G418. The cells that were reprogrammed cells by the candidate could then be selected with G418 (Fig1.A).

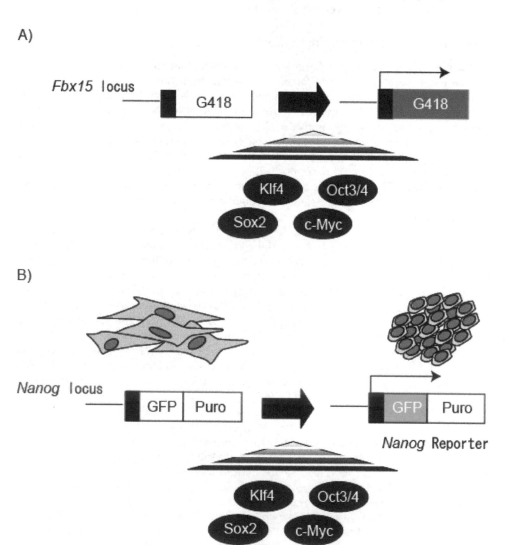

C)

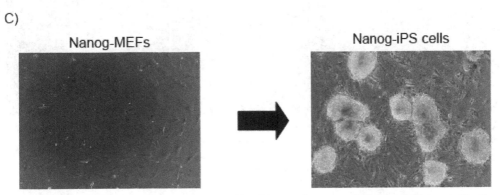

Nanog-MEFs

Nanog-iPS cells

A - An illustration of the Fbx15 reporter system. Fbx15 is a marker gene of ES cells which is specifically expressed in ES cells. Fbx15 is not expressed in fibroblasts. If fibroblasts are reprogrammed by reprogramming factors, then the Fbx15 locus is activated in the cells. These reprogrammed cells thereafter demonstrate resistance for G418; a tocix antibiotic to mammalian cells.
B - An illustration of the Nanog reporter system. The Nanog locus is inactivated in somatic cells. On the other hand, the Nanog locus is activated in reprogrammed cells. The reprogrammed cells are positive for GFP (green fluorescent protein) and also show resistance for Puromycin ,
C- MEFs and iPS cells carrying the Nanog reporter system. The iPS cells are positive for GFP driven by the Nanog reporter system.

Fig. 1. Reporter system

5. Creating the world's first iPS cells

Candidate reprogramming genes were introduced into mouse embryonic fibroblasts (MEF) carrying a Fbx15 reporter system. When 24 candidates were introduced into MEF at the same time, G418 resistant mouse ES-like colonies appeared about 2 weeks later. The 24 candidates were narrowed down to just 4 factors: Oct3/4, Sox2, klf4 and c-Myc. The cells reprogrammed from somatic cells by these four factors were named "induced pluripotent stem cells" (iPS cells). Their global gene expression patterns were similar to those of mouse ES cells. The proliferation of iPS cells was also similar to ES cells. The iPS cells can differentiate into all 3 germ layers in vitro and in vivo. The iPS cells generated using the Fbx15 reporter system could also contribute to mouse embryos, but the chimeric embryos did not survive until birth (Takahashi & Yamanaka, 2006). These data indicated that these first iPS cells had many features like ES cells, but were not completely ES cell like. These iPS cells were considered to be only partially reprogrammed, so the reporter system was improved to facilitate the development of completely reprogrammed iPS cells. Nanog and Oct3/4 are more tightly associated with pluripotency in ES cells than Fbx15. The iPS cells established using a Nanog or Oct3/4 reporter system (Fig1.B,C) contributed to chimeric mouse embryos which survived beyond birth, and these improved iPS cells contribute to the germline of chimeric mice (Okita et al.,2007; Wernig et al.,2007; Maherali et al., 2007) (Fig,2). Moreover, it was reported that cloned live pups could be generated using iPS cells by tetraploid complementation (Kang et al., 2009). These studies strongly suggest that mouse iPS cells are substantially comparable to mouse ES cells, at least in terms of their differentiation potential.

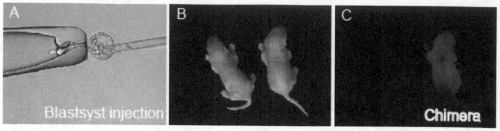

A - iPS cells are injected into blastocysts to make chimera mice. iPS cells are injected into mouse
blastocysts (middle) using a micro manipulation system consisting of a holding- (left) and a transfer
pipette (right)
B, C - Mouse iPS cells expressing red fluorescent proteins are injected into mouse blastocysts. The
mouse iPS cells contribute to all tissues in the mice bodies. The right mouse pup is the chimera.

Fig. 2. Contribution of iPS cell to all tissues in chimera mice

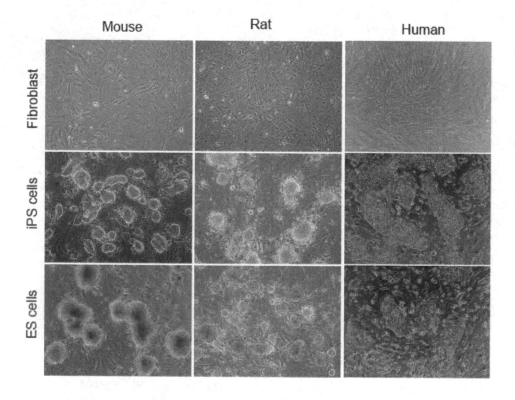

Fig. 3. Comparing the morphologies among the mouse, rat and human.
The mouse, rat and human morphologies of fibroblasts, iPS cells and ES cells. Mouse, rat
and human iPS cell colonies are morphologically very similar to ES cell colonies. Mouse and
at iPS and ES cell colonies are round shaped. On the other hand, human iPS and ES cell
colonies are flat shaped and different for many properties compared to mouse and rat.

In 2007, Human iPS cells were established (Takahashi et al., 2007; Yu et al., 2007). This was only one year after the establishment of mouse iPS cells, which is remarkable considering that it took about 15 years to establish human ES cells after establishing mouse ES cells. The establishment of the human iPS cells was the result of the accumulation of knowledge regarding human ES cells and mouse iPS cell induction. Human iPS cells were established using two different combinations of reprogramming factors. Our group used Oct3/4, Sox2, and Klf4 with or without c-Myc. Another group used Oct3/4, Sox2, and Nanog, with or without Lin28 (Takahashi et al., 2007; Yu et al., 2007). Therefore, Oct3/4 and Sox2 were common between our combinations and the other group's combinations. Human iPS cells can differentiate into all 3 germ layers in vitro (Fig.4) and in vivo (Fig.5). Up to now, rat, monkey, pig, dog and rabbit iPS cells have been established, however, the germline transmission of these iPS cells has not yet been reported (Liu et al., 2008; Jing et al., 2008; Wenlin etal., 2008; Esteban et al.,2009; Zhao et al.,2009; Shimada et al,. 2009; Wu et al., 2010; Honda et al., 2010).

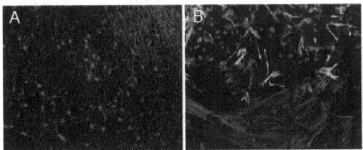

A - In vitro differentiation of human iPS cells into neurons (Red).
B - In vitro differentiation of human iPS cells into smooth (Red) and striated muscles (Green).
Fig. 4. Human iPS cells were differentiated in vitro.

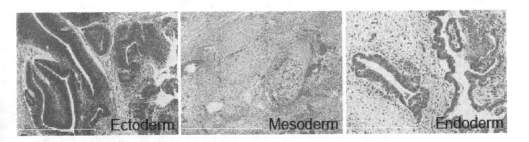

Fig. 5. In vivo differentiation of human iPS cells.

Human iPS cells are transplanted into testes of immunocompromised mice. After about 10 weeks, human iPS cells form teratomas. The teratomas are analysed histologically with haematoxylin and eosin staining. iPS cells are differentiated into all three germ layers.

6. Increasing the efficiency of generating iPS cells

In the beginning of iPS cell research, the generation efficiency was very low, when Oct3/4, Sox2 and klf4 were used. It was found that the addition of c-Myc increased the efficiency more than 100-fold. Although c-Myc is not essential for iPS cell induction, it is a very effective factor for increasing the efficiency. The stability of c-Myc is regulated by the glycogen synthase kinase 3 (GSK3), which negatively regulates the Wnt pathway. Phosphorylated c-Myc is rapidly degraded by the ubiquitin-proteosome pathway. Therefore, Wnt may enhance the generation efficiency of iPS cells with Oct3/4, Sox2 and klf4 (Marson et al., 2008). However, precisely role of c-Myc during iPS cell induction is still unclear. Even when iPS cells were induced with c-Myc, the overall efficiency calculated from the number of potentially reprogrammable cells was less than 1%. Therefore, further improvements in the reprogramming efficiency were needed. There are three main ways to increase this efficiency: inducing iPS cells with the help of chemicals, adding more reprogramming factors, and changing the combination of reprogramming factors.

6.1 Increasing the efficiency with chemical compounds
6.1.1 Chemicals affecting DNA and histone modifications

DNA and histone modifications regulate the gene expression patterns in cells. These modifications stably maintain the gene expression pattern to ensure the proper characteristics of the cells. During iPS cell generation, these modifications are changed dramatically (Deng et al., 2009). One of DNA methyltransferase inhibitors, 5-azacytidine, improved the efficiency of reprogramming by nuclear transfer. Several inhibitors of DNA methyltransferase, such as 5-azacytidine, BIX-01294, RG108, etc. improved the efficiency of iPS cell generation. Inhibitors of histone deacetylases, for example valproic acid (VPA), butyrate, and trichostatin A, also increased the iPS cell generation efficiency. iPS cells could be induced using just Oct3/4 and Sox2 with VPA (Xu et al., 2008; Shi et al., 2008; Huangfu et al., 2008; Danwei et al., 2008; Mali et al., 2010; Zhou et al., 2010). It was thought that the effects of these chemicals which change DNA and histone modifications was due to inhibition of genes expressed in somatic cells and the induction of those expressed in ES cells. However, these chemicals have low specificity. They change the global DNA and histone modifications. Therefore, they inhibit not only the expression of genes which define somatic cells, but also those which are important for ES and iPS cells. As a result, if the concentration of these chemicals, the length of the treatment, or the original somatic cells are different, these chemicals may either have no effect or may even decrease the efficiency of iPS cell generation.

6.1.2 Chemicals affecting molecular signaling pathways

The inhibition of the Tgf-β (transforming growth factor- β) pathway increases the efficiency of mouse iPS cell generation. This inhibition is effective during the early stage of iPS cell induction. It is thought that the mechanism of Tgf- β inhibition is as follows: Fibroblasts are mesenchymal cells, while iPS cells are epithelial cells. Fibroblasts need to be converted to epithelial cells during iPS cell induction (Payman et al., 2010). The Tgf- β pathway accelerates the epithelial-to-mesenchymal transition. Therefore, the inhibition of the Tgf- β pathway improves the iPS cell generation efficiency by accelerating the mesenchymal-to-epithelial transition (Maherali et al., 2009). The combined inhibition of the MAPK pathway and the Tgf- β pathway has a synergistic effect (Tongxiang et al., 2009) to generate human iPS cells. Moreover, using just an Oct3/4 transgene, mouse iPS cells can be generated from neonatal human epithelial keratinocytes with a combination of compounds including sodium butyrate (a histone deacetylase inhibitor), PS48 (an activator of 3'-phosphoinositide-dependent kinase-1), A-83-01 (a TGF-β inhibitor) and PD0325901 (a MAPK inhibitor) (Zhou et al., 2011). The use of 8-bromoadenosine 3', 5'-cyclic monophosphate (8-Br-cAMP), a cyclic AMP analog, also improves human iPS cell induction efficiency (Wang & Adjaye, 2010). It is thought that 8-Br-cAMP exerts its pro-induction effect by decreasing the expression of p53 and increasing the expression of Cyclins.

6.2 Promoting the efficiency by adding more reprogramming factors

Suppressing p53 gene (TP53) expression enhances the efficiency of generating both mouse and human iPS cells (Kawamura et al., 2009; Rowland et al., 2009; Hong et al., 2009; Li et al., 2009; Marión et al., 2009; Utikal Banito et al., 2009). The p21 gene is one of the p53 downstream targets. The p21 protein binds and inactivates the G1/S-cyclin dependent kinase (cdk) and S-Cdk complexes to stop the cell cycle. Overexpression of p21 negated the amplifying effect of p53 suppression during iPS cell transduction. Inhibition of the retinoblastoma protein (RB) also improves the efficiency of iPS cell generation. RB inhibits E2F, which accelerates the transcription of S-phase genes such as Cyclin E and Cyclin A. The complex of G1-cdk and Cyclin D1 phosphorylate RB. Phosphorylated RB cannot bind and inhibit E2F, allowing the cell cycle to progress from the G1 phase to the S phase. Cyclin D1 also increases the iPS cell generation efficiency. Rem2 GTPase is one of the suppressors of the p53 pathway. Rem2 is an important player to maintain human ES cells. Rem2 enhances the reprogramming by regulating p53 and cyclinD1 (Edel et al., 2010). These data suggest that accelerating cell proliferation enhances the iPS cell generation efficiency. Promoting cell proliferation accelerates the stochastic process of reprogramming. However it is thought that the amplifying effect of p53 inhibition does not only result from the acceleration of cell cycle. It is known that p53 directly binds to the promoter region of the Nanog gene and suppresses its expression in mouse ES cells (Sabapathy et al., 1997; Qin et al., 2007). There is a possibility that p53 directly regulates the gene expression pattern during iPS cell generation.

Lin28 is also effective for increasing the efficiency of reprogramming. Lin28 was used to generate some of the first human iPS cells. Like c-Myc, Lin28 is effective, but not essential, for the generation of human iPS cells. Lin28 is also effective in combination with Oct3/4, Sox2, Klf4 and c-Myc. Lin28 can interfere with the maturation of miRNA and promote their degradation by uridylation of miRNA (Heo et all., 2008 2009). Let-7 is one of the Lin28-associated miRNAs, and regulates the translation of several genes including c-Myc, K-Ras, Cyclin D1 and Hmga2. However, the mechanism(s) underlying the effects of Lin28 are still unclear (Kim et al., 2009; Viswanathan et al., 2009).

Tbx3 also improves the efficiency of mouse iPS cell generation. The association between Tbx3, Nanog and Tcf3 is important for pluripotency and self-renew of ES cells. Moreover, the efficiency of germline transmission of mouse iPS cells with Tbx-3 is higher than that with just Oct3/4, Sox2 and Klf4 (Jianyong et al ., 2010).

E-Cadherin also enhanced the mouse reprogramming efficiency in combination with Oct3/4, Sox2 and Klf4 or Oct3/4, Sox2, Klf4 and c-Myc. E-Cadherin is a molecule that mediates cell-cell interactions, and is upregulated during iPS cell induction. An antibody against the extracellular domain of E-cadherin reduced the efficiency of iPS cell generation. These data indicated that the cell-cell contact mediated by E-cadherin plays an important role in reprogramming (Chen et al., 2010).

In addition, some micro RNAs also enhance the efficiency of iPS cell generation. The mir-290 cluster is highly expressed in mouse ES cells. The efficiency of mouse iPS cell generation with Oct3/4, Sox2 and klf4 was improved by miR-291-3p, miR-294, miR-295, which are included in the cluster of mir-290. However, they are not effective with c-Myc. While c-Myc binds to the promoter of the mir-290 cluster, introducing c-Myc could not induce the expression of the mir-290 cluster in fibroblasts. The promoter of the mir-290 cluster is regulated negatively by histone modifications in fibroblasts. These data suggest that the mir-290 cluster is one of targets which are regulated by histone modification (Robert et al., 2009).

6.3 Promoting the efficiency by using different combinations of reprogramming factors

L-Myc is one of Myc family members. L-Myc is more effective for iPS cell induction than c-Myc. Moreover, mouse iPS cells established with L-Myc contribute to the germline more efficiently than iPS cells with c-Myc (Nakagawa et al., 2010).

Utf1 also improves the efficiency of mouse iPS cell generation. The number of mouse iPS colonies generated using a combination of Oct3/4, Sox2, klf4 and Utf1 was 10 times higher than that with Oct3/4, Sox2, Klf4 and c-Myc (Zhao et al., 2008).

Recently, both human and mouse iPS cells were established using just the miR-302/367 cluster in the absence of any other reprogramming factors. The miR-302/367 cluster is highly expressed in ES and iPS cells, and is one of the target of Oct3/4 and Sox2. The use of just the miR302/367 cluster reprogrammed both human and mouse cells more efficiently and rapidly than the combination of Oct3/4, Sox2, Klf4 and c-Myc (Anokye-Danso et al., 2011).

7. The methods for generating iPS cells

There are two main methods to generate iPS cells. These are the genomic integration method and the genomic integration-free method.

7.1 The Genomic integration method
7.1.1 Retrovirus systems

Retrovirus systems were used to generate the world's first mouse and human iPS cells (Takahashi et al., 2006, 2007). The reprogramming factors introduced by a retrovirus system are strongly and stably expressed in somatic cells. The retrovirus system can efficiently introduce several reprogramming factors into cells at the same time. For these reasons, a retrovirus system efficiently generates iPS cells. Therefore, retrovirus systems are suitable for investigating the mechanism of iPS cell induction. Moreover, reprogramming factors introduced into somatic cells by the retrovirus system are gradually silenced during the reprogramming progress (Okita et al., 2007). This is good for iPS cell generation, because the expression of reprogramming factors in reprogrammed cells sometimes induces differentiation and cell death. Moreover, expressing transgenic reprogramming factors into reprogrammed cells can induce tumorigenicity.

7.1.2 Lentivirus systems

Lentiviral vectors were also used to generate some of the first human iPS cells (Yu et al., 2007). Lentivirus can infect not only the dividing cells, but also non-dividing cells. Lentivirus infection therefore occurs independent of cell division. The reprogramming factors introduced by lentiviruses are stably expressed and less silenced than those introduced by retroviruses. Thus, drug-inducible transgene expression systems were made because of these characteristics of lentiviral vectors to investigate the mechanism of iPS cell induction (Hockemeyer et al., 2008; Maherali et al., 2008).

7.2 Genomic integration-free method
The genes introduced by either retroviral or lentiviral vectors permanently integrate into the genome. Such integration increases the risk of tumorigenicity for two reasons: the first reason is that the integration can interrupt genes and gene promoters; the second reason is that the integrated factors could be reactivated unexpectedly by nearby promoters. For clinical applications, these issues will need to be overcome. Recently, two principal ways to generate iPS cells without genomic integration were developed. One of them is removing the genomic integration after establishing iPS cells. The other is establishing iPS cells without integration vectors.

7.2.1 Removing genomic integration after establishing iPS cells
Cre-mediated recombination can be used to remove transgenes from the iPS cell genome. Human iPS cells have been established using lentiviral constructs including loxP sequences in their long terminal repeat (LTR). Established iPS cells can be treated with Cre recombinase in order to excise the lentiviral cassettes. However, the LTR sequence still remains in the genome (Soldner et al., 2009).

A "piggybac" transposon vector system can also solve this problem. Using this system, the integrated reprogramming factor can be removed seamlessly. Transposase has activities for both the insertion and excision of transposon vectors by recognizing the TTAA tetra-nucleotide sequence in the host genome (Kaji et al., 2009 Woltjen et al., 2009 Yusa et al., 2009).

7.2.2 Generating iPS cells without genomic integration of reprogramming factors
The first integration-free iPS cells were generated from mouse somatic cells with adenoviral vectors or conventional expression vectors (Okita et al, 2008; Stadtfeld et al, 2008). Recently, episomal vectors were used to generate human iPS cells (Yu et al., 2009). Episomal vectors consist of the replication origin and an Epstein-Barr nuclear antigen (EBNA). The EBNA vector can self-replicate and maintain the expression of transgenic reprogramming factors without genomic integration. However, the efficiency of reprogramming with episomal vectors was 10 times less than that with integration vectors. However, the efficiency was recently improved using episomal vectors encoding Oct3/4, Sox2, Klf4, L-Myc, Lin28 and a short hairpin RNA against p53 (Okita et al., 2011). This method is very promising for clinical application because the possibility of episomal vector genomic integration is very low, although it is still not zero. There is a little possibility that this vector may accidentally integrate into the genome accidentally. This possibility should be kept in mind when planning trial for clinical application.

The Sendai RNA virus is also a promising vector that can be used to generate clinical-grade iPS cells. This virus does not enter into the nucleus for replication, transcription or translation. Therefore, there are no risks of insertion of reprogramming factors introduced by this virus. The transduction efficiency using this virus is comparable to that using retrovirus system. iPS cells were also established from less than 1 ml of peripheral blood using this system(Seki et al. 2010). If deficient sendai viral vectors are used for iPS induction, the vectors can be removed by siRNA (Nishimura et al., 2011).

There are also other ways to establish iPS cells virus-free. In one study, the Oct3/4, Sox2, Klf4 and c-Myc proteins were modified so that they could easily pass through the cell membrane. Both human and mouse iPS cells were established using these proteins (Hongyan et al., 2009; Dohoon et al., 2009). Another recent method used synthetic modified mRNA to generate iPS cells. RNA usually is unstable, and cells with foreign RNA are usually destroyed by the interferon response. The authors modified the medium and RNA to reduce the interferon response and improve RNA stability. The reprogramming factor from the introduced RNA was expressed stably and highly in the cells. Using this method, the possibility of genomic integration is very low, because of the nature of RNA. However, the possibility of cell damage in iPS cells generated using this method is slightly increased through the stressful induction method that requires consecutive introduction of RNA into cells for 2 weeks and artificial inhibition of the cell interferon response. A newer method to establish both human and mouse iPS cells used just miRNA, miR-200c, 302 and 369. These iPS cells were named mi-iPS cells (Miyoshi et al., 2011).

Regardless of the method used to generate iPS cells, the quality of the cells should be examined from various points of view and in depth before using the iPS cells for clinical applications.

8. Applications of iPS cells

The major benefit of iPS cells is that they make it possible to obtain differentiated cells in the required quantities. It is expected that iPS cells can be used for regenerative medicine and drug discovery (Fig. 6).

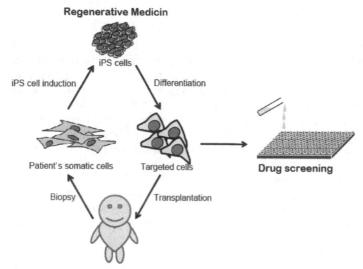

Fig. 6. A Schematic illustration for the application of iPS cells

iPS cells derived from patients are useful for regenerative medicine and drug discovery. Somatic cells are taken by biopsy from patients. Patient specific iPS cells are then established from the somatic cells and differentiated into targeted cells. If the targeted cells are transplanted into a disease site, then this would bethat is very promising for regenerative medicine. Moreover, if disease phenotypes are reproduced using patient specific iPS cells in vitro, patient specific responses to drugs could be evaluated for individual therapies.

8.1 Using iPS cells for regenerative medicine

Differentiated cells from iPS cells derived from the recipients are not rejected by the immune system upon transplantation, because they have the same immune markers as the recipient. Hence, it is expected that it will be possible to use iPS cells for cell therapy and regenerative medicine. Under this scheme, iPS cells are differentiated into the targeted cells, and the differentiated cells are then implanted into the diseased area where they can improve the patient's symptoms. Experiment procedures utilizing lab animals have already proven the effectiveness of this scheme for cell therapy. For example, in a rat model of Parkinson's disease, the implantation of dopamine-producing neurons that were differentiated from iPS cells led to a clear improvement in the symptoms (Hargus et al., 2010).

It is also possible to use an approach which is a combination of cell therapy and gene therapy. Sickle cell anemia is a genetic blood disorder. The patient's red blood cells are abnormally sickle-shaped, thus decreasing the oxygen transport ability of these patients' red blood cells compared to unaffected individuals. This abnormality is caused by a mutation in one gene. The mutation was repaired using gene therapy technology in iPS cells derived from model mice. The repaired iPS cells were differentiated into hematopoietic stem cells. The hematopoietic stem cells transplanted into the model mice started to generate normal red blood cells and cure the disease (Hanna et al., 2007). The effectiveness of these procedures has not yet been examined in humans. However, Geron and Advanced Cell Technology announced that they plan to start clinical trials of transplantation of cells derived from ES cells for spinal cord injury and muscular degeneration, respectively. The current advances in the differentiation induction technology are likely to facilitate human studies. For example, the three dimensional structure of the neural retina differentiated from mouse ES cells was recently demonstrated (Eiraku et al., 2011). The combinations of the various differentiation technologies will likely provide new sources and methods for regenerative medicine.

8.2 Concerns about using iPS cells for regenerative medicine

Before using iPS cells for clinical applications, the safety of iPS cells should be sufficiently verified. In the paper introduced previously about curing Parkinson disease model mice, the authors suggested several problems that need to be overcome before this strategy can be clinically used. The major problem was that the model mice transplanted with the cells differentiated from iPS cells eventually developed teratomas (Hargus et al., 2010). The formation of teratomas in donor mice was caused by the undifferentiated cells that were present in the differentiated cells used for transplantation. It will therefore be necessary to develop an efficient differentiation system that allows for the invariably selection of targeted somatic cells and complete removal of all residual undifferentiated cells. In fact, attempts have already been made to select or generate iPS cells which can easily be differentiated into targeted cells. Recently, our group demonstrated that iPS cells have various differentiation potentials, and we found that several iPS cell clones were highly resistant to neural differentiation (Miura et al., 2009). Additional, studies to identify the genes responsible for the resistance are currently underway.

In addition, it was reported iPS cells carry epigenetic memory of the original somatic cells during early passages. This memory affects their differentiation potential. For example, iPS cells from B cells differentiated into blood progenitor cells more efficiently than iPS cells derived from fibroblasts (Kim et al., 2010; Polo et al., 2010). The origin of iPS cells was therefore reflected in the differentiation potential of the iPS cells. Further accumulation of this knowledge will help create smooth path toward the clinical application of iPS cells.

8.3 Using iPS cells to understand pathological conditions and for drug discovery

Utilizing the advantages provided by the iPS cell technology, differentiated cells which are difficult to harvest from patients and culture in vitro can now be obtained in sufficient quantities for researchers to study the pathogenesis of diseases and to perform drug screening.

The first disease-specific iPS cells were established from patients with familial amyotrophic lateral sclerosis (ALS). However, the authors could not reproduce disease phenotypes using differentiated cells from ALS-iPS cells in vitro (Dimos et al., 2008). The first in vitro reproduction of a disease phenotype was achieved with iPS cells derived from a spinal muscular atrophy (SMA) patient. The motor neurons differentiated from SMA iPS cells exhibited the specific phenotype, such as a decreased number and size of neurons (Ebert et al., 2009). Recently, many disease models have been generated in vitro with iPS cells from patients with Familial dysautonomia (FD), myeloproliferative disorders, Dyskeratosis congenital, Leopard syndrome, Rett syndrome (REFS) and further diseases (Lee et al., 2009; Ye et al., 2009; Suneet et al., 2010; Carvajal et al., 2010; Marchetto et al., 2010).

The effects and side effects of drugs are generally tested using laboratory animals, primarily rodents. However, the effects of drugs are different between humans and animals, and such studies were one of obstacle to developing new therapeutic agents. Moreover, using laboratory animals is cost- and time-intensive. The ability to test new agents on specific types of cells will greatly facilitate research on drug effects and toxicity.

It was previously very difficult to collect sufficient amounts of targeted cells from patients for analyses until the iPS cell breakthrough. Many disease models using iPS cells will likely be established in the near future, because the safety of iPS cells (with regard to teratoma formation) is not an issue affecting basic research involving these cells. Therefore, iPS cell technologies will greatly facilitate our understanding of the pathogenesis of various diseases and will help in the development of novel treatments.

9. Conclusion

About sixty years ago, humans started to deeply and systematically investigate living things from a molecular point of view. The major purposes were to achieve a better understanding of the basic function of living things and to try to regulate and use these findings to enhance human lives. The biological systems improved by nature for several billion years are much more efficient than the engineered systems developed by humans. For example, fireflies emit thermal free light while producing their fluorescence, while electric lights produce heat. This indicates that biological systems are very efficient. Understanding and using these biological systems can therefore have a major impact on the quality of human life.

The development of iPS cells is a prime example of using such biological systems for human benefit. The development of iPS cells has demonstrated that the characteristics of differentiated cells could be changed artificially by employing appropriate factors and methods. Recently, new direct reprogramming technologies have been developed, which allowed somatic cells to be directly reprogrammed into targeted somatic cells without involving iPS cells.

However, precisely what occurs during iPS cell inductionstill remains unclear. Human fertilized eggs differentiate into somatic cells for several months in the mother's womb. During the induction of iPS cells, the somatic cells are artificially induced to regress into pluripotent stem cells within just a few weeks. There is a possibility that abnormalities are accumulated in iPS cells due to artificial reprogramming stresses. It will be necessary to uncover the full mechanism of iPS cell induction, and many questions remain to be answered, including: Exactly what is happening during iPS cell induction? Can abnormalities of cells be caused by what is happening during iPS induction? Moreover, it is also important to evaluate the established iPS cells in comparison to ES cells. Such research will help pave the way for iPS cells to move from a scientific finding to a medical revolution.

10. Acknowledgments

We would like to thank the members in the Yamanaka laboratory and CiRA. We especially appreciate Yuji Mochizuki's and Birger Voigt's help with the revision of this review.

11. References

Anokye-Danso F, Trivedi CM, Juhr D, Gupta M, Cui Z, Tian Y, Zhang Y, Yang W, Gruber PJ, Epstein JA, Morrisey EE. (2011). Highly Efficient miRNA-Mediated Reprogramming of Mouse and Human Somatic Cells to Pluripotency. Cell Stem Cell, Vol,8, pp. 376-388

Banito, A., Rashid, ST., Acosta, JC., Li, S., Pereira, CF., Geti, I., Pinho, S., Silva, JC., Azuara, V., Walsh, M., Vallier, L. & Gil, J. (2009) Senescence impairs successful reprogramming to pluripotent stem cells. Genes. Dev., Vol.23, pp.2134-2139.

Boiani, M. & Schöler, HR. (2005) Regulatory networks in embryo-derived pluripotent stem cells. Nat. Rev. Mol. Cell. Biol. Vol.6 pp872-884.

Briggs, R. & King, T. J. (1952). Transplantation of living nuclei from blastula cell into enucleated frog's egg . Proc. Natl. Acad. Sci. USA, Vol.38, pp.455-463

Byrne, JA., Pedersen, DA., Clepper, LL., Nelson, M., Sanger, WG., Gokhale, S., Wolf, DP. & Mitalipov, SM. (2007). Producing primate embryonic stem cells by somatic cell nuclear transfer. Nature, vol. 450, pp.497-502.

Carvajal-Vergara X, Sevilla A, D'Souza SL, Ang YS, Schaniel C, Lee DF, Yang L, Kaplan AD, Adler ED, Rozov R, Ge Y, Cohen N, Edelmann LJ, Chang B, Waghray A, Su J, Pardo S, Lichtenbelt KD, Tartaglia M, Gelb BD, Lemischka IR.(2010). Patient-specific induced pluripotent stem-cell-derived models of LEOPARD syndrome. Nature, 465, pp.808-12

Chambers I, Colby D, Robertson M, Nichols J, Lee S, Tweedie S and Smith A. (2003).Functional expression cloning of nanog, a pluripotency sustaining factor in embryonic stem cells. Cell, Vlo.113, pp. 643–655.

Chen T, Yuan D, Wei B, Jiang J, Kang J, Ling K, Gu Y, Li J, Xiao L and Pei G. (2010). E-cadherin-Mediated Cell-Cell Contact is Critical for Induced Pluripotent Stem Cell Generation. Stem Cells, Vol.28, pp.1315-25.

Chung, Y., Klimanskaya, I., Becker, S., Li, T., Maserati, M., Lu, SJ., Zdravkovic, T., Ilic, D., Genbacev, O., Fisher, S., Krtolica, A. & Lanza, R. (2008). Human embryonic stem cell lines generated without embryo destruction. Cell Stem Cell, Vol.2, pp.113-117.

Chung, Y., Klimanskaya, I., Becker, S., Marh, J., Lu, SJ., Johnson, J., Meisner, L. & Lanza, R. (2006). Embryonic and extraembryonic stem cell lines derived from single mouse blastomeres. Nature, Vol. 439, pp.216-219.

Danwei H, Kenji O, René M, Wenjun G, Astrid E, Shuibing C, Whitney M and Douglas A M. Induction of pluripotent stem cells from primary human fibroblasts with only Oct4 and Sox2. (2008). Nat Biotechnol. Vol. 26, 1269 – 1275

Deng J, Shoemaker R, Xie B, Gore A, Leproust EM, Antosiewicz-Bourget J, Egli D, Maherali N, Park IH, Yu J, Daley GQ, Eggan K, Hochedlinger K, Thomson J, Wang W, Gao Y and Zhang K. Targeted bisulfite sequencing reveals changes in DNA methylation associated with nuclear reprogramming. (2009). Nat Biotechnol, Vol.27, Issue.4, pp. 353-60

Dimos, JT., Rodolfa, KT., Niakan, KK., Weisenthal, LM., Mitsumoto, H., Chung, W., Croft, GF., Saphier, G., Leibel, R., Goland, R., Wichterle, H., Henderson, CE. & Eggan, K. (2008) Induced Pluripotent Stem Cells Generated from Patients with ALS Can Be Differentiated into Motor Neurons. Science, Vol.321, pp.1218-1221.

Dimos, JT., Rodolfa, KT., Niakan, KK., Weisenthal, LM., Mitsumoto, H., Chung, W., Croft, GF., Saphier, G., Leibel, R., Goland, R., Wichterle, H., Henderson, CE. & Eggan, K. (2008) Induced Pluripotent Stem Cells Generated from Patients with ALS Can Be Differentiated into Motor Neurons. Science, Vol.321, pp.1218-1221.

Dohoon Kim, Chun-Hyung Kim, Jung-Il Moon, Young-Gie Chung, Mi-Yoon Chang, Baek-Soo Han, Sanghyeok Ko, Eungi Yang, Kwang Yul Cha, Robert Lanza and Kwang-Soo Kim. (2009). Generation of Human Induced Pluripotent Stem Cells by Direct Delivery of Reprogramming Proteins.

Ebert, AD., Yu, J., Rose, FF., Mattis, VB., Lorson, CL., Thomson, JA. & Svendsen, CN. (2009) Induced pluripotent stem cells from a spinal muscular atrophy patient. Nature, 457, 277-280.

Edel MJ, Menchon C, Menendez S, Consiglio A, Raya A and Izpisua Belmonte JC. (2010)Rem2 GTPase maintains survival of human embryonic stem cells as well as enhancing reprogramming by regulating p53 and cyclin D1. Genes Dev, Vol.24, pp.561-573

Eiraku M, Takata T, Ishibashi H, Kawada M, Sakakura E, Okuda S, Sekiguchi K, Adachi T, & Sasai Y. (2011) Self-organizing optic-cupmorphogenesisin three-dimensional culture. Nature, Vol.472, pp.51–56

Esteban MA, Xu J, Yang J, Peng M, Qin D, Li W, Jiang Z, Chen J, Deng K, Zhong M, Cai J, Lai L, Pei G and Pei D. Generation of induced pluripotent stem cell lines from tibetan miniature pig.(2009). J Biol Chem, Vol.284, Issue.26, pp. 17634-40

Evans, M.J. and Kaufman, M.H. (1981). Establishment in culture of pluripotent cells from mouse embryos. Nature, Vol.292, pp.154–156

Gurdon, JB. (1962). The developmental capacity of nuclei taken from intestinal epithelium cells of feeding tadpoles. J. Embryol. Exp. Morphol, Vol.10, pp.622–40

Hanna J, Wernig M, Markoulaki S, Sun CW, Meissner A, Cassady JP, Beard C, Brambrink T, Wu LC, Townes TM, Jaenisch R.(2007). Treatment of sickle cell anemia mouse model with iPS cells generated from autologous skin. Science. Vol.318, pp.1920-3.

Hargus G, Cooper O, Deleidi M, Levy A, Lee K, Marlow E, Yow A, Soldner F, Hockemeye D, Hallett PJ, Osborn T, Jaenisch R and Isacson O. (2010). Differentiated Parkinson patient derived induced pluripotent stem cells grow in the adult rodent brain and reduce motor asymmetry in Parkinsonian rats. Proc Natl Acad Sci U S A. Vol.107, pp.15921-15926

Heo, I., Joo, C., Cho, J., Ha, M., Han, J. & Kim, VN. (2008) Lin28 mediates the terminal uridylation of let-7 precursor MicroRNA. Mol. Cell, Vol.32, pp.276-284.

Heo, I., Joo, C., Kim, YK., Ha, M., Yoon, MJ., Cho, J., Yeom, KH., Han, J. & Kim, VN. (2009) TUT4 in concert with Lin28 suppresses microRNA biogenesis through pre-microRNA uridylation. Cell, Vo.138, pp.696-708.

Hockemeyer, D., Soldner, F., Cook, EG., Gao, Q., Mitalipova, M. & Jaenisch, R. (2008). A Drug-Inducible System for Direct Reprogramming of Human Somatic Cells to Pluripotency. Cell Stem Cell, Vol.3, pp.346-353.

Honda A, Hirose M, Hatori M, Matoba S, Miyoshi H, Inoue K, Ogura A. Generation of induced pluripotent stem cells in rabbits: potential experimental models for human regenerative medicine. (2010). J Biol Chem, Vol.285, Issue.41, pp. 31362-31369

Hong, H., Takahashi, K., Ichisaka, T., Aoi, T., Kanagawa, O., Nakagawa, M., Okita, K. & Yamanaka, S. (2009) Suppression of induced pluripotent stem cell generation by the p53-p21 pathway. Nature, Vol.460, pp.1132-1135.

Hongyan Zhou, Shili Wu, Jin Young Joo, Saiyong Zhu, Dong Wook Han, Tongxiang Lin, Sunia Trauger, Geoffery Bien, Susan Yao, Yong Zhu, Gary Siuzdak, Hans R. Schöler, Lingxun Duan and Sheng Ding.(2009). Generation of Induced Pluripotent Stem Cells Using Recombinant Proteins. Cell stem cell, Vol.4, pp.381-384

Huangfu D, Maehr R, Guo W, Eijkelenboom A, Snitow M, Chen AE, Melton DA. (2008) Induction of pluripotent stem cells by defined factors is greatly improved by small-molecule compounds. Nat Biotechnol. Vol.26. pp.795-7

Jianyong H, Ping Y, Henry Y, Jinqiu Z, Boon S S, Pin L, Siew L L, Suying C, Junliang T, Yuriy L. O, Thomas L, Huck-Hui N, Wai-Leong Tand Bing L. (2010).Tbx3 improves the germ-line competency of induced pluripotent stem cells. Nature, Vol.463, pp.1096-1100

Jing Liao, Chun Cui, Siye Chen, Jiangtao Ren, Jijun Chen, Yuan Gao, Hui Li, Nannan Jia, Lu Cheng, Huasheng Xiao, and Lei Xiao. Generation of induced pluripotent stem cell lines from adult rat cells. (2008). Cell stem cell, Vol.4, pp.11-15

Kaji, K., Norrby, K., Paca, A., Mileikovsky, M., Mohseni, P. & Woltjen, K. (2009) Virus-free induction of pluripotency and subsequent excision of reprogramming factors. Nature, vol.458, pp.771-775.

Kang, L., Wang, J., Zhang, Y., Kou, Z. & Gao, S. (2009). iPS cells can support full-term development of tetraploid blastocyst-complemented embryos. Cell Stem Cell, Vol.5, pp.135-138.

Kawamura, T., Suzuki, J., Wang, YV., Menendez, S., Morera, LB., Raya, A., Wahl, GM. & Izpisúa Belmonte, JC. (2009) Linking the p53 tumour suppressor pathway to somatic cell reprogramming. Nature, Vol. 460, pp.1140-1144.

Kim K, Doi A, Wen B, Ng K, Zhao R, Cahan P, Kim J, Aryee MJ, Ji H, Ehrlich LI, YabuuchiA, Takeuchi A, Cunniff KC, Hongguang H, McKinney-Freeman S, Naveiras O, Yoon TJ, Irizarry RA, Jung N, Seita J, Hanna J, Murakami P, Jaenisch R, Weissleder R,

Orkin SH, Weissman IL, Feinberg AP and Daley GQ. (2010) Epigenetic memory in induced pluripotent stem cells. Nature, Vol.467, pp. 285-290

Kim, HH., Kuwano, Y., Srikantan, S., Lee, EK., Martindale, JL. & Gorospe, M. (2009) HuR recruits let-7/RISC to repress c-Myc expression. Genes. Dev, Vol.23, pp.1743-1748.

Klimanskaya, I., Chung, Y., Becker, S., Lu, SJ. & Lanza, R. (2006). Human embryonic stem cell lines derived from single blastomeres. Nature, 444, 481-485.

Lee G, Papapetrou EP, Kim H, Chambers SM, Tomishima MJ, Fasano CA, Ganat YM, Menon J, Shimizu F, Viale A, Tabar V, Sadelain M and Studer L.(2009) Modelling pathogenesis and treatment of familial dysautonomia using patient-specific iPSCs. Nature,vol.461, pp.402-6

Li, H., Collado, M., Villasante, A., Strati, K., Ortega, S., Cañamero, M., Blasco, MA. & Serrano, M. (2009) The Ink4/Arf locus is a barrier for iPS cell reprogramming. Nature, Vol.460, pp.1136-1139.

Liu H, Zhu F, Yong J, Zhang P, Hou P, Li H, Jiang W, Cai J, Liu M, Cui K, Qu X, Xiang T, Lu D, Chi X, Gao G, Ji W, Ding M and Deng H. Generation of Induced Pluripotent Stem Cells from Adult Rhesus Monkey Fibroblasts. (2008). Cell Stem Cell, Vol.3, pp.587-590

Maherali N, Hochedlinger K. (2009).Tgfbeta Signal Inhibition Cooperates in the Induction of iPSCs and Replaces Sox2 and cMyc. Curr Biol, Vol.19, pp.1718-23

Maherali, N., Ahfeldt, T., Rigamonti, A., Utikal, J., Cowan, C. & Hochedlinger, K. (2008) A High-Efficiency System for the Generation and Study of Human Induced Pluripotent Stem Cells. Cell Stem Cell, Vol.3, pp.340-345.

Maherali, N., Sridharan, R., Xie, W., Utikal, J., Eminli, S., Arnold, K., Stadtfeld, M., Yachechko, R., Tchieu, J., Jaenisch, R., Plath, K. & Hochedlinger, K. (2007) Directly reprogrammed fibroblasts show global epigenetic remodeling and widespread tissue contribution. Cell Stem Cell, vol.1, pp.55-70.

Mali P, Chou BK, Yen J, Ye Z, Zou J, Dowey S, Brodsky RA, Ohm JE, Yu W, Baylin SB, Yusa K, Bradley A, Meyers DJ, Mukherjee C, Cole PA and Cheng L. (2010)Butyrate Greatly Enhances Derivation of Human Induced Pluripotent Stem Cells by Promoting Epigenetic Remodeling and the Expression of Pluripotency-Associated Genes. Stem Cells,Vol.28, pp.713-20.

Marchetto MC, Carromeu C, Acab A, Yu D, Yeo GW, Mu Y, Chen G, Gage FH and Muotri AR. (2010). A model for neural development and treatment of rett syndrome using human induced pluripotent stem cells. Cell, Vol.143, pp.527-39

Marión, RM., Strati, K., Li, H., Murga, M., Blanco, R., Ortega, S., Fernandez-Capetillo, O., Serrano, M. & Blasco, MA. (2009) A p53-mediated DNA damage response limits reprogramming to ensure iPS cell genomic integrity. Nature, Vol.460, pp.1149-1153.

Marson, A., Foreman, R., Chevalier, B., Bilodeau, S., Kahn, M., Young, RA. and Jaenisch, R. Wnt signaling promotes reprogramming of somatic cells to pluripotency. (2008). Cell Stem Cell, Vol.3, 132-135.

Mitsui, K., Tokuzawa, Y., Itoh, H., Segawa, K., Murakami, M., Takahashi, K., Maruyama, M., Maeda, M., and Yamanaka, S. (2003). The homeoprotein Nanog is required for maintenance of pluripotency in mouse epiblast and ES cells. Cell Vol.113, pp.631-642

Miura, K., Okada, Y., Aoi, T., Okada. A., Takahashi, K., Okita, K., Nakagawa, M., Koyanagi, M., Tanabe, K., Ohnuki, M., Ogawa, D., Ikeda, E., Okano, H., Yamanaka, S. (2009).

Variation in the safety of induced pluripotent stem cell lines.Nat Biotechnol 27, 743-745.

Miyoshi N, Ishii H, Nagano H, Haraguchi N, Dewi D L, Kano Y, Nishikawa S, Tanemura M, Mimori K, Tanaka F, Saito T, Nishimura J, Takemasa I, Mizushima T, Ikeda M, Yamamoto H, Sekimoto M, Doki Y and Mori M. Reprogramming of Mouse and Human Cells to Pluripotency Using Mature MicroRNAs. Cell stem cell,

Nakagawa, M., Takizawa, N., Narita, M., Ichisaka, T. & Yamanaka, S. (2010) Promotion of direct reprogramming by transformation-deficient Myc. Proc. Natl. Acad. Sci.U. S. A., vol.107, pp.14152-14157.

Nishimura K, Sano M, Ohtaka M, Furuta B, Umemura Y, Nakajima Y, Ikehara Y, Kobayashi T, Segawa H, Takayasu S, Sato H, Motomura K, Uchida E, Kanayasu-ToyodaT, Asashima M, Nakauchi H, Yamaguchi T and Nakanishi M. (2011).Development of Defective and Persistent Sendai Virus Vector: A UNIQUE GENE DELIVERY/EXPRESSION SYSTEM IDEAL FOR CELL REPROGRAMMING. J Biol Chem, Vol.286, pp.4760-71

Niwa, H., Miyazaki, J. & Smith, A.G. Nature Genet. Quantitative expression of Oct-3/4 defines differentiation, dedifferentiation or self-renewal of ES cells. (2000)Nature gene. Vol.24, pp.372–376.

Okita, K., Ichisaka, T. & Yamanaka, S. (2007). Generation of germline-competent induced pluripotent stem cells. Nature, Vol.448, pp.313-317.

Okita, K., Matsumura, Y., Sato, Y., Okada, A., Morizane, A., Okamoto, S., Hong, H., Nakagawa, M., Tanabe, K., Tezuka, K., Shibata, T., Kunisada, T., Takahashi,M., Takahashi, JB, Saji, H. & Yamanaka, S. (2011). Efficient and Simple Method to Generate Integration-Free Human iPS Cells. Nature methods, NatureMethods, Vol.8, pp. 409–412

Okita, K., Nakagawa, M., Hong, H., Ichisaka, T. & Yamanaka, S. (2008) Generation of Mouse Induced Pluripotent Stem Cells Without Viral Vectors. Science, Vol.322, pp.949-953.

Payman S.T., Azadeh G, Laurent D, Hoon-ki S, Tobias A. B, Alessandro D, Knut W, Andras Nagy, J and L. W.Beyer, A.D., Knut W, Andras N, Jeffrey L. W. (2010). Functional Genomics Reveals a BMP-Driven Mesenchymal-to-Epithelial Transition in the Initiation of Somatic Cell Reprogramming. Cell Stem Cell, Vol 7, Issue 1, pp.64-77

Polo JM, Liu S, Figueroa ME, Kulalert W, Eminli S, Tan KY, Apostolou E, Stadtfeld M, Li Y, Shioda T, Natesan S, Wagers AJ, Melnick A, Evans T and Hochedlinger K. (2010).Cell type of origin influences the molecular and functional properties of mouse induced pluripotent stem cells. Nat Biotechnol, Vol.28, pp. 848-55.

Qin, H., Yu, T., Qing, T., Liu, Y., Zhao, Y., Cai, J., Li, J., Song, Z., Qu, X., Zhou, P., Wu, J., Ding, M. & Deng, H. (2007). Regulation of apoptosis and differentiation by p53 in human embryonic stem cells. J. Biol. Chem, Vol.282, pp.5842-5852.

Rideout, WM. 3rd., Wakayama, T., Wutz, A., Eggan, K., Jackson-Grusby, L., Dausman, J., Yanagimachi, R. & Jaenisch, R. (2000). Generation of mice from wild-type and targeted ES cells by nuclear cloning. Nat. Genet., Vol. 24, pp.109-110.

Robert L. J, Joshua E. B, Monica V and Robert B. (2009). Embryonic stem cell–specific microRNAs promote induced pluripotency. Nature Biotechnology, Vol.27, pp.459 – 461

Rowland, BD., Bernards, R. & Peeper, DS. (2005) The KLF4 tumour suppressor is a transcriptional repressor of p53 that acts as a context-dependent oncogene. Nat. Cell. Biol., Vol.7, pp.1074-1082.

Sabapathy, K., Klemm, M., Jaenisch, R. & Wagner, EF. (1997) Regulation of ES cell differentiation by functional and conformational modulation of p53. EMBO J, vol.16, pp.6217-6229.

Seki, T., Yuasa, S., Oda, M., Egashira, T., Yae, K., Kusumoto, D., Nakata, H., Tohyama, S., Hashimoto, H., Kodaira, M., Okada, Y., Seimiya, H., Fusaki, N., Hasegawa, M. and Fukuda, K. (2010). Generation of induced pluripotent stem cells from human terminally differentiated circulating T cells. Cell Stem Cell, vol.7, pp.11-14.

Shi Y, Desponts C, Do JT, Hahm HS, Schöler HR and Ding S. (2008) Induction of pluripotent stem cells from mouse embryonic fibroblasts by Oct4 and Klf4 with small-molecule compounds. Cell stem cell, Vol.3, pp. 568-74.

Shimada H, Nakada A, Hashimoto Y, Shigeno K, Shionoya Y, Nakamura and T. Generation of canine induced pluripotent stem cells by retroviral transduction and chemical inhibitors. (2009) Mol Reprod Dev. Vol.77,issue1, pp.2

Soldner, F., Hockemeyer, D., Beard, C., Gao, Q., Bell, GW., Cook, EG., Hargus, G., Blak, A., Cooper, O., Mitalipova, M., Isacson, O. & Jaenisch, R. (2009) Parkinson's Disease Patient-Derived Induced Pluripotent Stem Cells Free of Viral Reprogramming Factors. Cell, Vo.136, pp.964-977.

Spemann (1983) Embryonic Development and Induction. Hofner Publishing

Stadtfeld, M., Nagaya, M., Utikal, J., Weir, G. & Hochedlinger, K. (2008) Induced Pluripotent Stem Cells Generated Without Viral Integration. Science, Vol.322, pp.945-949.

Suneet Agarwal, Yuin-Han Loh, Erin M. McLoughlin, Junjiu Huang, In-Hyun Park, Justine D. Miller, Hongguang Huo, Maja Okuka, Rosana Maria dos Reis, Sabine Loewer, Huck-Hui Ng, David L. Keefe, Frederick D. Goldman, Aloysius J. Klingelhutz, Lin Liu & George Q. Daley (2010). Telomere elongation in induced pluripotent stem cells from dyskeratosis congenita patients. Nature, Vol.464, pp.292-296

Takahashi, K. & Yamanaka, S. (2006) Induction of pluripotent stem cells from mouse embryonic and adult fibroblast cultures by defined factors. Cell, Vol.126, pp.663-676.

Takahashi, K., Tanabe, K., Ohnuki, M., Narita, M., Ichisaka, T., Tomoda, K. & Yamanaka, S. (2007) Induction of pluripotent stem cells from adult human fibroblasts by defined factors. Cell, 131, 861-872.

Thomson, J.A., Itskovitz-Eldor, J., Shapiro, S.S., Waknitz, M.A., Swiergiel, J.J., Marshall, V.S., and Jones, J.M. (1998). Embryonic stem cell lines derived from human blastocysts. Science, Vol.282, pp.1145–1147.

Tongxiang Lin, Rajesh Ambasudhan, Xu Yuan, Wenlin Li, Simon Hilcove, Ramzey Abujarour, Xiangyi Lin, Heung Sik Hahm, Ergeng Hao, Alberto Hayek & Sheng Ding. (2009) A chemical platform for improved induction of human iPSCs. Nature Methods, vol.6, pp.805 – 808

Utikal, J., Polo, JM., Stadtfeld, M., Maherali, N., Kulalert, W., Walsh, RM., Khalil, A., Rheinwald, JG. & Hochedlinger, K. (2009) Immortalization eliminates a roadblock during cellular reprogramming into iPS cells. Nature, Vol.460, pp.1145-1148.

Viswanathan, SR., Powers, JT., Einhorn, W., Hoshida, Y., Ng, TL., Toffanin, S., O'Sullivan, M., Lu, J., Phillips, LA., Lockhart, VL., Shah, SP., Tanwar, PS., Mermel, CH.,

Beroukhim, R., Azam, M., Teixeira, J., Meyerson, M., Hughes, TP., Llovet, JM., Radich, J., Mullighan, CG., Golub, TR., Sorensen, PH. & Daley, GQ. (2009) Lin28 promotes transformation and is associated with advanced human malignancies. Nat. Genet, Vol.41, pp.843-848.

Wang Y and Adjaye J. (2010)A Cyclic AMP Analog, 8-Br-cAMP, Enhances the Induction of Pluripotency in Human Fibroblast Cells. Stem Cell Rev., vol.7, pp.331-41.

Wenlin Li, Wei Wei, Saiyong Zhu, Jinliang Zhu, Yan Shi, Tongxiang Lin, Ergeng Hao, Alberto Hayek, Hongkui Deng, and Sheng Ding. Generation of rat and human induced pluripotent stem cells by combining genetic reprogramming and chemical inhibitors. (2008). Cell stem cell, Vol.4, Issue.1 p16-19

Wernig, M., Meissner, A., Foreman, R., Brambrink, T., Ku, M., Hochedlinger, K., Bernstein. BE.& Jaenisch R. (2007) In vitro reprogramming of fibroblasts into a pluripotent ES-cell-like state. Nature, 448, 318-324.

Wilmut, I, Schnieke AE, McWhir J, Kind AJ and Campbell KH. (1997). Viable offspring derived from fetal and adult mammalian cells. Nature Vol.385 pp.810–13

Woltjen, K., Michael, IP., Mohseni, P., Desai, R., Mileikovsky, M., Hämäläinen, R., Cowling, R., Wang, W., Liu, P., Gertsenstein, M., Kaji, K., Sung, HK. & Nagy, A. (2009) piggyBac transposition reprograms fibroblasts to induced pluripotent stem cells. Nature, Vol.458, pp.766-770.

Wu Y, Zhang Y, Mishra A, Tardif SD and Hornsby PJ. Generation of induced pluripotent stem cells from newborn marmoset skin fibroblasts. (2010). Stem Cell Res, Vol.4, Issue.3, pp.180-188.

Xu Y, Shi Y and Ding S. (2008) A chemical approach to stem-cell biology and regenerative medicine. Nature, vol.453, pp.338-344

Ye Z, Zhan H, Mali P, Dowey S, Williams DM, Jang YY, Dang CV, Spivak JL, Moliterno AR, and Cheng L. (2009). Human induced pluripotent stem cells from blood cells of healthy donors and patients with acquired blood disorders. Blood,Vol 114, pp.5473-80

Yu, J., Hu, K., Smuga-Otto, K., Tian, S., Stewart, R., Slukvin, II. & Thomson, JA. (2009). Human induced pluripotent stem cells free of vector and transgene sequences. Science, Vol.324, pp.797-801.

Yu, J., Vodyanik, MA., Smuga-Otto, K., Antosiewicz-Bourget, J., Frane, JL., Tian, S., Nie. J., Jonsdottir, GA., Ruotti, V., Stewart, R., Slukvin, II. & Thomson, JA. (2007) Induced pluripotent stem cell lines derived from human somatic cells. Science, 318, 1917-1920.

Yusa, K., Rad, R., Takeda, J. & Bradley, A. (2009) Generation of transgene-free induced pluripotent mouse stem cells by the piggyBac transposon. Nat. Methods, Vol.6, pp.363-369.

Zhao Wu, Jijun Chen, Jiangtao Ren, Lei Bao, Jing Liao, Chun Cui, Linjun Rao, Hui Li, Yijun Gu, Huiming Dai, Hui Zhu, Xiaokun Teng, Lu Cheng, and Lei Xiao. Generation of Pig-Induced Pluripotent Stem Cells with a Drug-Inducible System. (2009). Journal of Molecular Cell Biology. Vol.1, pp.46-54

Zhao Y, Yin X, Qin H, Zhu F, Liu H, Yang W, Zhang Q, Xiang C, Hou P, Song Z, Liu Y, Yong J, Zhang P, Cai J, Liu M, Li H, Li Y, Qu X, Cui K, Zhang W, Xiang T, Wu Y, Zhao Y, Liu C, Yu C, Yuan K, Lou J, Ding M, Deng H. (2008) Two supporting factors greatly improve the efficiency of human iPSC generation. Cell Stem Cell, vol.3, pp. 475-9.

Zhou, H., Li, W., Zhu, S., Joo, JY., Do, JT., Xiong, W., Kim, JB., Zhang, K., Scholer, HR. and
    Ding, S. (2010) Conversion of mouse epiblast stem cells to an earlier pluripotency
    state by small molecules. J. Biol. Chem., Vol.285, pp.29676-29680.
Zhou, H., Li, W., Zhu, S., Joo, JY., Do, JT., Xiong, W., Kim, JB., Zhang, K., Scholer, HR. and
    Ding, S. (2010). Conversion of mouse epiblast stem cells to an earlier pluripotency
    state by small molecules. J. Biol. Chem, Vol.285, pp.29676-29680.

8

Generation of ICM-Type Human iPS Cells from CD34⁺ Cord Blood Cells

Naoki Nishishita[1,2], Noemi Fusaki[3,4] and Shin Kawamata[1,2]
[1]Foundation for Biomedical Research and Innovation
TRI308, 1-5-4 Minatojima,-Minamimachi, Chuo-ku,
[2]Riken Center for Developmental Biology, 2-2-3, Minatojima-Minamimachi, Chuo-ku,
[3]DNAVEC Corporation 6, Okubo, Tsukuba,
[4]Japan Science and Technology Agency (JST) ,
PRESTO, 4-1-8 Honcho, Kawaguchi, Saitama,
Japan

1. Introduction

One of the major technical hurdles for clinical application of embryonic stem (ES) cells or induced pluripotent stem (iPS) cells is formation of teratomas by undifferentiated cells after transplantation. In addition, iPS cells have their own safety concerns such as an increased chance of tumorigenicity caused by chromosomal instability or alteration during the reprogramming process (1). Since the first report of mouse iPS cell generation by retroviral vectors (2), several non-integrating vector systems have been examined in pursuit of "safer" iPS cell generation methods. These approaches include adenoviruses (3), Sendai viruses (SeV) (4, 5), Cre-excisable viruses (6), the piggyBac transposition system (7, 8) conventional plasmids (9), the oriP/EBNA1-episomal vector (10), direct protein delivery methods (11, 12) or small molecule delivery methods (13, 14).

A number of cell sources for generating human iPS cells have been reported, including dermal fibroblasts (15), keratinocytes (16), peripheral blood cells (17), adipose tissue (18), and cord blood (CB) cells (19). The three germ layer differentiation potential of these established iPS cells has been demonstrated. However, it is not clear which cell source is best for generating "standard" iPS cells, as differentiation preferences of established iPS cells reflect the epigenetic status of the original cells (called "epigenetic memory") (20).

Recently, several groups reported new insights into two distinct stages of pluripotency in ES cells. These stem cell stages consist of the inner cell mass (ICM) of blastocyst type (ICM type-cells or naïve cells), and epiblast type stem cells (EpiSCs or prime cells) (21). Mouse 129 or C57/BL6 mouse ES cells are the ICM type: "true" pluripotent stem cells representing pre-implantation blastocysts that contribute to chimerism and demonstrate germ line transmission when placed back into blastocysts. They can also be grown in single cell suspension. In contrast, the "EpiSCs" or "prime" ES cells represent post-implantation stage epiblasts. They retain the potential of three germ line differentiation in vitro, but are incapable of contributing to chimerism and cannot survive after single cell cloning. Human ES cells or iPS cells seem to correspond to the EpiSCs with respect to colony morphology and gene expression prolife (22, 23), but can be converted to the naïve stem cell stage by cultivation (24) or constitutive activation of *KLF2/KLF4* genes (25). In this report, we demonstrate an easier and safer reprogramming method for the direct establishment of ICM-type human iPS cells from fresh or frozen CB cells using temperature-sensitive SeV vectors, which facilitates confirmation of removal of the SeV construct at a single cell level.

2. Experimental procedures, materials, and methods

All experimental protocols were reviewed and approved by the ethical committee of the Riken Center for Developmental Biology (CDB), the Foundation for Biomedical Research and Innovation (FBRI), Asagiri Hospital, and the animal experiment committee of FBRI.

Fresh CB was supplied by Asagiri Hospital. CD34+ cells were purified from mononuclear cells (isolated from fresh CB with Lymphoprep TM (Cosmo Bio Co., Tokyo, Japan)) using a human CD34 Micro Bead kit and Auto Macs columns (Miltenyi Biotec) in accordance with the manufacturer's instruction. We also used frozen CD34+ CB cells obtained from Riken RBC (Tsukuba, Japan). CD34+ cells were cultured in hematopoietic culture medium (HC media) [serum free X-VIVO 10 (Lonza, Basel Switzerland) containing 50 ng/mL IL-6 (Peprotech, London UK), 50 ng/mL sIL-6R (Peprotech), 50 ng/mL SCF (Peprotech), 10 ng/mL TPO (Peprotech), 20 ng/mL Flt3-ligand (R&D system, MN)] (4) for one day prior to viral infection. SNL76/7 feeder cells (European Collection of Cell Culture, Salisbury, UK) were treated with 100 µL of mitomycin C solution (1 mg/mL) (Nacalai Tesque, Kyoto, Japan) in 10 cm dishes for three hours to generate mitomycin C treated-SNL 76/7 feeder cells (MMC-SNL). They were seeded on 24-well plates (Becton Dickinson, Tokyo, Japan), or in six-well plates, or in 60 mm dishes in naïve human ES cell culture medium. Fifty mL of naïve human ES cell medium was prepared by mixing 24 mL DMEM/F12 (Invitrogen; 11320), 24 mL Neurobasal (Invitrogen; 21103), 0.5 mL of x100 nonessential amino acids (Invitrogen), 1 mL B27 supplement (Invitrogen; 17504044), and 0.5 mL N2 supplement (Invitrogen; 17502048). The medium also contained 0.5 mg/mL of BSA Fraction V (Sigma), penicillin-streptomycin (final x 1, Invitrogen), 1 mM glutamine (Invitrogen), 0.1 mM β-mercaptoethanol (Invitrogen), 1.0 µM PD0325901 (Stemgent), 3.0 µM CHIR99021 (Stemgent), 10 µM forskolin (Sigma) and 20 ng/mL of recombinant human LIF (Millipore; LIF1005). Prime human iPS cells were cultured with prime human ES cell medium [DMEM/F-12 (SIGMA) containing 20% KSR (Invitrogen), 2 mM L-glutamine (Invitrogen), 1% NEAA (Invitrogen), 0.1 mM 2-ME (Invitrogen), and 4 ng/mL bFGF (Peprotech)]. The medium was changed every day. Passage of human ES cell-like cells was previously described (26). The split ratio was routinely 1:3 or 1:4.

2.1 Viral infection and generation of ICM-type iPS cells

Temperature-sensitive Sendai viral vector constructs integrating the four Yamanaka factors (SeV18+OCT3/4/TS7, SeV18+SOX2/TS7, SeV18+KLF4/TS7, and SeV(HNL)c-MYC/TS7) were supplied by DNAVEC Corp. The CD34+ cells were thawed and cultured for one day in HC media in six-well plates at a density of 2×10^4 cells/two mL/well before the infection with SeV. The thawed CD34+ cells (1×10^4), or an equivalent number of freshly isolated CD34+ cells, were transferred to 96-well plates in 180 µL of hematopoietic cell culture medium with 20 µL of viral supernatant containing two m.o.i. each of the five SeV constructs (SeVTS7-OCT3/4, -SOX2, -KLF4, -c-MYC, -GFP). The medium was replaced by fresh medium the following day and infected cells were cultured another four days. At this point, 1×10^4

infected CB cells were seeded and cultured on confluent MMC-SNL cells in six-well plates in human naïve ES cell medium supplemented with PD0325901, CHIR99021, recombinant human LIF (rhLIF) and forskolin under hypoxic conditions (MCO-5M, SANYO Japan, 5% O_2, 5% CO_2 at 37° C). Dome-shaped naive ES cell like-colonies were picked up between fourteen and nineteen days, suspended as single cells, seeded on MMC-SNL and cultured with naïve ES cell medium. The second passage colonies were subjected to heat treatment (38° C for three days) and then passaged again for detection of remaining SeV constructs by RT-PCR and immunostaining with anti-SeV (HN) antibody. SeV-free colonies were transferred to a normal oxygen environment (MCO-5M, SANYO Japan, 20% O_2, 5% CO_2 at 37° C) and cultured on MMC-SNL cells with prime human ES cell medium shown in Fig 1.

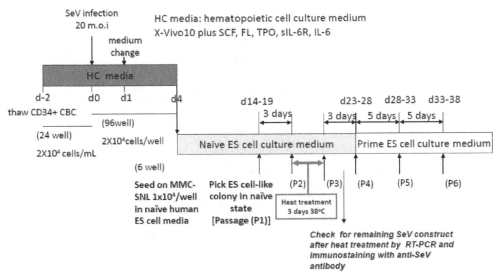

Fig. 1. Schema for generating naive and prime iPS cell from CB cells with SeV vectors.

2.1.1 Optimized culture conditions for naïve iPS cells

$1X10^4$ SeV-infected CD34⁺ CB cells were transferred onto various numbers of pre-seeded MMC-SNL cells in 60 mm dishes (from 1.0×10^5 to 2.0×10^6). Cells were cultured for 14 days in naïve human ES cell medium either under hypoxic or normoxic conditions. The emergent colonies were fixed and stained for ALP activities. The number of colonies stained positively for ALP activities was scored.

The naïve ES cell-like colonies were picked up 14 to 19 days after seeding on SNL in naïve ES cell medium under 5% O_2 culture conditions. These cells were subjected to heat treatment at 38 °C for three days at passage two in the naive state. After heat treatment, prime ES cell-like colonies were passaged (passage three) and checked for residual SeV constructs by RT-PCR and immunostaining with anti-SeV antibody. Then, the virus-free cell clumps from passage three were cultured in prime human ES cell medium under 20% O_2 culture conditions. Viral-Free (VF) iPS cell colonies were passaged two or three times and then tested for further appraisal of differentiation potential of the reprogrammed cell clones. We tried to induce pluripotency in adherent cells derived from CD34⁺ cells in Table 1.

Cell source	Vector	Infected cell numbers	Infectivity	Substrate on cuture plate	Numbers of ES-like colony	iPS cell clones characterized
Fresh CD34+ CB	SeV	1.0×10^4	20	MMC-SNL cells	5	5

Clone #	RT-PCT (undifferentiation)	RT-PCT (differentiation)	IHC	Teratoma	Karyotype
#24	✓				
#30	✓		✓		
#35	✓	✓	✓	✓	
#36	✓				
#37	✓	✓	✓	✓	✓

✓: performed

Table 1. Efficiency of induction of iPSC clones from cord blood cells with SeV vectors.

2.1.2 Alkaline phosphatase and immunohistological staining

Naive ES cell like- and prime ES cell like-colonies were stained with leukocyte alkaline phosphatase kit (VECTOR, Burlingame, CA) in accordance with the manufacturer's instructions. Cells were fixed with 4% paraformaldehyde followed by immunostaining with a series of antibodies. Nuclei were stained with DAPI (1:1000, SIGMA). Photomicrographs were taken with a fluorescent microscope (Olympus BX51, IX71, Tokyo) and a visible light microscope (Olympus CKX31).

Expression of CD34 and CD45 in mononuclear cells (MNC) from CB was determined by flow cytometry (middle). CD34+CD45^{low+} cells (0.2%) and CD34- CD45+ cells were fractionated by cell sorting and both were infected with SeV carrying four factors and GFP. Phase contrast microscopic and fluorescence photographs of CD34+ cells (right) and CD34- mononuclear cells (left) the day after infection are shown in lower panels.

We found that the GFP+ population was selectively found in the CD34+ fraction the day after SeV infection (Fig. 2). This fraction corresponds to hematopoietic stem cells or progenitors, as reported elsewhere (27).

2.1.3 Determination of SeV construct in naïve ES cell-like cells

The remaining SeV constructs in naïve ES cell-like colonies were determined by RT-PCR and immunostaining. Using four temperature-sensitive Sendai viral constructs (SeV TS7) integrating Yamanaka's transcription factor quartet (c-MYC, KLF4, OCT3/4 and SOX2), we were able to generate ES cell-like colonies from CD34+ CD45^{low+} CB cells. The protocol for generating iPS cells from CB cells with temperature-sensitive SeV vector is shown in Fig. 1. Naïve ES cell-like colonies were generated by culturing cells in naïve human ES cell medium under hypoxic conditions (5% O_2). Merged dome-like colonies were picked up three weeks after SeV infection and subjected to heat treatment at 38°C to reduce the amount of residual SeV constructs. Remaining SeV constructs were detected by RT-PCR and immunostaining with anti-SeV antibody. Then, the cell clumps of "naïve" virus-free cell clones were transferred to conventional prime human ES cell medium and cultured under normoxic

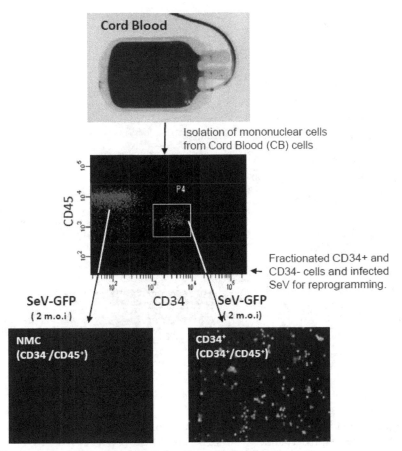

Fig. 2. SeV selectively infects the CD34⁺ fraction of CB cells.

conditions (20% O_2) to convert cells to "prime" virus-free ES cell-like cells. We cannot maintain the naïve state for more than five passages due to the instability of pluripotency in naïve culture conditions and the tendency for spontaneous differentiation. In contrast, pluripotency in the prime state (like conventional human ES cells) was stable and we could maintain prime ES or iPS cells for more than 50 passages. Therefore, further appraisal of the differentiation potential of the reprogrammed cells was done in the prime state (Fig. 4A,B).

Naïve ES cell-like clones from a single cell suspension were examined. Like mouse ES cells, emergent dome-like colonies (P = 1) started to express SSEA-1 in the naïve stage (Fig. 3C, lower left), but its expression ceased after shifting to the prime state (Fig. 3C, lower right). Expression of pluripotency-related molecules in the prime state was examined by immunostaining with a set of antibodies (Table 2). The presence of SeV constructs in the naïve reprogrammed cells was examined by RT-PCR at the single cell level (Fig. 3D). Heat-treated naïve clones that were free of SeV constructs under hypoxic conditions (5% O_2) were transferred to prime culture with a normoxic atmosphere (20% O_2). These virus-free ES cell like-clones were expanded in conventional prime human ES cell culture for further appraisal of the differentiation potential.

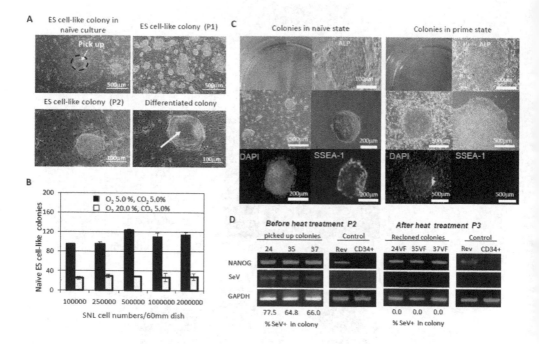

Fig. 3. Elimination of SeV constructs as determined by RT-PCR and generation of naïve or prime iPS cells.

A: Emerging naïve ES cell–like colony. Dome-like colonies emerged and were picked up (top left). Naïve ES cell-like colonies were seeded on MMC-SNL cells (passage one: P = 1, top right). Naïve ES cell-like colony (P = 2, lower left). Cells in the center of the naïve colony (white arrow) started to differentiate at later passages (P = 6, lower right). **B**: The efficiency of generation of naïve ES cell-like colonies under hypoxic (black) and normoxic (white) conditions. The number of MMC-SNL cells seeded on 60 mm dishes and the number of ES cell-like colonies which emerged are scored on the X-axis and Y-axis, respectively. **C**: Staining of naïve ES cell-like colonies (left panels) and prime ES cell-like colonies (right panels). ALP staining of colonies on MMC-SNL (top left and right), phase contract observations of colonies on MMC-SNL (middle left) or Matrigel (middle right), colonies stained with DAPI (lower left) or immunostained with anti-SSEA-1 antibody (lower right). **D**: Detection of SeV construct in heat-treated clones by PCR. Picked colonies #24, #35, and #37 were subject to heat treatment (passage 2: P = 2) and subcloned. Subclones were named #24VF, #35VF, or #37VF (passage 3: P = 3). iPS cells generated from CB by retrovirus (ReV) and parent CD34+ CB cell were used as negative controls. % SeV+ in colony is the area positively stained with anti-SeV antibody divided by the total area of the colony calculated by two value recognition software (Adobe Photoshop). There was no difference in the frequency of emerging dome-shaped ES cell-like colonies in the naïve state from freshly isolated CD34+ cells and from frozen CD34+ cells.

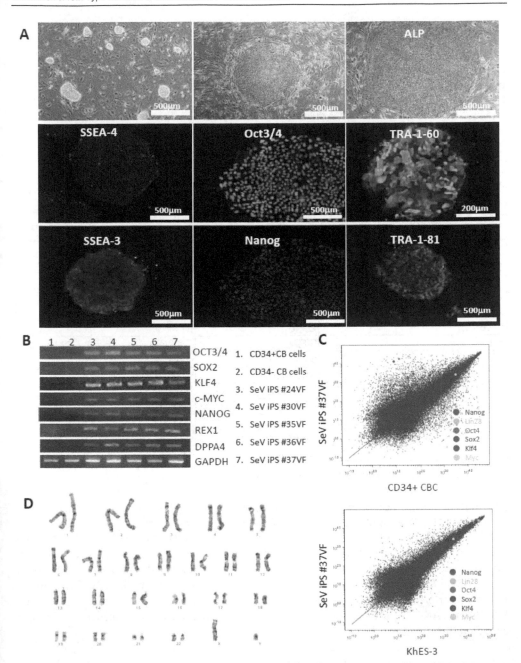

Fig. 4. Expression of pluripotency-associated genes and molecules in established SeV-free iPS cell clones.

A: Phase contrast images of a representative naive ES cell-like colony on MMC-SNL (P = 1: top left), after heat-treatment and recloning of a prime clone (SeV iPS #37VF, top middle) and its

ALP staining (top right). The expression of SSEA-4, Oct3/4, TRA-1-60, SSEA-3, Nanog and TRA-1-81 in the same prime clone (SeV iPS #37VF) was detected by immunohistochemistry. Alexa 594 (red) and Alexa 488 (green) conjugated secondary antibodies were used to visualize expression. **B**: Endogenous gene expression determined by RT-PCR. Sample description, pluripotency-associated genes, and lanes are indicated. CD34$^+$ and CD34$^-$ CB cells were used for controls. **C**: Gene expression comparison of SeV iPS #37VF vs CD34$^+$ CBC (upper panel) and SeV iPS #37VF vs human ES cell line KhES-3 (lower panel). Expression levels of pluripotency-related genes are marked in the panels. **D**: Karyotyping of SeV iPS #37VF.

Antibodies	supplier	Cat No	Dilution
anti-Oct4	Santa Cruz	sc-5279	1/ 100
anti-TRA-1-81	Chemicon	MAB4381	1/ 200
anti-TRA-1-60	Chemicon	MAB4360	1/ 200
anti-SSEA-3	Chemicon	MAB4303	1/ 200
anti-SSEA-4	Chemicon	MAB4304	1/ 200
anti-Nanog	Reprocell	RCAB0003P	1/ 1000
α-fetoprotein(AFP)	R&D	MAB1368	1/ 100
vimentin	Santa Cruz	sc-5565	1/ 200
α-smooth muscle actin(SMA)	SIGMA	A-2547	1/ 400
desmin	Dako	M0760	1/ 50
beta-III tubulin	SIGMA	T4026	1/ 200
GFAP	Santa Cruz	sc-6170	1/ 50
anti-SSEA-1	Santa Cruz	sc-21702	1/100
anti SeV HN	DNAVEC	IL4.1	1/100
Alexa Fluor 488 goat anti mouse	Invitrogen	A11001	1/ 1000
Alexa Fluor 594 rabbit anti mouse	Invitrogen	A11005	1/ 1000
Alexa Fluor 594 goat anti rabbit	Invitrogen	A11037	1/ 1000
DAPI	Invitrogen	D1306	5ug/ml

Table 2. List of antibodies used for immunostaining

2.2 Characterization of virus-free ES cell-like clones
2.2.1 Reverse transcriptase polymerase chain reaction (RT-PCR)
Total RNA was purified with RNeasy Mini kit (QIAGEN), according to the manufacturer's instructions. One μg of total RNA was used for reverse transcription reactions with PrimeScript RT reagent kit (TAKARA, Japan). PCR was performed with EXTaq (TAKARA, Japan). Total RNA from cell clones was extracted with the RNeasy minikit (QIAGEN). q-RT-PCR was performed with an ABI PRISM 7000 (Life Technologies Japan) using SYBR Premix EX Taq™ (TAKARA, RR041A) in accordance with the manufacturer's instructions. Primers are listed in Table 3.

2.2.2 Gene Chip analysis and karyotyping
Total RNAs from several established iPS cell clones, human ES cell line KhES-1, CD34$^-$ CB cells and CD34$^+$ CB cells were purified with RNeasy Mini kit (QIAGEN) and hybridized with human Gene Chip (U133 plus 2.0 Array Affymetrix) according to the manufacturer's

Primers			Size (bp)
hOCT3/4-F1165	GAC AGG GGG AGG GGA GGA GCT AGG	undifferentiated ES cell (endo)	144
hOCT3/4-R1283	CTT CCC TCC AAC CAG TTG CCC CAA AC		
hSOX2-F1430	GGG AAA TGG GAG GGG TGC AAA AGA GG	undifferentiated ES cell (endo)	151
hSOX2-R1555	TTG CGT GAG TGT GGA TGG GAT TGG TG		
hMYC-F253	GCG TCC TGG GAA GGG AGA TCC GGA GC	undifferentiated ES cell (endo)	328
hMYC-R555	TTG AGG GGC ATC GTC GCG GGA GGC TG		
hKLF4-F1128	ACG ATC GTG GCC CCG GAA AAG GAC C	undifferentiated ES cell (endo)	397
hKLF4-R1826	TGA TTG TAG TGC TTT CTG GCT GGG CTC C		
DPPA4-F	GGAGCCGCCTGCCCTGGAAAATTC	undifferentiated ES cell	408
DPPA4-R	TTT TTC CTG ATA TTC TAT TCC CAT		
REX1-F	CAG ATC CTA AAC AGC TCG CAG AAT	undifferentiated ES cell	306
REX1-R	GCG TAC GCA AAT TAA AGT CCA GA		
NANOG-F	CAG CCC CGA TTC TTC CAC CAG TCC C	undifferentiated ES cell	391
NANOG-R	CGG AAG ATT CCC AGT CGG GTT CAC C		
hGAPDH F	AAC AGC CTC AAG ATC ATC AGC	control	337
hGAPDH R	TTG GCA GGT TTT TCT AGA CGG		
hBRACHYURY-F1292	GCC CTC TCC CTC CCC TCC ACG CAC AG	mesoderm	274
hBRACHYURY-R1540	CGG CGC CGT TGC TCA CAG ACC ACA GG		
hPAX6-F1206	ACC CAT TAT CCA GAT GTG TTT GCC CGA G	ectoderm	317
hPAX6-R1497	ATG GTG AAG CTG GGC ATA GGC GGC AG		
hSOX17-F423	CGC TTT CAT GGT GTG GGC TAA GGA CG	endoderm	608
hSOX17-R583	TAG TTG GGG TGG TCC TGC ATG TGC TG		
SeV vector F15204	GGATCACTAGGTGATATCGAGC	SeV vectors	193
SeV vector R15397e	CATATGGACAAGTCCAAGACTTC		

Table 3. List of primers used to detect pluripotency-associated genes in reprogrammed cells.

instructions. Karyotyping of established iPS cells was reported by Nihon Gene Research Laboratories, Inc. (Sendai, Japan).

The expression of pluripotency-related molecules in the prime stage such as SSEA-4, SSEA-3, TRA-1-60, TRA-1-81, Oct3/4 and Nanog were detected by immunostaining (Fig. 4A). Endogenous expression of pluripotency-related genes was determined by RT-PCR (Fig. 4B). Total gene expression profiles of the established iPS clone SeV iPS #37VF are compared with human ES cell line KhES-3 or CD34⁺ cord blood cells (Fig. 4C). Karyotype of the established iPS cell clone SeV iPS #37VF is presented (Fig. 4D).

2.3 Differentiation assays of virus-free iPS cells *in vitro* and *in vivo*
2.3.1 *In vitro* differentiation assay
Established human ES cell-like clones were harvested using collagenase IV. Cells were transferred to six-well ultra-low attachment plates (Corning) and cultured in human prime ES cell medium without bFGF to form embryoid bodies (EB). The medium was changed every other day. The resulting EBs were transferred to gelatin-coated plates after eight days and cultured in the same fresh medium for another eight days. Three cell lines were tested for differentiation potential on gelatin coated dishes after EB formation (Fig. 5a). All of these

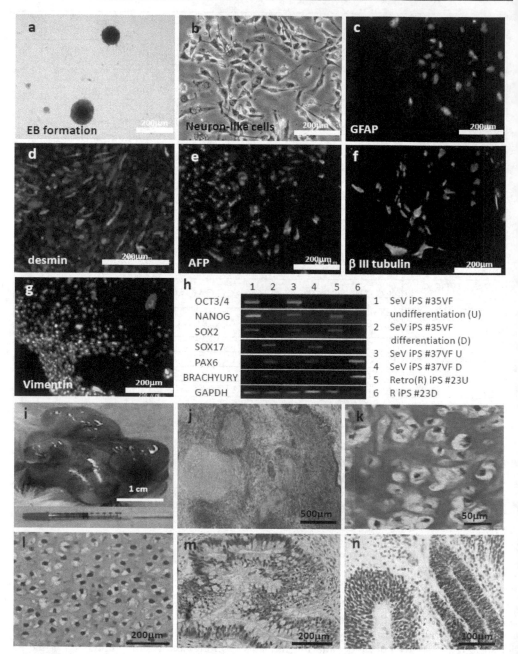

Fig. 5. *In vitro* and *in vivo* differentiation potentials of established iPS cell lines.
(**a-g**) Embryoid body-mediated differentiation of established iPS cells. All images shown are from cells derived from clone SeV iPS #35VF. Bright field images of embryoid bodies generated after eight days of culture (**a**). Embryoid bodies were transferred to gelatin dishes

and differentiated for a further eight days to induce either un-directed or guided differentiation (**b-g**). Phase contrast images of neuron-like cells (**b**) after differentiation on gelatin. Cells were fixed and stained with antibodies against GFAP (**c**), desmin (**d**), AFP (**e**), βIII-tubulin (**f**), and vimentin (**g**) to determine lineage-specific differentiation potential. (**h**) RT-PCR for lineage-specific differentiation of established iPS cell lines, SeV clones #35VF and #37VF. Retrovirally generated iPS cell clone R#23 from CD34+ CB cells was used for a control. (**i**) Teratoma formed from SeV iPS #35VF was injected into testis capsule. Teratoma had a cystic structure. The content of cysts is shown in the 1 mL syringe. (**j**) Hematoxylin and eosin staining of teratoma derived from iPS cells at low magnification. Histology showed derivatives of all three embryonic germ layers including bone-like (**k**: mesoderm), cartilage-like (**l**: mesoderm), gut-like epithelium (**m**: endoderm) and neural rosette-like (**n**: ectoderm) tissue.

clones were able to give rise to cells from all three germ layers as evidenced by cell morphology (Fig. 5b) and immunocytochemistry (Fig. 5c-g). Upon differentiation, the presence of gene expression characteristic of all three germ layers was determined by RT-PCR (Fig. 5h).

2.3.2 *In vivo* differentiation assay
One million iPS cells were injected beneath the testicular capsule of SCID mice (SLC Japan) for teratoma formation. Tumor formation was observed 60 - 80 days after cell transplantation. Tumor tissues were fixed with 4% formalin followed by hematoxylin and eosin staining. Two lines were tested for teratoma formation and both cell lines formed teratomas with a cystic structure (Fig. 5i). HE staining of teratoma tissues (Fig. 5j - 5n) showed differentiated tissues corresponding to all three germ layers.

3. Conclusions

Reprogramming of somatic cells with SeV vector without DNA integration is advantageous, as it reduces the chance for tumorigenicity caused by random genomic integration. Advantages of using SeV vector over other non-integrating reprogramming methods such as using adenovirus, episomal plasmid vectors, conventional plasmid vectors, or small molecule delivery systems include superior reprogramming capability with potent protein expression potential (13). The remaining concern in using SeV vector is how we can confirm the removal of potent SeV vectors from reprogrammed cells. In this report, we used the temperature-sensitive SeV vector TS7 to reduce the number of SeV-infected cells. In addition, we made use of a single cell cloning technique in the naïve state to confirm the absence of SeV vector constructs in the reprogrammed cells at a single cell level. Therefore, this cloning technique provides an ultimate solution for RNA virus vector-based reprogramming methodology.

The benefits of reprogramming somatic cells in the naïve state are not limited to a single cell cloning technology. It may provide answers to interesting questions like whether "standard" human iPS cells, having the correct epigenetic memory, can be generated by reprogramming somatic cells in the naïve state. Accumulation of epigenetic information before and after transferring to the naïve state would provide an answer to this question.

Several reports showed that iPS cells can be preferentially generated from the CD34+ fraction of CB cells and peripheral blood cells with retroviral vectors (19, 26). In our experiment, we also showed that the SeV TS7-GFP vector selectively infects freshly isolated

$CD34^+$ $CD45^{low+}$ cells and is able to reprogram this fraction. These data suggested that the use of SeV would facilitate the effective generation of iPS cells from CB cells. However, the molecule(s) responsible for SeV viral entry into the cell is elusive. Hemagglutinin-neuraminidase (HN), an envelope protein of Sev is reported to bind to sialomucin (28) and facilitate the cellular entry of virus. CD34 belongs to the sialomucin family. Although SeV is not able to infect $CD34^-$ cells from freshly isolated (non-cultured) CB cells, SeV is able to infect $CD34^-$ cells that have differentiated from $CD34^+$ CB cells after seven days of culture in hematopoietic cell culture media. With limited information, we cannot conclude that CD34 is the SeV entry molecule. Rather, it appears that a set of molecules other than CD34, expressed in $CD45^{low+}$ cells, might be responsible for it.

As a cell source for generating iPS cells, CB cells have certain advantages over other somatic cells. Unlike cultured cells or those obtained by biopsy from a variety of tissues at various ages, freshly isolated (non-cultured) $CD34^+$ CB cells are the youngest stem cell population available following birth. They also have distinct genetic and epigenetic profiles as hematopoietic stem cells and progenitors and lack genetic alternations like rearrangements or possible post-natal genomic damage caused by UV irradiation or chemical irritants. Furthermore, generating iPS cells from this fraction would facilitate our understanding of the reprogramming process, since the genetic profiles of the cell source and the reprogrammed cells are known. Another advantage of using cord blood cells would be the possibility of collaborating with the existing world-wide network of public cord blood banks. Extensive discussions concerning the conditions and ethical issues are necessary before such clinical applications are pursued. Nonetheless, the use of CB as a source for iPS cells is a realistic option for generating "bona fide" iPS cells for future clinical use.

4. Acknowledgment

We thank Satomi Nishikawa and K. Kobayashi for useful discussions. We also thank M. Miyako for editorial help. This work was partly supported by the grant from Regional consortium project 19K5510 from the Ministry of Industry and Economy Tokyo Japan (2007-2009) and Grant-in-Aid for JSPS Fellows 2210853. S-Innovation project JST Tokyo Japan (2009-2011) and "Tests for Safety Issue of Pluripotent Stem Cell" JST Tokyo Japan (2010-14). Riken BCR and Asagiri Hospital for supplying cord blood cells.

5. References

[1] Nakagawa, M., Koyanagi, M., Tanabe, K., Takahashi, K., Ichisaka, T., Aoi, T., Okita, K., Mochiduki, Y., Takizawa, N., and Yamanaka, S. (2008). Generation of induced pluripotent stem cells without Myc from mouse and human fibroblasts. Nat Biotechnol 26, 101-106.

[2] Takahashi, K., Yamanaka, S. (2006). Induction of pluripotent stem cells from mouse embryonic and adult fibroblast cultures by defined factors. Cell 126, 663-76.

[3] Stadtfeld, M., Nagaya, M., Utikal, J., Weir, G., and Hochedlinger, K. (2008). Induced pluripotent stem cells generated without viral integration. Science 322, 945-949.

[4] Fusaki, N., Ban, H., Nishiyama, A., Saeki, K., and Hasegawa, M. (2009). Efficient induction of transgene-free human pluripotent stem cells using a vector based on Sendai virus, an RNA virus that does not integrate into the host genome. Proc Jpn Acad Ser B Phys Biol Sci 85, 348-362.

[5] Seki, T., Yuasa, S., Oda, M., Egashira, T., Yae, K., Kusumoto, D., Nakata, H., Tohyama, S., Hashimoto, H., Kodaira, M., et al. (2010). Generation of induced pluripotent stem cells from human terminally differentiated circulating T cells. Cell Stem Cell 7, 11-14.

[6] Huangfu, D., Maehr, R., Guo, W., Eijkelenboom, A., Snitow, M., Chen, A. E., and Melton, D. A. (2008). Induction of pluripotent stem cells by defined factors is greatly improved by small-molecule compounds. Nat Biotechnol 26, 795-797.

[7] Soldner, F., Hockemeyer, D., Beard, C., Gao, Q., Bell, G. W., Cook, E. G., Hargus, G., Blak, A., Cooper, O., Mitalipova, M., et al. (2009). Parkinson's disease patient-derived induced pluripotent stem cells free of viral reprogramming factors. Cell 136, 964-977.

[8] Woltjen, K., Michael, I. P., Mohseni, P., Desai, R., Mileikovsky, M., Hamalainen, R., Cowling, R., Wang, W., Liu, P., Gertsenstein, M., et al. (2009). piggyBac transposition reprograms fibroblasts to induced pluripotent stem cells. Nature 458, 766-770.

[9] Kaji, K., Norrby, K., Paca, A., Mileikovsky, M., Mohseni, P., and Woltjen, K. (2009). Virus-free induction of pluripotency and subsequent excision of reprogramming factors. Nature 458, 771-775.

[10] Okita, K., Nakagawa, M., Hyenjong, H., Ichisaka, T., and Yamanaka, S. (2008). Generation of mouse induced pluripotent stem cells without viral vectors. Science 322, 949-953.

[11] Yu, J., Hu, K., Smuga-Otto, K., Tian, S., Stewart, R., Slukvin, II, and Thomson, J. A. (2009). Human induced pluripotent stem cells free of vector and transgene sequences. Science 324, 797-801.

[12] Zhou, H., Wu, S., Joo, J. Y., Zhu, S., Han, D. W., Lin, T., Trauger, S., Bien, G., Yao, S., Zhu, Y., et al. (2009). Generation of induced pluripotent stem cells using recombinant proteins. Cell Stem Cell 4, 381-384.

[13] Kim, D., Kim, C. H., Moon, J. I., Chung, Y. G., Chang, M. Y., Han, B. S., Ko, S., Yang, E., Cha, K. Y., Lanza, R., and Kim, K. S. (2009). Generation of human induced pluripotent stem cells by direct delivery of reprogramming proteins. Cell Stem Cell 4, 472-476.

[14] Li, W., Wei, W., Zhu, S., Zhu, J., Shi, Y., Lin, T., Hao, E., Hayek, A., Deng, H., and Ding, S. (2009). Generation of rat and human induced pluripotent stem cells by combining genetic reprogramming and chemical inhibitors. Cell Stem Cell 4, 16-19.

[15] KAHN M, Hasegawa K, TEO J, Mcmillan M, Yasuda S, Method for formation of induced pluripotent stem cells. *Publication Number*: WO 2011/019957 A1, International Publication Date. 17 February 2011.

[16] Takahashi, K., Tanabe, K., Ohnuki, M., Narita, M., Ichisaka, T., Tomoda, K., and Yamanaka, S. (2007). Induction of pluripotent stem cells from adult human fibroblasts by defined factors. Cell 131, 861-872.

[17] Aasen, T., Raya, A., Barrero, M. J., Garreta, E., Consiglio, A., Gonzalez, F., Vassena, R., Bilic, J., Pekarik, V., Tiscornia, G., et al. (2008). Efficient and rapid generation of induced pluripotent stem cells from human keratinocytes. Nat Biotechnol 26, 1276-1284.

[18] Loh, Y. H., Agarwal, S., Park, I. H., Urbach, A., Huo, H., Heffner, G. C., Kim, K., Miller, J. D., Ng, K., and Daley, G. Q. (2009). Generation of induced pluripotent stem cells from human blood. Blood 113, 5476-5479.

[19] Sugii, S., Kida, Y., Kawamura, T., Suzuki, J., Vassena, R., Yin, Y. Q., Lutz, M. K., Berggren, W. T., Izpisua Belmonte, J. C., and Evans, R. M. (2010). Human and mouse adipose-derived cells support feeder-independent induction of pluripotent stem cells. Proc Natl Acad Sci U S A 107, 3558-3563.

[20] Giorgetti, A., Montserrat, N., Aasen, T., Gonzalez, F., Rodriguez-Piza, I., Vassena, R., Raya, A., Boue, S., Barrero, M. J., Corbella, B. A., et al. (2009). Generation of induced pluripotent stem cells from human cord blood using OCT4 and SOX2. Cell Stem Cell 5, 353-357.

[21] Kim, K., Doi, A., Wen, B., Ng, K., Zhao, R., Cahan, P., Kim, J., Aryee, M. J., Ji, H., Ehrlich, L. I., et al. (2010). Epigenetic memory in induced pluripotent stem cells. Nature 467, 285-90.

[22] Buecker, C., Chen, H. H., Polo, J. M., Daheron, L., Bu, L., Barakat, T. S., Okwieka, P., Porter, A., Gribnau, J., Hochedlinger, K., and Geijsen, N. (2010). A murine ESC-like state facilitates transgenesis and homologous recombination in human pluripotent stem cells. Cell Stem Cell 6, 535-546.

[23] Yang, J., van Oosten, A. L., Theunissen, T. W., Guo, G., Silva, J. C., and Smith, A. (2010). Stat3 Activation Is Limiting for Reprogramming to Ground State Pluripotency. Cell Stem Cell 7, 319-328.

[24] Hall, J., Guo, G., Wray, J., Eyres, I., Nichols, J., Grotewold, L., Morfopoulou, S., Humphreys, P., Mansfield, W., Walker, R., et al. (2009). Oct4 and LIF/Stat3 additively induce Kruppel factors to sustain embryonic stem cell self-renewal. Cell Stem Cell 5, 597-609.

[25] Zhou, H., Li, W., Zhu, S., Joo, J. Y., Do, J. T., Xiong, W., Kim, J. B., Zhang, K., Scholer, H. R., and Ding, S. (2010). Conversion of mouse epiblast stem cells to an earlier pluripotency state by small molecules. J Biol Chem. 285(39), 29676-80.

[26] Hanna, J., Cheng, A. W., Saha, K., Kim, J., Lengner, C. J., Soldner, F., Cassady, J. P., Muffat, J., Carey, B. W., and Jaenisch, R. (2010). Human embryonic stem cells with biological and epigenetic characteristics similar to those of mouse ESCs. Proc Natl Acad Sci U S A 107, 9222-9227.

[27] Takenaka, C., Nishishita, N., Takada, N., Jakt, L. M., and Kawamata, S. (2010). Effective generation of iPS cells from CD34+ cord blood cells by inhibition of p53. Exp Hematol 38, 154-162.

[28] Majeti, R., Park, C. Y., and Weissman, I. L. (2007). Identification of a hierarchy of multipotent hematopoietic progenitors in human cord blood. Cell Stem Cell 1, 635-645.

[29] Jin, C. H., Kusuhara, K., Yonemitsu, Y., Nomura, A., Okano, S., Takeshita, H., Hasegawa, M., Sueishi, K., and Hara, T. (2003). Recombinant Sendai virus provides a highly efficient gene transfer into human cord blood-derived hematopoietic stem cells. Gene Ther 10, 272-277.

[30] Nakatsuji, N., Nakajima, F., and Tokunaga, K. (2008). HLA-haplotype banking and iPS cells. Nat Biotechnol 26, 739-740.

9

Modelling of Neurological Diseases Using Induced Pluripotent Stem Cells

Oz Pomp, Chen Sok Lam, Hui Theng Gan,
Srinivas Ramasamy and Sohail Ahmed
Institute of Medical Biology, Agency for
Science Technology& Research
Singapore

1. Introduction

Human embryonic stem cells (hESCs) were first established as an *in vitro* culture system (Thomson et al., 1998). hESCs are pluripotent cells that are able to self-renew and can differentiate into the three primary germ layers; endoderm, ectoderm and mesoderm. Specifically, hESCs can be used to generate gut epithelium, cartilage, bone, muscle, neuroepithelium, and embryonic ganglia (Zhang et al., 2001, Itskovitz-Eldor et al., 2000, Sottile et al., 2003, Thomson et al., 1998, Green et al., 2003). Since these hESC cell lines can be maintained for months in an undifferentiated state, they can be used as a stable resource to model human development in vitro. The conversion of hESCs to neural progenitors and subsequently to the three main neural lineages: neurons, astrocytes and oligodendrocytes was first demonstrated in 2001 (Reubinoff et al., 2001).

The recent advent (Takahashi and Yamanaka, 2006) of induced pluripotent stem cells (iPSCs) makes it possible to derive pluripotent stem cells from somatic tissue. iPSCs are derived by transfecting somatic cells (e.g. skin fibroblasts) with a select group of transcription factors; Sox2, Oct4, Myc and Klf4 to induce reprogramming of the genome over a period of 3-4 weeks. This breakthrough by Yamanaka and colleagues enables the modelling of human disease by, for example, taking a patient's skin cells, converting them to iPSCs and then differentiating it to any desired cell-type. Thus iPSC technology opens a new era of patient-specific disease modelling. Here, we review diseases of the nervous system that have been modelled using iPSC which includes; RETT syndrome (RTT), Familial dysautonomia (FD), Parkinson's disease (PD), Huntingtons (HD) and Amyotrophic Lateral Sclerosis (ALS). To provide some background to the neurological disease modelling studies by iPSCs we begin by reviewing protocols for neural induction (differentiation) of hESC.

2. Neural induction and neuronal differentiation of human embryonic stem cells (hESCs)

2.1 Neural induction of human ESCs

Several protocols, based on knowledge from developmental studies of embryogenesis and neurogenesis, have been developed to optimize yield and purity of neural progenitors from hESCs (Fig1). They can be categorized into two broad approaches. The first involves a stepwise change of culture medium components followed by expansion of neural progenitors (Reubinoff et al., 2001). This protocol involves the long-term culture (3 weeks) of hESCs without replenishing the mouse embryonic fibroblast layer. These cells rapidly undergo morphological changes, forming neural rosettes. They are subsequently dissociated and replated in medium permissive for the growth and maintenance of NSCs (DMEM/F12, B27 supplement, EGF [epidermal growth factor], bFGF [basic fibroblast growth factor]). Similar to mouse ESCs, hESCs can also be differentiated as suspension cultures where they form cystic embryoid bodies (EBs). Formation of these three-dimensional spheres can recapitulate the microenvironment during embryo development, and are preferred over monolayer formats because it allows for up-scaling of differentiation cultures to a greater extent. However, differentiation of hESCs in this sphere format gives rise to issues such as heterogeneity (containing cell types pertaining to the three germ layers) and differential access to soluble factors, which translates to difficulties in optimizing the purity of the desired differentiated progenitors.

The second approach to induce neural lineage cells, is to co-culture hESCs with a variety of stromal cell types, such as the PA6 and MS5 (Kawasaki et al., 2000, Hong et al., 2008, Chimge and Bayarsaihan, 2010). Both PA6 and MS5 stromal cells were derived from murine bone marrow. This induction method is based on the knowledge that signals from mesodermal cells of the Spemann organizer (which develop into the notochord) can induce overlying ectoderm to neuroectodermal fate (Harland and Gerhart, 1997, Londin et al., 2005). This neural induction protocol was reported to generate up to 92% NCAM [neural cell adhesion molecule]–positive cells in 12 days. Given the ease and efficiency of this protocol it is not surprising that it is widely used. However, the neural-inducing effect of the stromal cells is not fully understood. PA6 cells can induce neural differentiation of hESCs in the absence of physical contact, but the conditioned medium of PA6 cells was unable to induce neural differentiation (Kawasaki et al., 2000). In addition, paraformalydehye-treated PA6 cells continued to exhibit neural-inducing activity, suggesting that the viability of these cells is not vital. In order to fine-tune the procedure to exclude animal products, a matrix material from the human amniotic membrane was found to support neural induction of hESCs with similar efficiencies to that of the mouse stromal cells (Ueno et al., 2006).

Given the caveats in the EB and co-culture methods, strategies were developed to maximize the induction of hESCs into neural lineage, using differentiating factors and monolayer subculture systems. The secretion of the bone morphogenic protein (BMP) antagonists, noggin and chordin, from the epidermal ectoderm of the *Xenopus* embryo was demonstrated to be essential for neural induction (Sasai et al., 1996). In addition, follistatin, an inhibitor of Activin signaling, was found to promote neural induction (Hemmati-Brivanlou and Melton, 1994). Hence, strategies used for increasing the yield of neural derivatives from hESCs include using inhibitors of BMP signaling such as Noggin (Itsykson et al., 2005), and the inhibitors of Activin/Nodal signaling such as the pharmacological inhibitor of Nodal signaling, SB431542 (Smith et al., 2008). Since both signaling pathways converge to downstream SMAD proteins, subsequent work further optimized the induction of neural lineage cells by using the inhibitors of both BMP and Nodal signaling (Chambers et al., 2009). However, Noggin, as a protein is expensive and may exhibit batch-to-batch variability. Recent findings report that substituting noggin with a small-molecule inhibitor of BMP, Dorsomorphin, can efficiently promote neural differentiation of hESCs and iPSCs (Morizane et al., 2010, Zhou et al., 2010). Other methods rely on genetic manipulations such as generating nestin-EGFP hESC reporter lines to allow purification of hESC-derived neural progenitors (Noisa et al., 2010).

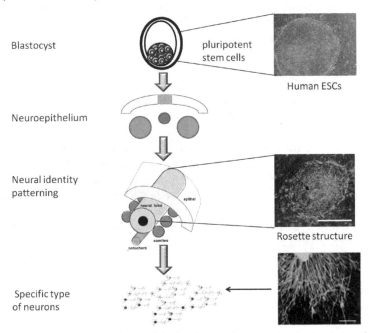

Fig. 1. Schematic representation of neural induction and patterning in *in vivo* and *in vitro*. 1) At early gastrulation, the notochord (orange) secretes BMP-antagonists, such as Noggin and Chordin to create a *gradient of BMP* activity (yellow). 2) Neuroepithelial (NE) cells that are proximal to the notochord become neural precursors (grey) as a consequence of low BMP activity; and the rest of the ectoderm becomes epithelial (yellow) or neural crest (not shown). The NE is patterned by many signals including Shh, RA, Noggin and Chordin (orange) that are secreted from the notochord; BMP (yellow) from the epithelium and FGF (blue) from the somites. 3) The cells in the NE differentiate to specific subtypes of neurons depending on the location in the neural tube and the factors that influence the differentiation. Neural induction and patterning of human ESCs can be induced *in vitro* as shown in the right panels (bright field micrograph or GFP labeled neuronal sub type).

The next aim, upon obtaining neural progenitors/stem cells, is to coax these cells into differentiation of various neuronal subtypes including the cholinergic neurons, dopaminergic neurons, motorneurons, and peripheral sensory neurons. Several methods using various combination of protein factors, co-culture systems and small molecules have successfully been utilized to obtain individual neuronal subtypes. The basic strategy for developing culture cocktails to obtain neuronal subtypes is to mimic signals from early developmental events during specification of the body axis of the embryo. Factors frequently used to induce neural progenitor differentiation include retinoic acid (RA), FGFs and Wingless-Int (Wnts) that can poise cells to differentiate to the neural lineage along the the anterior/posterior (A-P) axis (Hendrickx et al., 2009, Onai et al., 2009). Similarly, Sonic Hedgehog (Shh) and BMPs secreted from the ventral and dorsal neural tube respectively are important for the precise patterning of multiple neuronal progenitors (Furuta et al., 1997, Litingtung and Chiang, 2000). Hence, the efficiency of deriving specific neuronal subtypes can be influenced by the mode of neural induction. The selection of the appropriate neural differentiation protocol is pertinent for the maximization of desired neuronal subtype.

2.2 Neuronal differentiation of human ESCs

Many neuronal subtypes have successfully been derived from hESCs (Fig1). Amongst them are the dopaminergic neurons, serotonergic neurons, peripheral sensory neurons, and cholinergic neurons (Bissonnette et al., 2011). Dopaminergic neurons are progressively lost in Parkinson's disease (PD), while the motorneurons are lost in amyotrophic lateral sclerosis (ALS). The factors and conditions used for successful derivation of dopaminegic neurons, motoneurons as well as other neuronal subtypes can be found in Table 1.

Shh and FGF8 were identified to be crucial for the specification of dopaminergic neurons *in vivo* (Ye et al., 1998) but were not directly effective *in vitro* (Stull and Iacovitti, 2001). This led to the search for other signals in promoting dopaminergic neuron differentiation. Currently, differentiation of human ESCs into midbrain dopaminergic neurons can be achieved through the formation of EBs and the use of various factors such as serum-free conditioned-medium from human hepatocarcinoma cell line HepG2, brain-derived neurotrophic factor (BDNF), ascorbic acid, transforming growth factor (TGF), and glial cell line-derived Neurotrophic factor (GDNF) (Cho et al., 2008a, Cho et al., 2008b, Park et al., 2004, Schulz et al., 2004, Yan et al., 2001). Particularly, TGFß can cooperate with Shh and FGF8 to increase the yield of dopaminergic neurons by enhancing their survival (Roussa et al., 2004); and GDNF was found to be important for the maintenance of motoneurons in the striatum proper (Nevalainen et al., 2010). Large-scale production of dopaminergic neurons from hESC was reported using the EB format with addition of Shh, FGF8 and ascorbic acid. 86% of totally differntiated cells were dopaminergic neurons. Secretion of factors by PA6 cells is important for dopaminergic differentiation (Vazin et al., 2008). PA6 secreted factors include stromal cell-derived factor 1 (SDF-1/CXCL12), pleiotrophin (PTN), insulin-like growth factor 2 (IGF2), and ephrin B1 (EFNB1).

The protocols used for the specification of spinal motoneurons from hESCs were derived from developmental studies. Here motoneurons were found to be induced by signals such as retionic acid from the caudal paraxial mesoderm (Guidato et al., 2003). Shh signaling from the notochord is also required for the induction of motoneurons (Lewis and Eisen, 2001). Neural induction is predominantly performed through the formation of EBs, using defined medium conditions. Because neuroectodermal cells differentiated from hESCs generally have a rostral character, motoneuron differentiation is then achieved by the caudalizing factor retinoic acid followed by the ventralizing factor Shh (Li et al., 2005). Small molecules that can activate the Shh signaling, purmorphamine and SAG (*a* chlorobenzothiophene-containing Hh pathway agonist), have been shown to be effective as substitutes of Shh in motoneuron differentiation (Li et al., 2008, Hu and Zhang, 2009, Wada et al., 2009). The use of Hb9 (homeobox gene selectively expressed in motoneurons) promoter driven GFP hESCs allows isolation of a fairly pure population of motoneurons (Singh Roy et al., 2005). Enrichment of derived motoneurons, up to 80%, was also shown to be achieved by gradient centrifugation in Biocoll (Wada et al., 2009), alleviating the need for genetic manipulations.

Neuronal Subtypes	Neural Induction Method	Factors for Final Differentiation	Done with iPS?	Reference
Dopaminergic neurons	50%-MedIIconditionedmedium, bFGF or DMEM/N2	DMEM/N2, GDNF, BDNF, 5% serum		(Schulz et al., 2004)
	EB with RA and bFGF	BDNF, TGF-α		(Park et al., 2004)
	EB, followed by bFGF and N2 supplement	Shh, FGF8		(Cho et al., 2008)
	PA6 co-culture	PA6, Shh, FGF8, GDNF		(Vazin et al., 2008)
	PA6 co-culture	PA6 co-culture or SDF-1/CXCL12, PTN, IGF2, EFNB1		(Vazin et al., 2009)
	MS5 co-culture	RA, Shh, FGF8, Wnt1	√	(Cooper et al., 2010)
Motoneurons	EB, then adherent in F12/DMEM, N2 supplement, heparin and bFGF	RA, then Shh		(Li et al., 2005)
	EB, bFGF	RA in DMEM/F12,N2, heparin, cAMP. Then Shh/purmorphamine, then GDNF, BDNF, IGF1		(Li et al., 2008)
	EB	RA, then Shh/purmophamine, then BDNF, GDNF, IGF, cAMP	√	(Hu and Zhang, 2009)
Peripheral sensory neurons	PA6 co-culture	Co-culture with PA6 stromal cells		(Pomp et al., 2008)
	MS-5 co-culture, followed by Shh, FGF8, BDNF, ascorbic acid	BDNF, GDNF, NGF (nerve growth factor), Dibutyryl-cAMP	√	(Lee et al., 2009)
Cholinergic neurons	Free-floating aggregates	BDNF, NT3, CNTF, NGF		(Nilbratt et al., 2010)
	RA, followed by free-floating aggregates	FGF8, Shh, BMP9		(Bissonnette et al., 2011)
Serotonergic neurons	RA with EB formation	5-HT, forskolin, acidic FGF, BDNF, GDNF		(Kumar et al., 2009)

Table 1. Factors used in differentiation of hESC-induced NSCs into the various neuronal subtypes.

2.3 Glial differentiation of hESCs

The two glial cell types of the nervous system, the astrocytes and oligodendrocytes, play supporting roles in the brain and peripheral nervous system. Astrocytes secrete various neurotrophic factors, are known to modulate oligodendrocyte myelination of neuronal axons (Moore et al., 2011), and modulate neurotransmitter levels through re-uptake and release mechanisms (Voutsinos-Porche et al., 2003). Evidence is emerging that implicates astrocytes in the pathogenesis of neurological disorders such as Rett syndrome (Maezawa et al., 2009) and ALS (Nagai et al., 2007). A protocol to obtain astrocytes includes exposure of adherent hESCs to cyclopamine, an inhibitor of hedgehog signaling, and subsequent culture in human astrocyte medium to generate a high percentage of nestin and glial fibrillary acidic protein (GFAP)-expressing cells (Lee et al., 2006).

Oligodendrocytes are cells that produce myelin sheaths that insulate axons of neurons, enabling saltatory conduction between the Nodes of Ranvier for rapid propogation of action potential. These cells are targets of severe developmental diseases such as Pelizaeus-Merzbacher disease, and demyelinating diseases such as multiple sclerosis and Charcot-Marie-Tooth (Bramow et al., 2010, Garbern, 2007, Sargiannidou et al., 2009). Dysfunctional oligodendrocytes in these diseases lead to disruptions in axonal transport. In spinal cord injury, demyelination of nerve fibres attributes to functional loss of neurons. So, myelin formation and insulation of neurons is crucial to restore functional network. Hence, it is important to source for pure poulation of glial (oligodendrocyte precursor) cells that can restore function of neurons by remyelination. A few reports and studies from Geron trial have shown the feasibility of using functional OPCs or neurotrophin expressing GRPs from directed differentiation of hESCs and their therapeutic potential at early time points after spinal cord injury (Keirstead et al., 2005, Cao et al., 2005).

Oligodendrocytes undergo multiple stages of differentiation, from oligodendrocyte progenitors, to pro-oligodendrocytes, to non-myelinating oligodendrocytes, and finally myelinating oligodendrocytes (Reviewed in Miller, 2000). A protocol by Hu *et al.* 2009 provides an excellent example of the procedure for obtaining oligodendrocyte progenitors. Briefly, hESC-derived neural progenitors are treated with RA and Shh for patterning into the ventral spinal progenitors, followed by FGF2 for inhibition of differentiation into motoneurons. Oligodendrocyte progenitors were induced with the addition of factors promoting for survival and proliferation of oligodendrocytes – transferrin, progesterone, sodium selenite, putrescine, triiodothyronine (T3), neurotrophin 3 (NT3), platelet-derived growth factor (PDGF), cyclic adenosine-monophosphate (cAMP), insulin growth factor-1 (IGF-1) and biotin. Other factors shown to promote oligodendrocyte differentiation of hESCs include hepatocyte growth factor (Hu et al., 2009) and extracellular matrix protein vitronectin (Gil et al., 2009). Oligodendrocytes have also been shown to be derived from iPS cells (Czepiel et al., 2011).

3. iPSC technology and implications for neurodegenerative diseases

Neurological diseases are conditions that affect the central and peripheral nervous system. At present pharmacological interventions for many neurological diseases, especially the degenerative conditions, are limited and predominantly restricted to alleviation of symptoms. Finding drugs for treatment of neurological disorders represents one of the critical goals of medical research today. The recent discovery of iPSC technology (Takahashi and Yamanaka, 2006) opens the possibility to generate patient specific models of human disease. The generation of patient specific cells using iPSC technology will be a powerful resource for both cell therapy and drug screening (Fig2). iPSC is particulary important for neurological diseases as there are limited cellular models of the nervous system.

3.1 X-linked diseases

A disproportionately large number of disease conditions have been associated with the X chromosome because the phenotypic consequence of a recessive mutation is revealed directly in males for any gene that has no active counterpart on the Y chromosome. Thus, although the X chromosome contains only 4% of all human genes, almost 10% of diseases with a mendelian pattern of inheritance have been assigned to the X chromosome (307 out of 3,199). 168 X-link diseases have been explained by mutations in 113 X-linked genes(Ross et al., 2005).

While males carry a single X chromosome, females have two and hence two copies of each gene. Yet, as one of their X chromosomes is inactive in each cell, females also have only one working X chromosome in each cell. Thus, females havea mosaic of cells that express either the paternal X allele or the maternal X allele. This cellular mosaicism gives females a big advantage over males in the context of X-linked diseases. When an X-linked gene is mutated, the normal cells can partly compensate for the cells that express the mutant allele as a result from cell elimination or by functional compensation (Migeon, 2007). In males, on the other hand, all cells express the mutant gene and therefore usually show much more severe symptoms.

Because the process that inactivates X chromosomes is random with respect to parental origin of the X, usually half of the female cells contain a working X chromosome from the father while the other half contain a working X chromosome from the mother. By reprogramming fibroblasts from female with X-linked disease one can generate both the perfect pair of control (expressing the normal allele) and experimental (expressing the mutant allele) cell types for investigation of the disease phenotype (see schematic Fig. 3). These isogenic control and mutant iPS-derived neurons represent a promising source for modelling X-linked diseases.

3.2 Rett syndrome (RTT)

RTT is one of the most common causes for mental retardation in females, affecting 1 in 10000 live female births. It was first reported in 1966 by the neurophysiologist Dr. Andreas Rett (Rett, 1966). The large majority of RTT cases are caused by sporadic or from germline mutations within the coding sequence of the X-linked methyl CpG binding protein 2 (MeCP2) gene (Amir et al., 1999) and therefore the mutation cannot be detected by simple screening of the parents. Females with classic RTT appear normal from birth until 6–18 months of age, but then they fail to acquire new milestones and enter a period of regression during which motor and language skills are lost. These females show a large diversity of symptoms, that appear progressively (reviewed in Chahrour and Zoghbi, 2007) until they reach a plateau, suggesting that the condition does not involve progressive neurodegeneration (Sun and Wu, 2006). The postnatal onset of symptoms might be explained by the increase in MeCP2 levels in cortical neurons throughout normal development (Akbarian et al., 2001, Balmer et al., 2003, Jung et al., 2003).

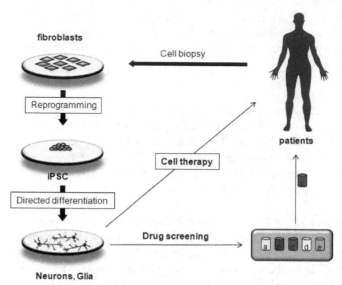

Fig. 2. The potential of iPSCs technology. Cell sample can be easily obtained from patients and cultured *in vitro*. These cells can then be reprogrammed into iPSCs and further be differentiated into the afflicted cells. Cellular phenotype is assessed by measuring cell properties (i.e. neural morphology, maturation of synapses, cell survival under stress, etc). Once a distinct disease related phenotype is identified, drug screening platform can be developed to test their potential to reverse these phenotypes (in this example, component 'c' is a potential candidate (see Fig. 3) and can be used for further tests *in vivo*). Another usage for this technology is cell therapy - transplantation of the cells back to the patient.

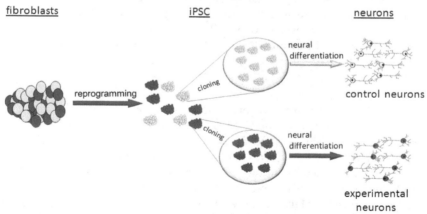

Fig. 3. *In vitro* disease modeling for X-linked diseases. Schematic explaining reprogramming of mosaic cell population from a female with X-linked disease, such as RTT, both iPSC clones expressing the mutant allele ($Xa^{mut} Xi^{wt}$) and iPSC clones expressing the wild-type ($Xa^{wt} Xi^{mut}$) can be expanded and further differentiated into the afflicted cells (i.e. neurons). The wild type neurons, can be used as a perfect control for the mutant neurons for further studies, such as screening of molecules that might potentially reverse the symptoms.

Although MeCP2 is expressed in a large variety of cells, the most afflicted cells in RTT are neurons. In agreement, a specific knockout in the central nervous system revealed the same spectrum of symptoms as the full mouse knockout. Several specific neurons were studied in the context of RTT. For example, pyramidal glutaminergic neurons, which show obvious morphological differences when they express the mutation (see Fig. 3), can account for the mental retardation seen in RTT; dopaminergic neurons can account for the motor function; neurons in the Amygdala can affect learning and memory; and hypothalamus neurons can affect feeding, aggression and stress.

In females, the major source for phenotypic variability is the pattern of X chromosome inactivation (XCI) (Bourdon et al., 2001). Females with classical RTT are usually a balanced mosaic with regard to MeCP2 expression (Adler et al., 1995), whereby half of their cells express the wild-type MeCP2 allele and the other half express the mutant MeCP2 allele (Shahbazian et al., 2002). However, sometimes, by chance, the XCI pattern favors expression of the wild-type allele. Such 'lucky' females might show milder symptoms and even to be asymptomatic(Sirianni et al., 1998). Another source for phenotypic variability is the type of mutation in the MeCP2 gene. Over 300 different mutations in the gene MeCP2 were identified, which are the major source of the phenotypic variability in males with RTT. Thus generation of iPSCs from multiple patients might shed more light on the correlation between mutation type and symptoms as well as the function of different domains in MeCP2 protein. In addition, there are important implications for drug screening, as some drugs might treat patients with certain mutations but not others. For example, aminoglycosides antibiotics, such as gentamicin, can increase wild type MeCP2 expression levels in affected neurons by skipping a premature stop codon by bind to the 16S rRNA, impairing ribosomal proofreading (Kellermayer, 2006, Marchetto et al., 2010). Thus, disease modeling for multiple patients will allow us to tailor specific drugs for each patient.

Initially, RTT was thought to be a neurodegenerative disease, however, the decrease in axondendritic arborization and impaired development of dendrites (Fig. 4) suggest that RTT is a disorder featuring an arrest in neuronal development (Hagberg, 1985, Belichenko et al., 1994, Armstrong, 1992, Armstrong, 2001). Furthermore, no obvious cell death is seen in RTT, and this therefore begs the question of whether restoring MeCP2 expression would restore normal neuronal function and reverse the resulting disease phenotypes. In a seminal work, Guy et al (2007) provide evidence supporting the feasibility of disease reversibility in mouse models of RTT (Guy et al., 2007). They created a mouse in which endogenous MeCP2 is silenced by insertion of a Lox-Stop cassette and can be conditionally activated through Cre-mediated deletion of the cassette. The MeCP2 lox-Stop allele behaved as a null mutation, and its activation was controlled by a tamoxifen-inducible Cre transgene. Gradual tamoxifen injection reversed the late-onset neurological phenotype of adult MeCP2-lox-Stop/+; cre heterozygotes, indicating that MeCP2-deficient neurons are not permanently damaged, since MeCP2 activation leads to robust abrogation of advanced neurological defects in both young and adult animals. This work establish that consequences of MeCP2 loss of function are reversible, and suggest that the neurological defects in RTT, and other MeCP2 disorders, are not impervious to therapeutic possibilities. Indeed, several molecules, have delayed the onset of RTT-like symptoms in animal models, and enhanced survival rates (Chang et al., 2006, Ogier et al., 2007). Potential molecules for treatment of RTT are BDNF, IGF-1 and NGF. A molecule with promise in RTT therapy is BDNF. There are phenotypic similarities between MeCP2- and BDNF-null mice, including a reduction in brain weight and hindlimb clasping. Over expression of BDNF in MeCP2-null mouse brains delayed the onset of RTT-like symptoms, and enhanced survival rates (Chang et al., 2006, Ogier et al., 2007). More specifically, BDNF overexpression rescued the hypoactivity in wheel running exhibited by MeCP2 knockout mouse, and the low frequency of action potential firing observed in their cortical neurons (Chang et al., 2006); and treatment of MeCP2 null mice with AMPAkines (which increases BDNF mRNA and protein levels) rescued the irregular respiratory patterns exhibited by MeCP2. However, the therapeutic utility of BDNF is hampered by its poor efficiency at crossing the blood–brain barrier. Nevertheless, a therapeutic intervention in humans might thus arise from identifying an agent similarly capable of stimulating synaptic maturation.

An *in vitro* disease modeling for RTT was established by Marchetto et al (2010). In this study they reprogrammed fibroblasts from RTT patients into iPSCs, and further differentiated them into neurons. When analyzed, these neurons showed lower synaptic density, simpler morphology with less branching and smaller cell body. Furthermore, by using electrophysiological methods they showed that RTT neurons have a significant decrease in frequency and amplitude. This is in agreement with studies on RTT mice models and on postmortem brain tissues from patients. This RTT disease model was used to screen molecules, such as IGF-1. Like BDNF, IGF-1 is widely expressed in the CNS during normal development (D'Ercole et al., 1996), strongly promotes neuronal cell survival and synaptic connections. Indeed, IGF-1 treatment leads to a partial rescue of RTT (Tropea et al., 2009).

In their study, Marchetto et al (2010) investigated the use of IGF1 and gentamicin in iPSC-derived neurons carrying a MeCP2 mutation. While IGF1 treatment increased synapse number in some clones, it stimulated glutamatergic RTT neurons above normal levels. Gentamicin was used to rescue neurons derived from iPSCs carrying a nonsense MeCP2 mutation by increasing full-length MeCP2 levels in RTT neurons, rescuing glutamatergic synapses. Thus, this *in vitro* disease model can be used to screen therapeutic candidate molecules.

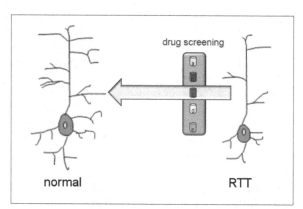

Fig. 4. Schematic representation of drug screening for pyramidal neurons carrying MeCP2 mutation. In RTT, the cell body is small and there is reduced dendritic branching (Armstrong 1995), fewer synapses, and reduced spine density compared to the control. These morphological differences can be an indicator for drug screening. In this example, component 'C' reverses the impaired morphology of the RTT neurons and therefore can be further studied in RTT animal models as a potential drug to reverse the RTT symptoms.

3.3 Familial dysautonomia

Familial dysautonomia (FD), also known as Riley–Day syndrome or HSAN-III is a neurodevelopmental disorder, caused by a mutation in the I-k-B kinase complex-associated protein (*IKBKAP*) gene on chromosome 9. This condition is affects 1 in 3,700 Eastern European Jewish ancestry (Ashkenazi Jews), but rare in the general population. The disease was first reported by Conrad Milton Riley and Richard Lawrence. It is a fatal autosomal recessive disease characterized by the degeneration of sensory and autonomic neurons (Slaugenhaupt et al., 2001, Axelrod et al., 2002), resulting in variable symptoms including: insensitivity to pain, inability to produce tears, poor growth, and labile blood pressure (episodic hypertension and postural hypotension). Future parents can be screened for the mutation and if both parents are shown to be carriers by genetic testing, there is a 25% chance that the child will produce FD. The point mutation in the *IKBKAP* gene results in a tissue-specific splicing defect with various levels of exon 20 skipping and reduced levels of normal IKBAP protein (Slaugenhaupt et al., 2001, Anderson et al., 2001). The ratio between the normal and mutant transcripts affects the severity of the disease.

An iPSC-based model for FD was established by Lee et al (Lee et al., 2009). FD-iPSC-derived neural crest showed reduced migration as well as decreased rate of neurogenesis. Furthermore, when they screened the afflicted cells with candidate drugs, they found that kinetin resulted in a marked reduction of the mutant *IKBKAP* splice form, associated with an increase in normal *IKBKAP* levels. This treatment increased the percentage of differentiating neurons but it did not affect the migration potential of the neural crest. Thus FD-iPSC model is an example of gaining insight about early progession of a neuro-developmental disease.

3.4 Parkinson's disease

Parkinson's disease (PD) is one of the most widely studied neurodegenerative disease caused by the progressive degeneration of midbrain dopaminergic neurons. Although the aetiology of PD remains enigmatic, partially attributed to complex environmental factors, and mutations in several genes (LRRK-2, Parkin, DJ-1, PINK1, ATP13A2, alpha-synuclein, GBA) have been found to give rise to PD-like pathogenesis. However, these genetic factors contribute to only a small fraction of PD cases, impeding significant progress in understanding PD pathogenesis completely. Moreover, it was found in PD patients who had received neuronal grafts through transplantation that the cells which were previously young and healthy developed α–synuclein and ubiquitin-positive Lewy bodies after more than a decade. This led to the proposal of several mechanisms such as inflammation, oxidative stress, excitotoxicity and growth-factor deprivation that may have substantial impact on the propagation of PD (Brundin et al., 2008). Thus, it would be necessary to re-examine the disease pathology by mimicking characteristics of the disease under these varied conditions or in combination with known genetic defects since the benefits of cell transplantation in PD trials is still uncertain. This objective may soon be achievable as Soldner et al (2009) demonstrated that iPSCs could be derived from patients with idiopathic PD. Furthermore, the iPSCs could be directed to differentiate into dopaminergic neurons through EB formation in the presence of FGF2, FGF8 and Shh. Coupled with the possibility of deriving large-scale functional dopaminergic neurons; via the generation of homogenous spherical neural masses (Cho et al., 2008), the ultimate goal of creating patient-specific neuronal cells for transplantation therapy may soon be in the pipeline. It is reassuring to note that neurons reprogrammed from mouse fibroblasts were able to integrate functionally into the fetal brain and improve the locomotor behavior in at least a rat model of PD upon transplantation into the adult brain (Wernig et al., 2008). However, whether these transplanted cells will succumb to the same fate in the long-term as observed in the post-mortem human PD trails remains to be investigated.

3.5 Huntington's disease

Huntington's disease (HD) is caused by CAG repeats in the N-terminus of the gene encoding Huntingtin protein. Like Lewy proteins in Parkinson's disease patients, the expression of aberrant polyglutamine-containing molecules in HD leads to massive loss of medium spiny neurons in the striatum and neurons in the cortex as the disease progresses. Despite substantial efforts invested in various cellular and animal models to understand the disease, the mechanisms implicated in the selective cell death of neurons remains unclear and there is no cure at present. One major hurdle is the lack of appropriate human samples carrying the genetic mutation for HD which would offer the most ideal system for investigating the process of neurodegeneration. With the advent of iPSC technology, HD-specific iPSCs were generated (Park et al., 2008). Thereafter, HD specific NSCs (nestin+/PAX6+/SOX1+/OCT4-) were obtained and these were subjected to differentiation conditions combining morhogens (SHH and DKK1) and neurotrophins (BDNF) to induce neurons of the striatal lineages (Zhang et al.,). Importantly, these neurons contained the same CAG expansion as the mutation in the HD patient in which the iPSC line was established. Thus, a valuable resource is now available to search for drugs that can reduce the toxicity of polyglutamine.

3.6 Amyotrophic lateral sclerosis

Another seminal study to interrogate a deliberating disease, arising from the progressive degeneration of motor neurons of the spinal cord using the iPSC technology is amyotrophic lateral sclerosis (ALS) (Dimos et al., 2008). In this landmark study, skin fibroblasts produced directly from an 82-year-old elderly woman patient, diagnosed clinically with ALS and a SOD1 mutation were reprogrammed successfully into the pluripotent state. These patient-specific iPSCs showed strong alkaline phosphatase activity and exhibited markers (SSEA-3, SSEA-4, TRA1-60 and TRA1-81) and a transcriptional profile (*REX1, FOXD3, TERT, NANOG* and *CRIPTO*) that are comparable to pluripotent hESCs. Furthermore, these cells could form EBs and were capable of differentiating into cells of the germ layers. Most importantly the iPSCs were directed specifically towards both motor neurons and glia fates, enabling further exploration of either a cell autonomous (such as the amount of SOD1 in motor neurons) or non-cell-autonomous (such as the role of neighboring astrocytes, microglia and oligodendrocytes) function of the disease as implicated in rodent models (Boillee et al., 2006, Yamanaka et al., 2008). Thus, the iPSC technology essentially reversed the patient's history to allow the onset and progression of ALS to be captured in culture for drawing mechanistic insights.

In addition to ALS, Park and co-workers (Park et al., 2008) managed to single-handedly generate reprogrammed cells from patients with a range of genetic diseases that were either Mendelian or complex in inheritance. The diseases in which iPSCs were derived include: adenosine deaminase deficiency-related severe combined immunodeficiency (ADA-SCID), Shwachman-Bodian-Diamond syndrome (SBDS), Gaucher disease (GD) type III, Duchenne

(DMD) and Becker muscular dystrophy (BMD), Parkinson disease, Huntington disease, juvenile-onset, type 1 diabetes mellitus (JDM), Down syndrome (DS)/trisomy 21 and the carrier state of Lesch-Nyhan syndrome. Similar to the set of assays used in the characterization of the ALS iPSCs, these disease-associated iPSC lines were all confirmed to be pluripotent and capable of multi-lineage differentiation. Moreover, these human iPSCs produced teratomas in immunodeficient Rag2−/−γC−/− mice, the golden standard for testing pluripotency. Taken together, these efforts undoubtedly demonstrated the feasibility of the iPSC technology to reprogram somatic cells from a variety of diseased patients. And in the process, provided valuable source of material that pave the way for unraveling disease mechanisms and customized cellular therapies tailored for the individual.

4. Conclusion

Research on hESCs has allowed the development of specific protocols for generation of neural progenitors and differentiated neural lineages. These protocols can now be applied to iPSCs to enable the generation of specific neurons, astrocytes and oligodendrocytes. The availability of samples from relevant donors carrying different mutations will also facilitate modelling of neuronal diseases by reprogramming somatic cells. A 'mutation library' for a particular disease can then serve as a platform for the tailoring of specific drugs for specific patients. Furthermore, disease modelling from multiple patients might provide additional insights on the pathogenesis of the disease; particularly RTT in which specific mutations are associated with variable severity in clinical symptoms. Another advantage in reprogramming is that the clinical history of every donor is known. This will allow us to model diseases in which the genetic component is not known such as Alzheimer and Parkinson's. Thus the use of iPSCs technology will herald a new era in the study of neurological diseases.

5. Acknowledgment

This work was funded by Agency for Science and Technology Research, Singapore.

6. References

Adler, D.A., Quaderi, N.A., Brown, S.D., Chapman, V.M., Moore, J., Tate, P. & Disteche, C.M. (1995). The X-linked methylated DNA binding protein, Mecp2, is subject to X inactivation in the mouse. *Mamm Genome*, Vol. 6, No. 8, pp. 491-2.

Akbarian, S., Chen, R.Z., Gribnau, J., Rasmussen, T.P., Fong, H., Jaenisch, R. & Jones, E.G. (2001). Expression pattern of the Rett syndrome gene MeCP2 in primate prefrontal cortex. *Neurobiol Dis*, Vol. 8, No. 5, pp. 784-91.

Amir, R.E., Van den Veyver, I.B., Wan, M., Tran, C.Q., Francke, U. & Zoghbi, H.Y. (1999). Rett syndrome is caused by mutations in X-linked MECP2, encoding methyl-CpG-binding protein 2. *Nat Genet*, Vol. 23, No. 2, pp. 185-8.

Balmer, D., Goldstine, J., Rao, Y.M. & LaSalle, J.M. (2003). Elevated methyl-CpG-binding protein 2 expression is acquired during postnatal human brain development and is correlated with alternative polyadenylation. *J Mol Med*, Vol. 81, No. 1, pp. 61-8.

Bissonnette, C.J., Lyass, L., Bhattacharyya, B.J., Belmadani, A., Miller, R.J. & Kessler, J.A. (2011). The controlled generation of functional Basal forebrain cholinergic neurons from human embryonic stem cells. *Stem Cells,* Vol. 29, No. 5, pp. 802-11.

Bourdon, V., Philippe, C., Bienvenu, T., Koenig, B., Tardieu, M., Chelly, J. & Jonveaux, P. (2001). Evidence of somatic mosaicism for a MECP2 mutation in females with Rett syndrome: diagnostic implications. *J Med Genet,* Vol. 38, No. 12, pp. 867-71.

Bramow, S., Frischer, J.M., Lassmann, H., Koch-Henriksen, N., Lucchinetti, C.F., Sorensen, P.S. & Laursen, H. (2010). Demyelination versus remyelination in progressive multiple sclerosis. *Brain,* Vol. 133, No. 10, pp. 2983-98.

Brundin, P., Li, J.Y., Holton, J.L., Lindvall, O. & Revesz, T. (2008). Research in motion: the enigma of Parkinson's disease pathology spread. *Nat Rev Neurosci,* Vol. 9, No. 10, pp. 741-5.

Cao, Q., Xu, X.M., Devries, W.H., Enzmann, G.U., Ping, P., Tsoulfas, P., Wood, P.M., Bunge, M.B. & Whittemore, S.R. (2005). Functional recovery in traumatic spinal cord injury after transplantation of multineurotrophin-expressing glial-restricted precursor cells. *J Neurosci,* Vol. 25, No. 30, pp. 6947-57.

Chambers, S.M., Fasano, C.A., Papapetrou, E.P., Tomishima, M., Sadelain, M. & Studer, L. (2009). Highly efficient neural conversion of human ES and iPS cells by dual inhibition of SMAD signaling. *Nat Biotechnol,* Vol. 27, No. 3, pp. 275-80.

Chimge, N.O. & Bayarsaihan, D. (2010). Generation of neural crest progenitors from human embryonic stem cells. *J Exp Zool B Mol Dev Evol,* Vol. 314, No. 2, pp. 95-103.

Cho, M.S., Hwang, D.Y. & Kim, D.W. (2008a). Efficient derivation of functional dopaminergic neurons from human embryonic stem cells on a large scale. *Nat Protoc,* Vol. 3, No. 12, pp. 1888-94.

Cho, M.S., Lee, Y.E., Kim, J.Y., Chung, S., Cho, Y.H., Kim, D.S., Kang, S.M., Lee, H., Kim, M.H., Kim, J.H., Leem, J.W., Oh, S.K., Choi, Y.M., Hwang, D.Y., Chang, J.W. & Kim, D.W. (2008b). Highly efficient and large-scale generation of functional dopamine neurons from human embryonic stem cells. *Proc Natl Acad Sci U S A,* Vol. 105, No. 9, pp. 3392-7.

Czepiel, M., Balasubramaniyan, V., Schaafsma, W., Stancic, M., Mikkers, H., Huisman, C., Boddeke, E. & Copray, S. (2011). Differentiation of induced pluripotent stem cells into functional oligodendrocytes. *Glia,* Vol. 59, No. 6, pp. 882-92.

Furuta, Y., Piston, D.W. & Hogan, B.L. (1997). Bone morphogenetic proteins (BMPs) as regulators of dorsal forebrain development. *Development,* Vol. 124, No. 11, pp. 2203-12.

Garbern, J.Y. (2007). Pelizaeus-Merzbacher disease: Genetic and cellular pathogenesis. *Cell Mol Life Sci,* Vol. 64, No. 1, pp. 50-65.

Gil, J.E., Woo, D.H., Shim, J.H., Kim, S.E., You, H.J., Park, S.H., Paek, S.H., Kim, S.K. & Kim, J.H. (2009). Vitronectin promotes oligodendrocyte differentiation during neurogenesis of human embryonic stem cells. *FEBS Lett,* Vol. 583, No. 3, pp. 561-7.

Green, H., Easley, K. & Iuchi, S. (2003). Marker succession during the development of keratinocytes from cultured human embryonic stem cells. *Proc Natl Acad Sci U S A,* Vol. 100, No. 26, pp. 15625-30.

Guidato, S., Prin, F. & Guthrie, S. (2003). Somatic motoneurone specification in the hindbrain: the influence of somite-derived signals, retinoic acid and Hoxa3. *Development,* Vol. 130, No. 13, pp. 2981-96.

Guy, J., Gan, J., Selfridge, J., Cobb, S. & Bird, A. (2007). Reversal of neurological defects in a mouse model of Rett syndrome. *Science,* Vol. 315, No. 5815, pp. 1143-7.

Harland, R. & Gerhart, J. (1997). Formation and function of Spemann's organizer. *Annu Rev Cell Dev Biol*, Vol. 13, pp. 611-67.

Hemmati-Brivanlou, A. & Melton, D.A. (1994). Inhibition of activin receptor signaling promotes neuralization in Xenopus. *Cell*, Vol. 77, No. 2, pp. 273-81.

Hendrickx, M., Van, X.H. & Leyns, L. (2009). Anterior-posterior patterning of neural differentiated embryonic stem cells by canonical Wnts, Fgfs, Bmp4 and their respective antagonists. *Dev Growth Differ*, Vol. 51, No. 8, pp. 687-98.

Hong, S., Kang, U.J., Isacson, O. & Kim, K.S. (2008). Neural precursors derived from human embryonic stem cells maintain long-term proliferation without losing the potential to differentiate into all three neural lineages, including dopaminergic neurons. *J Neurochem*, Vol. 104, No. 2, pp. 316-24.

Hu, B.Y. & Zhang, S.C. (2009). Differentiation of spinal motor neurons from pluripotent human stem cells. *Nat Protoc*, Vol. 4, No. 9, pp. 1295-304.

Hu, Z., Li, T., Zhang, X. & Chen, Y. (2009). Hepatocyte growth factor enhances the generation of high-purity oligodendrocytes from human embryonic stem cells. *Differentiation*, Vol. 78, No. 2-3, pp. 177-84.

Itskovitz-Eldor, J., Schuldiner, M., Karsenti, D., Eden, A., Yanuka, O., Amit, M., Soreq, H. & Benvenisty, N. (2000). Differentiation of human embryonic stem cells into embryoid bodies compromising the three embryonic germ layers. *Mol Med*, Vol. 6, No. 2, pp. 88-95.

Itsykson, P., Ilouz, N., Turetsky, T., Goldstein, R.S., Pera, M.F., Fishbein, I., Segal, M. & Reubinoff, B.E. (2005). Derivation of neural precursors from human embryonic stem cells in the presence of noggin. *Mol Cell Neurosci*, Vol. 30, No. 1, pp. 24-36.

Jung, B.P., Jugloff, D.G., Zhang, G., Logan, R., Brown, S. & Eubanks, J.H. (2003). The expression of methyl CpG binding factor MeCP2 correlates with cellular differentiation in the developing rat brain and in cultured cells. *J Neurobiol*, Vol. 55, No. 1, pp. 86-96.

Kawasaki, H., Mizuseki, K., Nishikawa, S., Kaneko, S., Kuwana, Y., Nakanishi, S., Nishikawa, S.I. & Sasai, Y. (2000). Induction of midbrain dopaminergic neurons from ES cells by stromal cell-derived inducing activity. *Neuron*, Vol. 28, No. 1, pp. 31-40.

Keirstead, H.S., Nistor, G., Bernal, G., Totoiu, M., Cloutier, F., Sharp, K. & Steward, O. (2005). Human embryonic stem cell-derived oligodendrocyte progenitor cell transplants remyelinate and restore locomotion after spinal cord injury. *J Neurosci*, Vol. 25, No. 19, pp. 4694-705.

Kellermayer, R. (2006). Translational readthrough induction of pathogenic nonsense mutations. *Eur J Med Genet*, Vol. 49, No. 6, pp. 445-50.

Kumar, M., Kaushalya, S.K., Gressens, P., Maiti, S. & Mani, S. (2009). Optimized derivation and functional characterization of 5-HT neurons from human embryonic stem cells. *Stem Cells Dev*, Vol. 18, No. 4, pp. 615-27.

Lee, D.S., Yu, K., Rho, J.Y., Lee, E., Han, J.S., Koo, D.B., Cho, Y.S., Kim, J., Lee, K.K. & Han, Y.M. (2006). Cyclopamine treatment of human embryonic stem cells followed by culture in human astrocyte medium promotes differentiation into nestin- and GFAP-expressing astrocytic lineage. *Life Sci*, Vol. 80, No. 2, pp. 154-9.

Lee, G., Papapetrou, E.P., Kim, H., Chambers, S.M., Tomishima, M.J., Fasano, C.A., Ganat, Y.M., Menon, J., Shimizu, F., Viale, A., Tabar, V., Sadelain, M. & Studer, L. (2009). Modelling pathogenesis and treatment of familial dysautonomia using patient-specific iPSCs. *Nature*, Vol. 461, No. 7262, pp. 402-6.

Lewis, K.E. & Eisen, J.S. (2001). Hedgehog signaling is required for primary motoneuron induction in zebrafish. *Development*, Vol. 128, No. 18, pp. 3485-95.

Li, X.J., Du, Z.W., Zarnowska, E.D., Pankratz, M., Hansen, L.O., Pearce, R.A. & Zhang, S.C. (2005). Specification of motoneurons from human embryonic stem cells. *Nat Biotechnol*, Vol. 23, No. 2, pp. 215-21.

Li, X.J., Hu, B.Y., Jones, S.A., Zhang, Y.S., Lavaute, T., Du, Z.W. & Zhang, S.C. (2008). Directed differentiation of ventral spinal progenitors and motor neurons from human embryonic stem cells by small molecules. *Stem Cells*, Vol. 26, No. 4, pp. 886-93.

Litingtung, Y. & Chiang, C. (2000). Control of Shh activity and signaling in the neural tube. *Dev Dyn*, Vol. 219, No. 2, pp. 143-54.

Londin, E.R., Niemiec, J. & Sirotkin, H.I. (2005). Chordin, FGF signaling, and mesodermal factors cooperate in zebrafish neural induction. *Dev Biol*, Vol. 279, No. 1, pp. 1-19.

Maezawa, I., Swanberg, S., Harvey, D., LaSalle, J.M. & Jin, L.W. (2009). Rett syndrome astrocytes are abnormal and spread MeCP2 deficiency through gap junctions. *J Neurosci*, Vol. 29, No. 16, pp. 5051-61.

Marchetto, M.C., Carromeu, C., Acab, A., Yu, D., Yeo, G.W., Mu, Y., Chen, G., Gage, F.H. & Muotri, A.R. (2010). A model for neural development and treatment of Rett syndrome using human induced pluripotent stem cells. *Cell*, Vol. 143, No. 4, pp. 527-39.

Migeon, B.R. (2007). Why females are mosaics, X-chromosome inactivation, and sex differences in disease. *Gend Med*, Vol. 4, No. 2, pp. 97-105.

Moore, C.S., Milner, R., Nishiyama, A., Frausto, R.F., Serwanski, D.R., Pagarigan, R.R., Whitton, J.L., Miller, R.H. & Crocker, S.J. (2011). Astrocytic Tissue Inhibitor of Metalloproteinase-1 (TIMP-1) Promotes Oligodendrocyte Differentiation and Enhances CNS Myelination. *J Neurosci*, Vol. 31, No. 16, pp. 6247-54.

Morizane, A., Doi, D., Kikuchi, T., Nishimura, K. & Takahashi, J. (2010). Small-molecule inhibitors of bone morphogenic protein and activin/nodal signals promote highly efficient neural induction from human pluripotent stem cells. *J Neurosci Res*.

Nagai, M., Re, D.B., Nagata, T., Chalazonitis, A., Jessell, T.M., Wichterle, H. & Przedborski, S. (2007). Astrocytes expressing ALS-linked mutated SOD1 release factors selectively toxic to motor neurons. *Nat Neurosci*, Vol. 10, No. 5, pp. 615-22.

Nevalainen, N., Chermenina, M., Rehnmark, A., Berglof, E., Marschinke, F. & Stromberg, I. (2010). Glial cell line-derived neurotrophic factor is crucial for long-term maintenance of the nigrostriatal system. *Neuroscience*, Vol. 171, No. 4, pp. 1357-66.

Nilbratt, M., Porras, O., Marutle, A., Hovatta, O. & Nordberg, A. (2010). Neurotrophic factors promote cholinergic differentiation in human embryonic stem cell-derived neurons. *J Cell Mol Med*, Vol. 14, No. 6B, pp. 1476-84.

Noisa, P., Urrutikoetxea-Uriguen, A., Li, M. & Cui, W. (2010). Generation of human embryonic stem cell reporter lines expressing GFP specifically in neural progenitors. *Stem Cell Rev*, Vol. 6, No. 3, pp. 438-49.

Onai, T., Lin, H.C., Schubert, M., Koop, D., Osborne, P.W., Alvarez, S., Alvarez, R., Holland, N.D. & Holland, L.Z. (2009). Retinoic acid and Wnt/beta-catenin have complementary roles in anterior/posterior patterning embryos of the basal chordate amphioxus. *Dev Biol*, Vol. 332, No. 2, pp. 223-33.

Park, I.H., Arora, N., Huo, H., Maherali, N., Ahfeldt, T., Shimamura, A., Lensch, M.W., Cowan, C., Hochedlinger, K. & Daley, G.Q. (2008). Disease-specific induced pluripotent stem cells. *Cell*, Vol. 134, No. 5, pp. 877-86.

Park, S., Lee, K.S., Lee, Y.J., Shin, H.A., Cho, H.Y., Wang, K.C., Kim, Y.S., Lee, H.T., Chung, K.S., Kim, E.Y. & Lim, J. (2004). Generation of dopaminergic neurons in vitro from human embryonic stem cells treated with neurotrophic factors. *Neurosci Lett,* Vol. 359, No. 1-2, pp. 99-103.

Pomp, O., Brokhman, I., Ziegler, L., Almog, M., Korngreen, A., Tavian, M. & Goldstein, R.S. (2008). PA6-induced human embryonic stem cell-derived neurospheres: a new source of human peripheral sensory neurons and neural crest cells. *Brain Res,* Vol. 1230, pp. 50-60.

Rett, A. (1966). [On a unusual brain atrophy syndrome in hyperammonemia in childhood]. *Wien Med Wochenschr,* Vol. 116, No. 37, pp. 723-6.

Reubinoff, B.E., Itsykson, P., Turetsky, T., Pera, M.F., Reinhartz, E., Itzik, A. & Ben-Hur, T. (2001). Neural progenitors from human embryonic stem cells. *Nat Biotechnol,* Vol. 19, No. 12, pp. 1134-40.

Ross, M.T., Grafham, D.V., Coffey, A.J., Scherer, S., McLay, K., Muzny, D., Platzer, M., Howell, G.R., Burrows, C., Bird, C.P., Frankish, A., Lovell, F.L., Howe, K.L., Ashurst, J.L., Fulton, R.S., Sudbrak, R., Wen, G., Jones, M.C., Hurles, M.E., Andrews, T.D., Scott, C.E., Searle, S., Ramser, J., Whittaker, A., Deadman, R., Carter, N.P., Hunt, S.E., Chen, R., Cree, A., Gunaratne, P., Havlak, P., Hodgson, A., Metzker, M.L., Richards, S., Scott, G., Steffen, D., Sodergren, E., Wheeler, D.A., Worley, K.C., Ainscough, R., Ambrose, K.D., Ansari-Lari, M.A., Aradhya, S., Ashwell, R.I., Babbage, A.K., Bagguley, C.L., Ballabio, A., Banerjee, R., Barker, G.E., Barlow, K.F., Barrett, I.P., Bates, K.N., Beare, D.M., Beasley, H., Beasley, O., Beck, A., Bethel, G., Blechschmidt, K., Brady, N., Bray-Allen, S., Bridgeman, A.M., Brown, A.J., Brown, M.J., Bonnin, D., Bruford, E.A., Buhay, C., Burch, P., Burford, D., Burgess, J., Burrill, W., Burton, J., Bye, J.M., Carder, C., Carrel, L., Chako, J., Chapman, J.C., Chavez, D., Chen, E., Chen, G., Chen, Y., Chen, Z., Chinault, C., Ciccodicola, A., Clark, S.Y., Clarke, G., Clee, C.M., Clegg, S., Clerc-Blankenburg, K., Clifford, K., Cobley, V., Cole, C.G., Conquer, J.S., Corby, N., Connor, R.E., David, R., Davies, J., Davis, C., Davis, J., Delgado, O., Deshazo, D., et al. (2005). The DNA sequence of the human X chromosome. *Nature,* Vol. 434, No. 7031, pp. 325-37.

Roussa, E., Farkas, L.M. & Krieglstein, K. (2004). TGF-beta promotes survival on mesencephalic dopaminergic neurons in cooperation with Shh and FGF-8. *Neurobiol Dis,* Vol. 16, No. 2, pp. 300-10.

Sargiannidou, I., Vavlitou, N., Aristodemou, S., Hadjisavvas, A., Kyriacou, K., Scherer, S.S. & Kleopa, K.A. (2009). Connexin32 mutations cause loss of function in Schwann cells and oligodendrocytes leading to PNS and CNS myelination defects. *J Neurosci,* Vol. 29, No. 15, pp. 4736-49.

Sasai, Y., Lu, B., Piccolo, S. & De Robertis, E.M. (1996). Endoderm induction by the organizer-secreted factors chordin and noggin in Xenopus animal caps. *EMBO J,* Vol. 15, No. 17, pp. 4547-55.

Schulz, T.C., Noggle, S.A., Palmarini, G.M., Weiler, D.A., Lyons, I.G., Pensa, K.A., Meedeniya, A.C., Davidson, B.P., Lambert, N.A. & Condie, B.G. (2004). Differentiation of human embryonic stem cells to dopaminergic neurons in serum-free suspension culture. *Stem Cells,* Vol. 22, No. 7, pp. 1218-38.

Shahbazian, M.D., Sun, Y. & Zoghbi, H.Y. (2002). Balanced X chromosome inactivation patterns in the Rett syndrome brain. *Am J Med Genet,* Vol. 111, No. 2, pp. 164-8.

Singh Roy, N., Nakano, T., Xuing, L., Kang, J., Nedergaard, M. & Goldman, S.A. (2005). Enhancer-specified GFP-based FACS purification of human spinal motor neurons from embryonic stem cells. *Exp Neurol,* Vol. 196, No. 2, pp. 224-34.

Sirianni, N., Naidu, S., Pereira, J., Pillotto, R.F. & Hoffman, E.P. (1998). Rett syndrome: confirmation of X-linked dominant inheritance, and localization of the gene to Xq28. *Am J Hum Genet*, Vol. 63, No. 5, pp. 1552-8.

Smith, J.R., Vallier, L., Lupo, G., Alexander, M., Harris, W.A. & Pedersen, R.A. (2008). Inhibition of Activin/Nodal signaling promotes specification of human embryonic stem cells into neuroectoderm. *Dev Biol*, Vol. 313, No. 1, pp. 107-17.

Sottile, V., Thomson, A. & McWhir, J. (2003). In vitro osteogenic differentiation of human ES cells. *Cloning Stem Cells*, Vol. 5, No. 2, pp. 149-55.

Stull, N.D. & Iacovitti, L. (2001). Sonic hedgehog and FGF8: inadequate signals for the differentiation of a dopamine phenotype in mouse and human neurons in culture. *Exp Neurol*, Vol. 169, No. 1, pp. 36-43.

Sun, Y.E. & Wu, H. (2006). The ups and downs of BDNF in Rett syndrome. *Neuron*, Vol. 49, No. 3, pp. 321-3.

Takahashi, K. & Yamanaka, S. (2006). Induction of pluripotent stem cells from mouse embryonic and adult fibroblast cultures by defined factors. *Cell*, Vol. 126, No. 4, pp. 663-76.

Thomson, J.A., Itskovitz-Eldor, J., Shapiro, S.S., Waknitz, M.A., Swiergiel, J.J., Marshall, V.S. & Jones, J.M. (1998). Embryonic stem cell lines derived from human blastocysts. *Science*, Vol. 282, No. 5391, pp. 1145-7.

Ueno, M., Matsumura, M., Watanabe, K., Nakamura, T., Osakada, F., Takahashi, M., Kawasaki, H., Kinoshita, S. & Sasai, Y. (2006). Neural conversion of ES cells by an inductive activity on human amniotic membrane matrix. *Proc Natl Acad Sci U S A*, Vol. 103, No. 25, pp. 9554-9.

Vazin, T., Chen, J., Lee, C.T., Amable, R. & Freed, W.J. (2008). Assessment of stromal-derived inducing activity in the generation of dopaminergic neurons from human embryonic stem cells. *Stem Cells*, Vol. 26, No. 6, pp. 1517-25.

Voutsinos-Porche, B., Bonvento, G., Tanaka, K., Steiner, P., Welker, E., Chatton, J.Y., Magistretti, P.J. & Pellerin, L. (2003). Glial glutamate transporters mediate a functional metabolic crosstalk between neurons and astrocytes in the mouse developing cortex. *Neuron*, Vol. 37, No. 2, pp. 275-86.

Wada, T., Honda, M., Minami, I., Tooi, N., Amagai, Y., Nakatsuji, N. & Aiba, K. (2009). Highly efficient differentiation and enrichment of spinal motor neurons derived from human and monkey embryonic stem cells. *PLoS One*, Vol. 4, No. 8, pp. e6722.

Yan, J., Studer, L. & McKay, R.D. (2001). Ascorbic acid increases the yield of dopaminergic neurons derived from basic fibroblast growth factor expanded mesencephalic precursors. *J Neurochem*, Vol. 76, No. 1, pp. 307-11.

Ye, W., Shimamura, K., Rubenstein, J.L., Hynes, M.A. & Rosenthal, A. (1998). FGF and Shh signals control dopaminergic and serotonergic cell fate in the anterior neural plate. *Cell*, Vol. 93, No. 5, pp. 755-66.

Zhang, N., An, M.C., Montoro, D. & Ellerby, L.M. Characterization of Human Huntington's Disease Cell Model from Induced Pluripotent Stem Cells. *PLoS Curr*, Vol. 2, pp. RRN1193.

Zhang, S.C., Wernig, M., Duncan, I.D., Brustle, O. & Thomson, J.A. (2001). In vitro differentiation of transplantable neural precursors from human embryonic stem cells. *Nat Biotechnol*, Vol. 19, No. 12, pp. 1129-33.

Zhou, J., Su, P., Li, D., Tsang, S., Duan, E. & Wang, F. (2010). High-efficiency induction of neural conversion in human ESCs and human induced pluripotent stem cells with a single chemical inhibitor of transforming growth factor beta superfamily receptors. *Stem Cells*, Vol. 28, No. 10, pp. 1741-50.

Part 5

Pluripotent Alternatives - Other Cell Sources

10

Pluripotent Stem Cells from Testis

Sandeep Goel[1] and Hiroshi Imai[2]
[1]Laboratory for the Conservation of Endangered Species,
Centre for Cellular and Molecular Biology, Hyderabad,
[2]Graduate School of Agriculture, Kyoto University, Kyoto,
[1]India
[2]Japan

1. Introduction

1.1 Importance of Spermatogonial Stem Cells (SSCs)

Spermatogonial stem cells (SSCs) are undifferentiated germ cells that balance self-renewing and differentiating divisions to maintain spermatogenesis throughout adult life. This is a productive stem cell system that produces millions of spermatozoa each day while also maintaining rigorous quality control to safeguard germline integrity. SSCs are the only adult stem cells that are capable of self renewal and that differentiate to produce haploid cells transmitting genes to next generation. In the recent years, derivation of multipotent embryonic stem (ES)-like cells, which are capable of differentiating to three germinal layers, from SSCs in the testis, has been reported. This is of immense importance in medicine, basic science and animal reproduction and overcomes ethical issues pertaining to the use of human embryos for research. Since the population of SSCs in the testis is very low (< 1%), the identification of markers that are specifically expressed in SSCs aids in their efficient isolation. The characteristics of SSCs and ES-like cells in culture, and differential expression of genes in both these cell types can provide better understanding. In the present chapter, we would describe and compare the expression of SSC-specific markers in vivo and in vitro. We will also review the in vitro culture conditions of SSCs and characteristics of ES-like cells that differentiate from SSCs. This would enhance our perceptive of these special cells that has opened new avenues for stem cell researchers.

1.2 Origin of Spermatogonial Stem Cell pool

SSCs arise from gonocytes in the postnatal testis, which originally derive from primordial germ cells (PGCs) during foetal development. PGCs are a transient cell population that is first observed as a small cluster of alkaline phosphatase-positive cells in the epiblast stage embryo at about 7–7.25 days post psot coitum (dpc) in mice (Phillips et al., 2010). The specification of PGC is dependent on the expression of BMP4 and BMP8b from the extraembryonic ectoderm (Ginsburg et al., 1990; Lawson et al., 1999; Ying et al., 2001). During the formation of the allantois, the PGCs are passively swept away from the original position before they start migrating via the hindgut to arrive at the indifferent gonad (genital ridge) between 8.5 and 12.5 dpc in mice. PGCs replicate during the migratory phase and approximately 3000 PGCs colonize the genital ridges (Bendel-Stenzel et al., 1998). In the male gonad at about 13.5 dpc, PGCs give rise to gonocytes, which become enclosed in testicular cords formed by Sertoli precursor cells and peritubular myoid cells. Gonocyte is a general term that can be subcategorized into mitotic (M)-prospermatogonia, T1-prospermatogonia and T2-propsermatogonia (McCarrey 1993). M-prospermatogonia are located in the centre of the testicular cords, away from the basal membrane and continue proliferating until about 16.5 dpc of mouse development when they become T1-prospermatogonia and enter the G0 stage of mitotic arrest (McLaren 2003; Tohonen et al., 2003). Gonocytes resume proliferation during the first week after birth (marking their transition to T2-prospermatogonia), concomitant with migration to the seminiferous tubules basement membrane (Clermont & Perey 1957). T2-prospermatogonia that colonize the basement membrane give rise to the first round of spermatogenesis as well as establish the initial pool of SSCs that maintains spermatogenesis throughout postpubertal life (Kluin & de Rooij 1981; McCarrey 1993; Yoshida et al., 2006).

1.3 Dynamics of SSCs

The kinetics of sperm production were first described in rodents (Oakberg 1956) with the knowledge of the presence of adult stem cells, such as hematopoietic stem cells (HSCs), researchers hypothesized that germ cell differentiation in the testis required a stem cell population. The presence of a stem cell population responsible for continual sperm production in the testis was demonstrated in 1994 (Brinster & Zimmermann). They documented the first successful spermatogonial stem cell (SSC) transplantation in mice resulting in donor-derived spermatogenesis. SSCs are part of a subset of male germ cells called undifferentiated spermatogonia (Caires et al., 2010). This subset includes A_{single} (As) spermatogonia that are thought to be the SSCs and their progeny cells A_{paired} (Apr) and $A_{aligned}$ (Aal) spermatogonia (figure 1). SSCs are a self-renewing population of adult stem cells capable of producing progeny for a continual production of sperm by sexually mature males. They help in maintaining a constant supply of undifferentiated spermatogonia, which are critical to the initiation of spermatogenesis and the long-term production of sperm. One must be careful to distinguish between spermatogonial stem cells (SSC) and spermatogonia in general. The term "spermatogonia" is used collectively to refer to a continuum of cells ranging from those resting on the basement membrane (known as either $A_{isolated}$ or A_{single} spermatogonia), to proliferating sub-populations (A_{paired} to $A_{aligned}$, spermatogonia) to differentiating sub-populations [A_{1-4}, Intermediate and Type B spermatogonia]. The differentiating stages are committed to enter spermatogenesis, but whether the $A_{isolated}$ cells represent the only spermatogonia with a true stem cell nature is not yet fully clear. The differentiation of germ cells from diploid undifferentiated spermatogonia to mature and haploid spermatozoa is supported by the Sertoli cells of the seminiferous epithelium. The formation of the SSC population is dependent on the associated niche in the microenvironment in the seminiferous tubules of the testis. This niche environment supplies factors and provides interactions crucial for the survival and development of SSCs. It is usually composed of adjacent differentiated cells, the stem cells themselves, and the extracellular matrix surrounding these cells. The somatic cells produce factors, which aid in the extrinsic regulation of the SSC self-renewal/differentiation process. SSCs represent a model for the investigation of adult stem cells because they can be maintained in culture, and the presence, proliferation and the loss of SSCs in a cell population can be determined with the use of a transplantation assay.

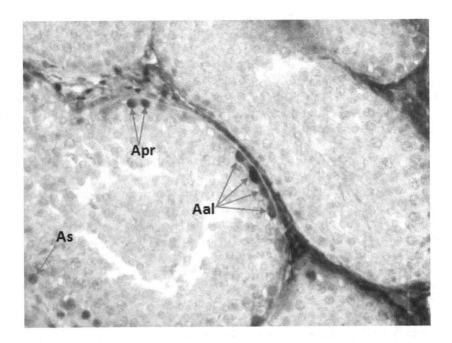

Fig. 1. Adult pig testis section stained with anti-UCHL-1 antibody. Spermatogonia are present as, A$_{single}$ (As), A$_{paired}$ (Apr) and A$_{aligned}$ (Aal) at the basement membrane of seminiferous tubule. The As spermatogonia are thought to be the spermatogonial stem cells (SSCs).

2. Identification of SSCs

2.1 Markers of SSCs

Exploring markers for spermatogonia help to identify the stem cell pool in the testis. Certain rodent markers for germ cells and SSCs such as VASA, DAZL, PLZF, and GFRα1are also of monkey (Hermann et al., 2007) and in other species. VASA expression marks spermatogonia in sheep (Borjigin et al., 2010), buffalo (Goel et al., 2010b) and bull (Fujihara et al., 2011) testis. It has been demonstrated that GFRα1 is a marker for mouse SSCs and probably their progeny (Meng et al., 2000; Buageaw et al., 2005; Hofmann et al., 2005; Naughton et al., 2006; He et al., 2007), and that KIT is a characteristic for the more differentiated spermatogonia, including type A$_{1-4}$ spermatogonia (Yoshinaga et al., 1991). KIT expression is shown to mark pig gonocytes (Goel et al., 2007) and spermatogonia (Dirami et al., 1999). PLZF marks pig (Goel et al., 2007) and sheep (Borjigin et al., 2010) gonocytes and type-A spermatogonia. Because there is not a unique marker available to distinguish the SSCs and other undifferentiated spermatogonia, called A$_{pr}$ and A$_{al}$, it is helpful to use two or three antibodies to characterize their phenotypes. The GFRα1 and POU5F1 antibodies stain the same subset of mouse spermatogonia (He et al., 2007). POU5F1 also marks spermatogonia in buffalo (Goel et al., 2010b) and bull (Fujihara et al., 2011). GPR125 is also believed to be a marker for mouse spermatogonial stem/progenitor cells (Seandel et al., 2007). It is speculated that some of these markers as mentioned above will also be applicable to human spermatogonia. It has been recently shown that GPR125 may be a marker for human SSCs, as it is for mouse SSCs (He et al., 2010).

A comparison of the markers for spermatogonia and their progenitors in human and rodents indicates that these spermatogonia share many but not all phenotypes. In rodents, α6-integrin (CD49f), β1-integrin (CD29), and Thy-1 (CD90) are surface markers for mouse spermatogonial stem/progenitor cells (Shinohara et al., 1999; Kubota et al., 2003). THY-1 also marks bovine spermatogonia (Reding et al., 2010). CD9 is a surface marker for mouse and rat spermatogonial stem/progenitor cells (Kanatsu-Shinohara et al., 2004a). GFRα1 and RET are co-receptors for GDNF and markers for spermatogonial stem/progenitor cells (Buaas et al., 2004; Costoya et al., 2004; Buageaw et al., 2005; Hofmann et al., 2005; Naughton et al., 2006). In human, α6-integrin is expressed in spermatogonia and their progenitors and was used to isolate and purify human spermatogonial cells by magnetic-activated cell separation (Conrad et al., 2008). Other rodent surface markers, such as CD90, GFRα1, and CD133, were also used to select human spermatogonia by magnetic-activated cell separation (MACS) and comparable results to α6-integrin were obtained (Conrad et al., 2008). PLZF is characterized as a hallmark for mouse spermatogonial stem/progenitor cells (Buaas et al., 2004; Costoya et al., 2004). In adult monkey, the expression of PLZF is confined to the A_{dark} and/or A_{pale} spermatogonia (Hermann et al., 2007). GPR125 has been demonstrated to be expressed in mouse spermatogonia and their progenitors (Seandel et al., 2007), and it is recently reported that GPR125 is also present in human spermatogonia (Dym et al., 2009). UCHL-1 is known to express in spermatogonia of mice (Kwon et al., 2004), monkey (Tokunaga et al., 1999) and humans (He et al., 2010). UCHL-1 protein expression is present specifically in the spermatogonia of domestic animal testes such as bull (Wrobel et al., 1995; Herrid et al., 2009), pig (Luo et al., 2006; Goel et al., 2007), sheep (Rodriguez-Sosa et al., 2006) and buffalo (Goel et al., 2010b). UCHL-1 protein expression is also specific to spermatogonia of wild bovids (Goel et al., 2010a). UCHL-1 also marks spermatogonia in the testis of Indian mouse deer (*Moschiola indica*) and slender loris (*Loris tardigradus*) (unpublished data). It is therefore likely that the expression of UCHL-1 is conserved in a variety of species. Collectively, the above studies suggest that some spermatogonial markers are conserved between rodents and humans and other species. In contrast, some other rodent markers for spermatogonia and their progenitors are not applicable to human and other species. This can be illustrated by the fact that α1-integrin (CD29), a marker for rodent spermatogonial stem/progenitor cells, is not expressed in human spermatogonia but present in spermatocytes, spermatids, and spermatozoa in normal human testis (Schaller et al., 1993). Another example is that POU5F1 (Oct-4), a marker for mouse spermatogonial stem/progenitor cells (Ohbo et al., 2003; Ohmura et al., 2004; Hofmann et al., 2005), is not detected in adult human spermatogonia (Looijenga et al., 2003). POU5F1 shows a rather unique expression pattern in pig testis where spermatogonia show a weak staining, however, strong expression is present in differentiating germ cells such as spermatocytes and spermatids (Goel et al., 2008). Similarly, KIT is regarded as a marker for mouse differentiating spermatogonia (Yoshinaga et al., 1991; Schrans-Stassen et al., 1999; Dolci et al., 2001), but it is undetected in human spermatogonia (Rajpert-De Meyts et al., 2003). Notably, some human markers for spermatogonia are also not applicable to rodents. As an example, the TSPY protein is preferentially expressed in elongated spermatids but not in spermatogonia of adult rat testis (Kido and Lau, 2006), unlike the expression pattern of the TSPY in adult human spermatogonia (Schnieders et al., 1996). Other rodent markers, including CD9 (Kanatsu- Shinohara et al., 2004b), CDH1 (Tokuda et al., 2007), neurogenin3 (Yoshida et al., 2004, 2007), RET (Naughton et al., 2006), and STRA8 (Giuili et al., 2002), were demonstrated to be expressed in spermatogonia and their progenitors; however, whether these rodent markers are present in human spermatogonia remains to be clarified. Similarly, some human markers, such as CD133 (Conrad et al., 2008), CHEK2 (also known as chk2 tumor suppressor protein) (Bartkova et al., 2001; Rajpert-De Meyts et al., 2003), and NSE (Neurone-specific enolase) (Rajpert-De Meyts et al., 2003), are also awaiting further studies to explore whether they are present in rodent spermatogonia and their progenitors. Such investigations would uncover further similarities and/or differences in spermatogonial phenotypes between human and rodents.

2.2 Functional assay of SSCs

Transplantation of isolated germ cells from a fertile donor male into the seminiferous tubules of infertile recipients can result in donor-derived sperm production. Therefore, this system represents a major development in the study of spermatogenesis and a unique functional assay to determine the developmental potential and relative abundance of spermatogonial stem cells in a given population of testis cells. The application of this method in farm animals has been the subject of an increasing number of studies, mostly because of its potential as an alternative strategy in producing transgenic livestock with higher efficiency and less time and capital requirement than the current methods such as microinjection of genes into fertilized eggs and somatic cell nuclear transfer.

Germ cell transplantation (GCT), also referred to as spermatogonial stem cell (SSC) transplantation, is a powerful technology first introduced in 1994 by Brinster and colleagues. Although initially developed using a mouse model, GCT has important applications in the study and manipulation of spermatogenesis in many species. In this method, testis cells obtained from a fertile donor male are transferred into the seminiferous tubules of infertile recipient testes, where donor-derived sperm production can occur, allowing the recipient to sire progeny (Brinster & Avarbock, 1994; Brinster & Zimmermann, 1994). In essence, donor SSCs deposited in the lumen of the recipient seminiferous tubules are allowed by the Sertoli cells to migrate to the basolateral compartment of the tubule, to proliferate, form new colonies and initiate donor-derived spermatogenesis (Nagano et al., 1999; Ohta et al, 2000). Following the original introduction of GCT in mice (Brinster & Avarbock, 1994; Brinster & Zimmermann, 1994), the technique was also successful in rats (Jiang & Short, 1995;Ogawa et al., 1999b), monkey (Schlatt et al., 2000a) and goat (Honaramooz et al., 2003). In laboratory rodents, GCT not only provides a unique opportunity for gaining a new insight into spermatogenesis and the biology of the stem cell niche, but also presents a unique functional bioassay to test the competence of putative SSCs. Furthermore, GCT also offers a new strategy for preservation of male fertility and an alternative approach for generation of transgenic animals (Brinster 2002, 2007).

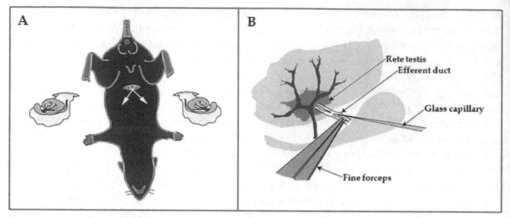

Fig. 2. Germ cell transplantation (GCT) in mice. (A) Germ cell depleted mice testes are extoriated through a ventral incision. (B) The testicular cell suspension is injected into seminiferous tubules through the efferent duct using a fine glass capillary.

Rather surprisingly, cross-species (xenogeneic/heterologous) transplantation of testis cells from donor rats and hamster into recipient mice resulted in complete rat (Clouthier et al., 1996) and hamster (Ogawa et al., 1999a) spermatogenesis. This development sparked an interest in the idea of using the laboratory mouse as a universal recipient model for testis cells from different donor species. However, GCT from genetically more distant donor species, including farm animals, into mice only resulted in colonization or proliferation of SSCs but not in complete spermatogenesis (Nagano et al., 2001, 2002; Dobrinski et al., 2000; Kim et al., 2006). We have recently shown that spermatogonia from endangered wild bovid (the Indian black buck; *Antelope cervecapra L.*) were able to colonize the recipient mice testis following GCT, however, showed no signs of proliferation or differentiation (Goel et al., 2011). This block in differentiation of donor germ cells is believed to be due to the incompatibility of donor germ cells and mouse Sertoli cells (Shinohara et al., 2003). Although GCT from nonrodent species into the mouse testis did not result in complete spermatogenesis, it is still the only available bioassay for detecting the colonization potential of SSCs in a given population of donor testis cells from any species (Dobrinski et al., 1999a, b, 2000). Interestingly, when (rather than transferring isolated testis cells into the seminiferous tubules) small fragments of testis tissue were transplanted under the back skin of recipient mice, complete donor-derived spermatogenesis was observed from a wide range of donor species, including farm animal species (Honaramooz et al., 2002, 2004; Schlatt et al., 2002b; Oatley et al., 2005; Rathi et al., 2006, 2008; Arregui et al., 2008; Ehmcke et al., 2008; Nakie et al., 2010).

3. Pluripotential ability of germ stem cells in testis

3.1 Introduction
In the years 2006 and 2007, many articles were published, where somatic skin cells could be reprogrammed to ES-like cells, the so-called induced pluripotent stem (iPS) cells. Each report on the induction of pluripotency in mouse and human skin fibroblasts used retroviral delivery of key pluripotent stem cell genes such as, Oct-4 (Pou5f1), Sox2, c-Myc, and Klf4

(Takahashi and Yamanaka, 2006; Hanna et al., 2007; Meissner et al., 2007; Okita et al., 2007; Takahashi et al., 2007; Wernig et al., 2007). In the second step, transformed iPS cells were identified and selected by expression of pluripotent markers including Nanog (Okita et al., 2007; Wernig et al., 2007) or Oct-4 (Wernig et al., 2007), or by ES-specific morphology (Meissner et al., 2007). These iPS cells had unique characteristics as they were germ-line competent and indistinguishable from ES cells derived from the embryo at the epigenetic level. Additionally, recent work has demonstrated that patient-autologous skin iPS cells can be genetically modified and used after differentiation by induction to cure a mouse model of sickle cell anemia (Hanna et al., 2007). Although this research paves the way toward stem cell therapy, it seems to be impractical for the iPS cells to be used in clinical application because of their instability and potential retroviral infections (Dym et al., 2009).

As a result, it is essential and necessary to figure out more physiological methods to induce pluripotency from adult somatic cells or adult stem cells. More recent efforts have been taken to generate iPS cells from neural stem cells using only two transcription factors, Oct-4 and either c-Myc or Klf4 (Kim et al., 2008). It has also been demonstrated that iPS cells can be produced from adult cells by non-integrating adenoviruses transiently expressing Oct-4, Sox2, Klf4, and c-Myc (Stadtfeld et al., 2008). However, it is still possible that these factors could somehow find their way into the genome of the iPS cells. Therefore, reprogramming of adult cells without the use of oncogenes would be very useful and safer as a means to produce ES-like cells. The proof of principle that spermatogonial stem cells/progenitor cells could be reprogrammed to pluripotent cells by biochemical means alone was first shown by Shinohara and colleagues (Kanatsu-Shinohara et al., 2004b). However, they could not derive ES-like cells from SSCs of adult mice. Guan et al. (2006) demonstrated that mouse adult spermatogonia, possibly the spermatogonial stem cells and/or their progeny, were able to reprogram biochemically to pluripotent ES-like cells. This was confirmed in mouse by (Seandel et al., 2007) showing that adult spermatogonia and/or their progenitors could indeed form pluripotent ES-like cells. Golestaneh and others (Conrad et al., 2008; Kossack et al., 2008; Golestaneh et al., 2009) have recently demonstrated a similar phenomenon in male germ cells and spermatogonia in the human testis. It is important to note that the SSCs/progenitor cells appear to reprogram spontaneously to pluripotency when the cells are removed from their niche and when ES cell media is added. Thus, SSCs/progenitor cells have a great potential to be used as a safe means to generate ES-like cells that eventually can be used for clinical therapies of human diseases. Human ES cells are pluripotent stem cells that have the potential to differentiate into all the types of cell lineages and tissues in the body, and thus they are ideal cell sources for cell transplantation and gene therapy. However, the major concern is the ethical issues associated with obtaining human ES cells from IVF clinics. The human iPS cells have major advantages over human ES cells because there are no ethical issues involved and, more importantly, the iPS cells appear to be similar to ES cells in morphology, proliferation, and pluripotency, as evaluated by teratoma formation and chimera contribution. In contrast, the iPS cells have some disadvantages, e.g., safety is a major concern due to the potential of cell transformation or tumor formation because of the oncogenes from the transfected iPS. It may be possible to overcome these issues by generating pluripotent stem cells without oncogene transfer directly from spermatogonial stem cells by testicular biopsy. Thus, the generation of human ES-like cells from SSCs may offer a safer means of obtaining pluripotent stem cells than from the iPS cells. The identification of human SSCs is now especially important in view of the discrepancy between the Skutella report (Conrad et al., 2008) and the report by the Reijo-

Pera group (Kossack et al., 2008). The Skutella group concluded that the ES-like cells derived from human spermatogonia (Spga) were in fact as pluripotent as true embryonic stem (ES) cells. The Reijo-Pera group noted that their cells differ from true ES cells in gene expression, methylation, and in their ability to form teratomas. Comparisons are difficult because the Skutella group used isolated Spga to get their ES-like cells, whereas the Reijo-Pera group used the entire testis biopsy without separating the Spga. It is possible that ES-like cells derived from isolated spermatogonial stem cells yield superior ES-like cells compared to using whole testis, but this remains to be determined. There are now three means to generate human pluripotent stem cells: (1) from a fertilized embryo as the traditional method; (2) from adult somatic cells through iPS technology; and (3) from adult SSCs and/or their progeny. One major advantage of the third approach is that the production of the ES-like cells is spontaneous, unlike method 2, where several genes, some cancer causing, is employed. Thus, human SSCs and/or their progeny have a great potential for cell- and tissue engineering-based medical regeneration for various human diseases. It is possible that in the near future men could be cured of their diseases using a biopsy from their own testes (Dym et al., 2009).

3.2 Culture of SSCs and induction of ES-like colonies

Kanatsu-Shinohara et al. (2004b) cultured SSCs in such a way that these cells propagated themselves, while retaining their capacity to repopulate a recipient mouse testis upon transplantation. A special medium, which was designed to culture hematopoietic stem cells, has been used for culture and contained several growth factors, including GDNF. In this culture system, a feeder layer is first formed that is composed of the contaminating somatic cells of the neonatal testis. Then, after 2 weeks and two passages, mitomycin-treated mouse embryonic fibroblasts (MEFs) are used as a feeder layer. During the first weeks of culture, the formed colonies consisted of SSCs, but, within 4-7 weeks, colonies that morphologically resembled ES cell colonies formed. Further work indicated that these colonies were indeed composed of multipotent ES-like cells. In order to maintain the multipotent character of these ES-like cells, they were subsequently cultured under a standard ES cell culture conditions in medium containing 15% fetal calf serum and LIF. Under these conditions, the cultured SSCs could not be propagated because of the lack of GDNF. ES-like colonies could only be obtained when the starting population of SSCs was derived from neonatal mice; when it was derived from older mice, ES-like colonies did not appear. However, cultures of SSCs derived from adult *p53* (*Trp53*)-null mice did produce ES-like colonies. P53 is involved in the cellular response to DNA damage and a lack of P53 increases the chances of teratoma development. Possibly, P53-deficient SSCs are more capable of undergoing the transition into ES-like cells.

An essentially similar protocol was followed by Seandel et al. (2007), except that this group used inactivated testicular stromal cells consisting of a mixture of CD34+ peritubular cells, α-smooth-muscle-actin-positive peritubular cells and cells positive for the Sertoli cell marker vimentin, as a feeder layer because they had less success using MEFs. By this method, ES-like colonies only appeared after more than 3 months in culture, more slowly than reported by Kanatsu-Shinohara et al. (2004b). A substantially different approach was taken by Guan et al. (2006). Their starting material was derived from 4- to 6-week-old mice and they did not use the stem cell medium described by Kanatsu-Shinohara et al. (2004b) but simply Dulbecco's Modified Eagle's Medium (DMEM) with serum and added GDNF, in which testicular cells were initially cultured for 4 to 7 days. These cells were then sorted for the expression of STRA8 and subsequently cultured in DMEM under various conditions, but without adding GDNF. Colonies of ES-like cells formed when LIF was added to the medium and/or when the cells were cultured on a feeder layer of MEFs. The ES-like cells were further expanded by culture on MEFs and the addition of LIF.

Hu et al. (2007) cultured germ cells of prepubertal mice under conditions that favour osteoblast differentiation and reported the emergence of cells that had characteristics of osteoblasts after several weeks in culture. In this system, there was no period of culture with added GDNF. Finally, Boulanger et al. (2007) employed no culture step at all. This group transplanted cells isolated from adult mouse seminiferous tubules, together with mammary cells, into mammary fat pads to obtain the differentiation of SSCs into mammary epithelial cells.

We have shown that gonocytes from neonatal pig testis can attain multipotency during short-term culture (Goel et al., 2009). Freshly isolated gonocytes were found to have either weak or no expression of pluripotency determining transcription factors, such as *POU5F1*, *SOX2* and *C-MYC*. Interestingly, the expression of these transcription factors, as well as other vital transcription factors, such as *NANOG*, *KLF4* and *DAZL*, were markedly upregulated in cultured cells. The formation of teratomas with tissues originating from the three germinal layers following the subcutaneous injection of cells into nude mice from primary cultures confirmed their multipotency.

Taken together, it does not seem that a very specific approach is required to obtain the transformation of SSCs into ES-like cells. This transformation can occur on different feeder layers and even without a feeder layer, if LIF is added to the culture medium. Furthermore, the culture medium also does not seem to play a decisive role in the transformation of SSCs into ES-like cells, as the groups of Kanatsu-Shinohara et al. (2004b) and Seandel et al. (2007) used a specific stem cell medium, whereas Guan et al. (Guan et al., 2006) used DMEM. All three groups added GDNF to the culture, either continuously (Kanatsu-Shinohara et al., 2004b; Seandel et al., 2007) or only at the start (Guan et al., 2006). However, to obtain the transformation of SSCs into cells of another lineage, it might not be necessary for them to become ES-like cells first. Putting the SSCs in an osteoblast-inductive environment in culture (Hu et al., 2007) or transplanting them into a mammary gland-inductive environment in vivo (Boulanger et al., 2007) might be enough for these cells to change their lineage. This rather suggests that SSCs are restricted to the spermatogenic lineage owing to the seminiferous tubular environment in which they reside. Once outside of this environment, they can switch to another lineage depending on the particular niche in which they are placed.

3.3 Gene expression in SSCs and ES-like cells

A crucial question is what changes in gene expression accompany the transition from a cultured SSC to an ES-like cell? In this respect, it is interesting to study the possible changes in the expression of those genes that can transform a fibroblast into an ES-like cell, that is *Myc, Oct4 (Pou5f1), Sox2* and *Klf4* (Takahashi and Yamanaka, 2006; Wernig et al., 2007), in SSCs and in the ES-like cells derived from them. Kanatsu-Shinohara et al. (2008b) found that all four pluripotency genes are already expressed at low levels in cultured SSCs, although no NANOG (Kanatsu-Shinohara et al., 2004b) or SOX2 protein expression was found in these cells. In ES-like cells, the expression of these four genes is much increased. In addition to these pluripotency genes, the ES cell markers such as stage-specific embryonic antigen-1

(SSEA-1; FUT4) and, to a low level, Forssman antigen (GBGT1), were induced in the ES-like cells and, as in ES cells, high levels of alkaline phosphatase (AP) were also found (Kanatsu-Shinohara et al., 2004b). Guan et al. (2006) assayed expression patterns in SSCs cultured under conditions that induced these cells to become ES-like cells. In this situation, it is difficult to categorize these cells as being either SSCs or ES-like cells as they might be in an in-between state. In these SSCs/early ES-like cells, *Oct4, Nanog* and *SSEA1* were expressed (Guan et al., 2006). Indeed, the level of expression of *Nanog* and *SSEA1* suggests that these cells were already on their way to becoming ES-like cells. Seandel et al. (2007) also studied gene expression levels before and after the transition of cultured SSCs to ES-like cells. *Oct4* was present in both cell types, but *Nanog* and *Sox2* were strongly induced in ES-like cells, whereas the early spermatogonial markers *Stra8, Plzf* (*Zbtb16*), *c-Ret* and *Dazl* became inhibited. Besides these specific studies, Kanatsu-Shinohara et al. (2008b) also carried out a microarray study and found that a great many genes changed their expression levels during the transition from being a cultured SSC to an ES-like cell. Among these genes, over a 100 were induced more than 5-fold in ES-like cells as compared with cultured SSCs, and another 100 were inhibited more than 5-fold in ES-like cells. Clear differences between the patterns of genomic imprinting are also seen between cultured SSCs and ES-like cells. Kanatsu-Shinohara et al. (2004b) studied the imprinting pattern of three paternally (*H19, Meg3* and *Rasgrf1*) and two maternally (*Igf2r* and *Peg10*) imprinted regions in cultured SSCs and in the ES-like cells derived from them. Cultured SSCs show a completely androgenetic (paternal) imprinting pattern at the differentially methylated regions (DMRs) of these genes and loci; the DMRs of *H19* and *Meg3* are completely methylated and that of *Igf2r* is demethylated. By contrast, in the ES-like cells, the paternally imprinted regions are methylated to different degrees and the maternally imprinted regions (*Igf2r* and *Peg10*) are rarely methylated. Interestingly, the methylation patterns that are seen in the ES-like cells are not the same as those seen in proper ES cells, as the DMRs in ES cells are generally more methylated than those in ES-like cells, including the maternally imprinted regions. Furthermore, both Kanatsu-Shinohara et al. (2004b) and Seandel et al. (2007) reported that most of the ES-like cells obtained had a normal karyotype and that there was no evidence of clonal cytogenetic abnormalities. However, recently, Takahashi et al. (2007) did find some SSC-derived ES-like cells that were trisomic for chromosomes 8 or 11, which is a common chromosomal abnormality in ES cells.

In conclusion, the transition from cultured SSCs to ES-like cells is accompanied by extensive changes in gene expression, during which three of the four pluripotency genes (the exception being *Oct4*, which is already expressed in mouse SSCs) become expressed at higher levels, along with many other genes. Furthermore, changes occur in the genomic imprinting patterns of these cells as they undergo this transition. Although the ES-like cells acquire the expression of ES cell-specific genes, the expression pattern of these genes in ES-like cells is not identical to that seen in normal ES cells, with differences evident, for example, in the expression of brachyury, *Gdf3*, Forssman antigen, *Nog* and *Stra8*.

4. Applications of SSCs

4.1 Restoration of fertility

SSC transplantation may have application for treating male infertility in some cases. For example, high-dose chemotherapy and total body radiation treatment of cancer can cause permanent infertility. While adult men can cryopreserve a semen sample prior to their oncologic treatment, this is not an option for pre-adolescent boys who are not yet making sperm. Using methods similar to those already established for other species, it may be possible for these young cancer patients to cryopreserve testis cells or tissue prior to cancer treatment and use those tissues to achieve fertility after they are cured (Orwig & Schlatt, 2005; Goossens et al., 2008; Hermann et al., 2009). Recently, a non-human primate model of cancer survivorship to test the safety and feasibility of SSC transplantation in a species that is relevant to human physiology has been established (Hermann et al., 2007). Although SSC transplantation is not yet ready for the human fertility clinic, it may be reasonable for young cancer patients, with no other options to preserve their fertility, to cryopreserve testicular cells (Schlatt et al., 2009). Ginsberg and co-workers have been cryopreserving testicular tissue for young cancer patients since 2008 and report that this intervention is acceptable to parents and that testicular biopsies caused no acute adverse effects (Ginsberg et al., 2010). A human SSC culture system would be particularly useful in this setting because a few SSCs could be obtained in a small biopsy and expanded to a number sufficient for transplantion therapy.

4.2 Genetic modification
4.2.1 Genetic modification of rodents
The establishment of SSCs led to the development of a new strategy for generating a genetically modified animal as an alternative or a potentially superior method to the conventional ES-based technology. First, SSCs are infected or transfected with a viral or plasmid vector carrying a drug-resistant gene. Individual clones of drug-resistant SSCs cells are selected and expanded in vitro. After DNA analysis, genetically modified SSCs are transplanted to infertile mice. In theory, half of spermatozoa that developed from the SSCs carry the transgene. Finally, recipient male mice are crossed with female mice to yield heterozygous transgenic mice with a theoretical success rate of 50%. In the conventional ES cell-based technology, the frequency of heterozygous transgenic mice depends on the properties of chimera mice. In some cases, no germline chimera can be found in the chimera population. In this respect, SSCs which are committed to spermatogenesis are advantageous. When SSCs were transfected with a plasmid vector bearing a drugresistant gene and used for the production of transgenic mice based on this method, approximately 50% of offspring derived from a drug-resistant clone maintained a transgene (Kanatsu-Shinohara et al., 2005). Mice lacking a specific gene (i.e. occludin) by homologous DNA recombination was then successfully produced (Kanatsu-Shinohara et al., 2006). Homozygous mutant mice showed signs of chronic gastritis, osteoporosis and a loss of acidic granule in the salivary glands, similar to the occludin knockout mice generated using ES cells (Saitou et al., 2000). From these finding, it was demonstrated that SSCs can be used for gene targeting in a similar manner to ES cells.

4.2.2 Application to generation of knockout animals in domestic species
The method for generating genetically modified mice based on ES cell technology has become a conventional experimental technique, and contributed to the functional analyses of many genes. Under current culture conditions, SSCs grow slower than ES cells. For example, clonal expansion from a single transfected SSCs requires mixing with non-transfected SSCs to maintain cell densities during drug selection. Thus, SSC-based transgenic technology is not yet useful as ES cell-based technology. However, SSC-based

technology is potentially applicable to animal species other than mouse, and this is the greatest advantage of this technology. At present, ES cell-based transgenesis is feasible only in mice, and cloning by somatic cell nuclear transfer is extremely difficult or impossible due to the low proliferation potential of somatic cells and the poor success rates of nuclear transfer. If SSC culture conditions specific for animal species are established, animal transgenesis may become feasible in other species. Specifically, SSCs are derived from the testes of rat, hamster and cattle (Hamra et al., 2005; Ryu et al., 2005; Aponte et al., 2008; Kanatsu- Shinohara et al., 2008c). Hamsters have been historically difficult to manipulate genetically; however, the SSC technology may provide a good animal model. Bovine SSCs may be useful for the cattle industry as an important application. In particular, rats are important experimental animals that are larger than mice and have been used in various research areas. Therefore, SSC technology will be highly beneficial if it allows unlimited transgenesis in rats. Transplantation of SSCs is an essential step in SSC-based animal transgenesis and is technically challenging. The efficiency of this method is low in large animals (Ogawa et al., 1999b). Development of technologies for xenogeneic transplantation and in vivo spermatogenesis, in addition to the determination of culture conditions, are anticipated for universal application to various species in the future. With regard to xenogeneic transplantation from rats to mice, normal rat offspring were successfully born after transferring rat spermatids and spermatozoa developed in the mouse testes into rat oocytes by in vitro microinsemination (Shinohara et al., 2006; Kanatsu-Shinohara et al., 2008a).

4.3 Regenerative therapy

Recent advances in cellular therapies have led to the emergence of a multidisciplinary scientific approach to developing therapeutics for a wide variety of diseases and genetic disorders. Although most cell-based therapies currently consist of heterogeneous cell populations, it is anticipated that the standard of care needs well-characterized stem cell lines that can be modified to meet the individual needs of the patient. Extensive research in the area of regenerative medicine is focused on the development of cells, tissues and organs for the purpose of restoring function through transplantation. The general belief is that replacement, repair and restoration of function is best accomplished by cells, tissues or organs that can provide the appropriate physiological/metabolic functions more efficiently than any mechanical devices, recombinant proteins or chemical compounds. Several cell-based strategies are currently being investigated, including cell preparations from autologous parenchyma or established cell lines, as well as cell therapies derived from a variety of stem cell sources such as bone marrow or cord blood stem cells, embryonic stem cells, as well as cells, tissues and organs from genetically modified animals. Several lines of evidence have suggested extensive proliferation activity and pluripotency of germline stem cells, including SSCs. These characteristics provide new and unprecedented opportunities for the therapeutic use of SSCs for regenerative medicine.

Guan et al. (2006) succeeded in developing a procedure for the isolation and purification of SSCs from adult mouse testis. They were able to isolate and culture these cells in culture medium containing the precise combination of cellular growth factors needed for the cells to reproduce themselves in vitro. These cells were characterized with regard to their molecular profiles and these were compared via molecular profiling of embryonic stem cells using a stem cell array which contains relevant genes related to stem cell metabolism. The results indicate that SSCs share many molecular characteristics with embryonic stem cells. On the cellular level, SSCs resemble embryonic stem cells; they form an embryoid body structure after 2 weeks of culture. Stem cell potential of isolated SSCs was examined using the transplantation technique. This method allowed SSCs to recolonize the seminiferous tubules of germ cell-depleted mice and regenerate spermatogenesis. These cells are able to differentiate into various cell types of three germ layers *in vitro* (Guan et al., 2006, 2007). In contrast to ESCs, the use of SSCs for cell transplantation will allow establishment of individual cell-based therapy, because the donor and recipient are identical. In addition, any ethical problems are avoided.This approach provides an accessible *in vitro* model system for studies of mammalian gametogenesis, as well as for developing new strategies for reproductive engineering, infertility treatment and establishment of regenerative therapy.

4.4 Conservation biology

Thus far, most works on technologies of assisted reproduction in males have focused on mature spermatozoa. Successful semen collection, cryopreservation, and thawing techniques have been determined for a number of species. Advancements in the handling and storage of mature sperm have revolutionized the practice of both human and veterinary clinical reproductive medicine. In addition, these innovations have changed the nature of agriculture and agricultural economics, as artificial insemination has often supplanted natural breeding in intensive production regimens. Research on mature sperm is limited in that there are no cell culture systems that support spermatogenesis *in vitro*; therefore, sperm can only be obtained as primary cells from reproductively mature individuals. The stem cells that will produce sperm, on the other hand, are present in early neonates. Soon after birth in most species, gonocytes migrate to the basement membrane of the seminiferous cords; at this point in time the gonocytes transition into spermatogonia.

The development of reproductive technologies based on SSCs could preserve the breeding potential of males that die prior to puberty. This can be of great importance when the genetic contribution of a single individual could have significant impact on a long-term viability of a population. Examples of this would include attempts to preserve the genetic information represented in offspring of founder individuals in captive breeding programs, or attempts to propagate individuals with diseases that preclude natural mating. In addition, because SSCs can be maintained in culture, these cells are similar to ESCs in providing an opportunity for genetic manipulation that is not present in the terminally-differentiated spermatozoa. Efforts to take advantage of the attributes of SSCs have thus far focused on two technologies: spermatogonial stem cell transplantation (SSCT) and testis xenografting.

5. Conclusions

SSCs are the novel source of pluripotent stem cells that have an advantage over the iPS cells in numerous ways. Firstly, pluripotent cells from SSCs do not require the addition of any foreign genes as they are spontaneously generated in culture. Secondly, since pluripotent cells from SSCs are derived without viral transduction, they provide a safer alternative to iPS cells. Finally, SSCs and SSC-derived pluripotent cells can find immediate application in the field of regenerative medicine, fertility restoration, and genetic modification of mice and large animals and in the conservation of endangered species.

6. References

Aponte, P. M., Soda, T., Teerds, K. J., Mizrak, S. C., van de Kant, H. J. & de Rooij, D. G. (2008). Propagation of bovine spermatogonial stem cells in vitro, *Reproduction* 136(5): 543-57.

Arregui, L., Rathi, R., Megee, S.O., Honaramooz, A., Gomendio, M., Roldan, E.R. & Dobrinski, I. (2008). Xenografting of sheep testis tissue and isolated cells as a model for preservation of genetic material from endangered ungulates, *Reproduction* 136(1): 85-93.

Bartkova, J., Falck , J., Rajpert-De Meyts E, Skakkebaek, N.E., Lukas , J. & Bartek J. (2001). Chk2 tumour suppressor protein in human spermatogenesis and testicular germ-cell tumours, *Oncogene* 20(41): 5897-902.

Bendel-Stenzel, M., Anderson, R., Heasman , J. & Wylie, C. (1998). The origin and migration of primordial germ cells in the mouse, *Semin Cell Dev Biol* 9 (4): 393–400.

Borjigin, U., Davey, R., Hutton, K. & Herrid, M. (2010). Expression of promyelocytic leukaemia zinc-finger in ovine testis and its application in evaluating the enrichment efficiency of differential plating, *Reprod Fertil Dev* 22(5):733-42.

Boulanger, C. A., Mack, D. L., Booth, B. W. & Smith, G. H. (2007). Interaction with the mammary bovine spermatogonial stem cells in vitro, *Reproduction* 136 (5): 543-57.

Brinster, R.L. & Avarbock, M.R. (1994). Germline transmission of donor haplotype following spermatogonial transplantation, *Proc Natl Acad Sci USA* 91(24): 11303-7.

Brinster, R.L. (2002). Germline stem cell transplantation and transgenesis, *Science* 296 (5576): 2174-6.

Brinster, R.L. (2007). Male germline stem cells: from mice to men, *Science* 316(5823): 404–5.

Brinster, R.L. & Zimmermann, J.W. (1994). Spermatogenesis following male germ-cell transplantation, *Proc Natl Acad Sci USA* 91(24): 11298-302.

Buaas, F.W., Kirsh, A.L., Sharma, M., McLean , D.J., Morris ,J.L., Griswold, M.D., de Rooij, D.G., Braun ,R.E. (2004). Plzf is required in adult male germ cells for stem cell self-renewal, *Nat Genet* 36(6): 647-52.

Buageaw, A., Sukhwani, M., Ben-Yehudah, A., Ehmcke, J., Rawe, V.Y., Pholpramool, C., Orwig, K.E., Schlatt, S. (2005). GDNF family receptor alpha1 phenotype of spermatogonial stem cells in immature mouse testes, *Biol Reprod* 73(5): 1011-6.

Caires, K., Broady, J. & McLean, D. (2010) Maintaining the male germline: regulation of spermatogonial stem cells. *J Endocrinol* 205(2): 133-45.

Clermont, Y. & Perey, B. (1957). Quantitative study of the cell population of the seminiferous tubules in immature rats, *Am J Anat* 100(2): 241-67.

Clouthier, D. E., Avarbock, M.R., Maika, S.D., Hammer, R.E. & Brinster, R.L. (1996). Rat spermatogenesis in mouse testis, *Nature* 381(6581): 418–21.

Conrad, S., Renninger, M., Hennenlotter, J., Wiesner, T., Just, L., Bonin, M., Aicher, W., Bühring, H.J., Mattheus, U., Mack, A., Wagner, H.J., Minger, S., Matzkies, M., Reppel, M., Hescheler, J., Sievert, K.D., Stenzl, A. & Skutella T. (2008). Generation of pluripotent stem cells from adult human testis, *Nature* 456 (7220): 344–9.

Costoya, J.A., Hobbs, R.M., Barna, M., Cattoretti, G., Manova, K., Sukhwani, M., Orwig, K.E., Wolgemuth, D.J., Pandolfi, P.P. (2004). Essential role of Plzf in maintenance of spermatogonial stem cells, *Nat Genet* 36(6): 653-9.

Dirami, G., Ravindranath, N., Pursel, V. & Dym, M. (1999). Effects of stem cell factor and granulocyte macrophage-colony stimulating factor on survival of porcine type A spermatogonia cultured in KSOM, *Biol Reprod* 61: 225-30.

Dobrinski, I., Avarbock, M.R. & Brinster, R.L. (1999a) Transplantation of germ cells from rabbits and dogs into mouse testes, *Biol Reprod* 61(5): 1331–9.

Dobrinski, I., Avarbock, M.R. & Brinster, R.L. (2000). Germ cell transplantation from large domestic animals into mouse testes, *Mol Reprod Dev* 57(3): 270–9.

Dobrinski, I., Ogawa, T., Avarbock, M.R. & Brinster, R.L. (1999b). Computer assisted image analysis to assess colonization of recipient seminiferous tubules by spermatogonial stem cells from transgenic donor mice, *Mol Reprod Dev* 53(2): 142–8.

Dolci, S., Pellegrini, M., Di Agostino, S., Geremia, R. & Rossi, P. (2001). Signaling through extracellular signal-regulated kinase is required for spermatogonial proliferative response to stem cell factor, *J Biol Chem* 276(43): 40225-33.

Dym, M., He, Z., Jiang, J., Pant, D. & Kokkinaki, M. (2009). Spermatogonial stem cells: unlimited potential, *Reprod Fertil Dev*. 21(1): 15-21.

Dym, M., Kokkinaki, M. & He, Z. (2009). Spermatogonial stem cells: mouse and humancomparisons. *Birth Defects Res C Embryo Today* 87(1): 27-34.

Ehmcke, J. & Schlatt, S. (2008). Animal models for fertility preservation in the male, *Reproduction*. 136(6): 717–23.

Fujihara, M., Kim, S.M., Minami, N., Yamada, M. & Imai, H. (2011). Characterization and In Vitro Culture of Male Germ Cells from Developing Bovine Testis, *J Reprod Dev*. 57(3): 355-64.

Ginsberg, J.P., Carlson, C.A., Lin, K., Hobbie, W.L., Wigo, E., Wu, X., Brinster, R.L. & Kolon, T.F. (2010). An experimental protocol for fertility preservation in prepubertal boys recently diagnosed with cancer: a report of acceptability and safety, *Hum Reprod* 25(1): 37-41.

Ginsburg, M., Snow, M.H. & McLaren, A. (1990). Primordial germ cells in the mouse embryo during gastrulation, *Development* 110(2): 521-8.

Giuili, G., Tomljenovic, A., Labrecque, N., Oulad-Abdelghani, M., Rassoulzadegan, M. & Cuzin, F. (2002). Murine spermatogonial stem cells: targeted transgene expression and purification in an active state, *EMBO Rep* 3(8): 753-9.

Goel, S., Sugimoto, M., Minami , N., Yamada, M., Kume, S. & Imai, H. (2007). Identification, isolation, and in vitro culture of porcine gonocytes, *Biol Reprod* 77(1): 127-37.

Goel, S., Fujihara, M., Minami, N., Yamada, M. & Imai, H. (2008). Expression of NANOG, but not POU5F1, points to the stem cell potential of primitive germ cells in neonatal pig testis, *Reproduction* 135(6): 785-95.

Goel, S., Fujihara, M., Tsuchiya, K., Takagi, Y., Minami, N., Yamada, M. & Imai, H. (2009). Multipotential ability of primitive germ cells from neonatal pig testis cultured in vitro, *Reprod Fertil Dev* 21(5): 696-708.

Goel, S., Mahla, R.S., Suman, S.K., Reddy, N. & Imai, H. (2010a). UCHL-1 Protein Expression Specifically Marks Spermatogonia in Wild Bovid Testis. *Euro J Wildlife Res* DOI: 10.1007/s10344-010-0454-1.

Goel, S., Reddy, N., Mandal, S., Fujihara, M., Kim, S.M. & Imai, H. (2010b). Spermatogonia-specific proteins expressed in prepubertal buffalo (Bubalus bubalis) testis and their utilization for isolation and in vitro cultivation of spermatogonia, *Theriogenology* 74 (7): 1221-32.

Goel, S., Reddy, N., Mahla, R.S., Suman, S.K., & Pawar, R.M. (2011). Spermatogonial stem cells in the testis of an endangered bovid: Indian Black buck (Antelope cervicapra L), *Animal Reproduction* Science DOI 10.1016/j.anireprosci.2011.05.012.

Golestaneh, N., Kokkinaki, M., Pant, D., Jiang, J., DeStefano, D., Fernandez-Bueno, C., Rone, J.D., Haddad, B.R., Gallicano, G.I. & Dym, M. (2009). Pluripotent stem cells derived from adult human testes. *Stem Cells Dev* 18(8): 1115-26.

Goossens, E., Geens, M., De Block, G. & Tournaye, H. (2008). Spermatogonial survival in long-term human prepubertal xenografts, *Fertil. Steril.* 90(5): 2019-22.

Guan, K., Wagner, S., Unsold , B. et al. (2007).Generation of functional cardiomyocytes from adult mouse spermatogonial stem cells, *Circ Res.* 100(11): 1615-25.

Guan, K., Nayernia, K., Maier, L. S., Wagner, S., Dressel, R., Lee, J. H., Nolte, J., Wolf, F., Li, M., Engel, W. & Hasenfuss, G. (2006). Pluripotency of spermatogonial stem cells from adult mouse testis, *Nature* 440(7088): 1199 -1203.

Hamra, F.K., Chapman, K.M., Nguyen, D. M.,Williams-Stephens, A. A., Hammer, R. E. & Garbers, D. L. (2005). Self renewal, expansion, and transfection of rat spermatogonial stem cells in culture, *Proc Natl Acad Sci USA* 102(48): 17430-5.

Hanna, J., Wernig, M., Markoulaki, S. Sun, C.W., Meissner, A., Cassady, J.P., Beard, C., Brambrink, T., Wu, L.C., Townes, T.M. & Jaenisch, R. (2007). Treatment of sickle cell anemia mouse model with iPS cells generated from autologous skin, *Science* 318(5858): 1920-3.

He, Z., Jiang, J., Hofmann, M.C. & Dym, M. (2007). Gfra1 silencing in mouse spermatogonial stem cells results in their differentiation via the inactivation of RET tyrosine kinase, *Biol Reprod* 77(4): 723-33.

He Z, Kokkinaki, M., Jiang, J., Dobrinski, I. & Dym, M. (2010).Isolation, characterization, and culture of human spermatogonia, *Biol Reprod* 82(2): 363-72.

Hermann, B. M., Sukhwani, M., Hansel, M. & Orwig, K. (2009). Spermatogonial stem cells in higher primates: are there differences to those in rodents? *Reproduction* 139: 479-493.

Hermann, B.P., Sukhwani, M., Lin, C.C., Sheng, Y., Tomko, J., Rodriguez, M., Shuttleworth, J.J., McFarland, D., Hobbs, R.M., Pandolfi, P.P., Schatten, G.P. & Orwig KE (2007). Characterization, cryopreservation and ablation of spermatogonial stem cells in adult rhesus macaques, *Stem Cells* 25(9): 2330-8.

Herrid, M., Davey, R.J., Hutton, K., Colditz, I.G. & Hill, J.R. (2009). A comparison of methods for preparing enriched populations of bovine spermatogonia, *Reprod Fertil Dev* 21(3): 393-9.

Hofmann, M.C., Braydich-Stolle, L., Dym, M. (2005 Mar). Isolation of male germ-line stem cells;influence of GDNF. *Dev Biol.* 279(1): 114-24.

Honaramooz, A., Behboodi, E., Blash, S., Megee, S.O. & Dobrinski, I. (2003). Germ cell transplantation in goats, *Mol Reprod Dev* 64(4): 422-8.

Honaramooz, A., Li, M.W., Penedo, M.C.T., Meyers, S. & Dobrinski, I. (2004). Accelerated maturation of primate testis by xenografting into mice, *Biol Reprod* 70(5): 1500-3.

Honaramooz, A., Megee, S.O. & Dobrinski, I. (2002). Germ cell transplantation in pigs, *Biol Reprod* 66(1): 21-8.

Honaramooz , A., Snedaker, A., Boiani , M., Schöler, H., Dobrinski, I. & Schlatt, S. (2002). Sperm from neonatal mammalia testes grafted in mice, *Nature* 418(6899): 778-81.

Hu, H. M., Xu, F. C., Li, W. & Wu, S. H. (2007). Biological characteristics of spermatogonial stem cells cultured in conditions for fibroblasts , *J Clin Rehab Tiss Engin Res* 11: 6611 -4.

Jiang, F.X. & Short, R.V. (1995). Male germ cell transplantation in rats: apparent synchronization of spermatogenesis between host and donor seminiferous epithelia, *Int J Androl* 18(6): 326-30.

Kanatsu-Shinohara, M., Toyokuni, S., Shinohara, T. (2004a). CD9 is a surface marker on mouse and rat male germline stem cells, *Biol Reprod* 70 (1): 70–5.

Kanatsu-Shinohara, M., Ikawa, M., Takehashi, M., Ogonuki, N., Miki, H., Inoue, K., Kazuki, Y., Lee, J., Toyokuni, S., Oshimura, M., Ogura, A. & Shinohara, T. (2006). Production of knockout mice by random and targeted mutagenesis in spermatogonial stem cells, *Proc. Natl Acad Sci USA* 103(21): 8018–23.

Kanatsu-Shinohara, M., Inoue, K., Lee, J., Yoshimoto, M., Ogonuki, N., Miki, H., Baba, S., Kato, T., Kazuki, Y., Toyokuni, S., Toyoshima M., Niwa O., Oshimura M., Heike T., Nakahata T., Ishino F., Ogura A., Shinohara T. (2004b). Generation of pluripotent stem cells from neonatal mouse testis, *Cell* 119(7): 1001 -12.

Kanatsu-Shinohara, M., Kato, M., Takehashi, M., Morimoto, H., Takashima, S., Chuma, S., Nakatsuji, N., Hirabayashi, M. & Shinohara, T. (2008a). Production of transgenic rats via lentiviral transduction and xenogeneic transplantation of spermatogonial stem cells, *Biol Reprod* 79(6): 1121–8.

Kanatsu-Shinohara, M., Lee, J., Inoue, K., Ogonuki, N., Miki, H., Toyokuni, S., Ikawa, M., Nakamura, T., Ogura, A. & Shinohara, T. (2008b). Pluripotency of a single spermatogonial stem cell in mice, *Biol Reprod* 78 (4): 681 -7.

Kanatsu-Shinohara, M., Toyokuni, S. & Shinohara, T. (2005). Genetic selection of mouse male germline stem cells in vitro: offspring from single stem cells, *Biol Reprod* 72(1): 236–40.

Kim, J.B., Zaehres, H., Wu, G., Gentile, L., Ko, K., Sebastiano, V., Araúzo-Bravo, M.J., Ruau, D., Han, D.W., Zenke, M. & Schöler, H.R. (2008). Pluripotent stem cells induced from adult neural stem cells by reprogramming with two factors, *Nature* 454(7204): 646-50.

Kim,Y., Selvaraj, V., Dobrinski, I., Lee, H., Mcentee, M.C. & Travis, A.J. (2006).Recipient preparation and mixed germ cell isolation for spermatogonial stem cell transplantation in domestic cats, *J Androl* 27(2): 248–56.

Kluin, P. M. & de Rooij, D. G. (1981). A comparison between the morphology and cell kinetics of gonocytes and adult type undifferentiated spermatogonia in the mouse, *Int J Androl* 4: 475–493.

Kossack, N., Meneses, J. & Shefi, S., Nguyen, H.N., Chavez, S., Nicholas, C., Gromoll, J., Turek, P.J., Reijo-Pera, R.A. (2009). Isolation and characterization of pluripotent human spermatogonial stem cell-derived cells, *Stem Cells* 27(1): 138–49.

Kubota, H., Avarbock, M.R. & Brinster, R.L. (2003). Spermatogonial stem cells share some, but not all, phenotypic and functional characteristics with other stem cells, *Proc Natl Acad Sci USA*100(11): 6487-92.

Kwon, J., Wang, Y.L., Setsuie, R., Sekiguchi, S., Sakurai, M., Sato, Y., Lee, W.W., Ishii, Y., Kyuwa, S., Noda, M., Wada, K. & Yoshikawa, Y. (2004). Developmental regulation of ubiquitinC-terminal hydrolase isozyme expression during spermatogenesis in mice, *Biol Reprod.* 71(2): 515-21.

Lawson, K.A., Dunn, N.R., Roelen, B.A., Zeinstra, L.M., Davis, A.M., Wright, C.V., Korving, J.P. & Hogan, B.L. (1999). Bmp4 is required for the generation of primordial germ cells in the mouse embryo, *Genes Dev* 13(4): 424–36.

Looijenga, L.H., Stoop, H., de Leeuw, H.P., de Gouveia Brazao, C.A., Gillis, A.J., van Roozendaal, K.E., van Zoelen, E.J., Weber, R.F., Wolffenbuttel, K.P., van Dekken, H., Honecker, F., Bokemeyer, C., Perlman, E.J., Schneider,D.T., Kononen, J., Sauter, G.& Oosterhuis, J.W. (2003). POU5F1 (OCT3/4) identifies cells with pluripotent potential in human germ cell tumors, *Cancer Res* 63(9): 2244-50.

Luo, J., Megee, S., Rathi, R. & Dobrinski, I. (2006). Protein gene product 9.5 is a spermatogonia-specific marker in the pig testis: application to enrichment and culture of porcine spermatogonia, *Mol Reprod Dev* 73(12): 1531-40.

McCarrey, J. (1993). Development of the germ cell, In: *Cell and molecular biology of the testis* (eds Desjardins, C. & Ewing, L. L.), (pp. 58–89), Oxford University Press , ISBN13: 9780195062694 , New York.

McLaren, A. (2003). Primordial germ cells in the mouse, *Dev. Biol.* 262(1): 1–15.

Meissner, A., Wernig, M. & Jaenisch, R. (2007). Direct reprogramming of genetically unmodified fibroblasts into pluripotent stem cells, *Nat Biotechnol* 25(10):1177–81.

Meng, X., Lindahl, M., Hyvönen, M.E., Parvinen, M., de Rooij, D.G., Hess, M.W., Raatikainen-Ahokas, A., Sainio K., Rauvala , H., Lakso, M., Pichel ,J.G., Westphal, H., Saarma, M. & Sariola, H. (2000). Regulation of cell fate decision of undifferentiated spermatogonia by GDNF, *Science* 287(5457): 1489-93.

Boulanger, C.A., Mack, D.L., Booth, B.W. & Smith, G.H. (2007) Interaction with the mammary microenvironment redirects spermatogenic cell fate in vivo, *Proc Natl Acad Sci USA* 104 (10): 3871 -6.

Nagano, M., Avarbock, M.R. & Brinster, R.L. (1999). Pattern and kinetics of mouse donor spermatogonial stem cell colonization in recipient testes, *Biol Reprod* 60(6): 1429–36.

Nagano, M., McCarrey, J.R. & Brinster, R.L. (2001). Primate spermatogonial stem cells colonize mouse testes, *Biol. Reprod.* 64(5): 1409–16.

Nagano, M., Patrizio, P. & Brinster, R.L. (2002). Long-term survival of human spermatogonial stem cells in mouse testes, *Fertility and Sterility* 78(6): 1225–33.

Nakai, M., Kaneko, H., Somfai,T., Maedomari, N., Ozawa, M., Noguchi, J., Ito, J., Kashiwazaki, N. & Kikuchi, K. (2010). Production of viable piglets for the first time using sperm derived from ectopic testicular xenografts, *Reproduction* 139(2): 331–5.

Naughton, C.K., Jain, S., Strickland, A.M., Gupta, A. & Milbrandt, J. (2006). Glial cell-line derived neurotrophic factor-mediated RET signaling regulates spermatogonial stem cell fate, *Biol Reprod* 74(2): 314-21.

Oakberg, E.F. (1956). Duration of spermatogenesis in the mouse and timing of stages of the cycle of the seminiferous epithelium, *Am J Anat* 99(3): 507-16.

Oatley, J.M., Reeves, J.J. & McLean, D.J. (2005). Establishment of spermatogenesis in neonatal bovine testicular tissue following ectopic xenografting varies with donor age, *Biol Reprod* 72(2): 358–64.

Ogawa, T., Dobrinski, I., Avarbock, M.R. & Brinster, R.L. (1999a). Xenogeneic spermatogenesis following transplantation of hamster germ cells to mouse testes, *Biol Reprod* 60(2): 515-21.

Ogawa, T., Dobrinski, I. & Brinster, R.L. (1999b). Recipient preparation is critical for spermatogonial transplantation in the rat, *Tissue and Cell* 31(5):461–72.

Ohbo, K., Yoshida, S., Ohmura, M., Ohneda, O., Ogawa, T., Tsuchiya, H., Kuwana, T., Kehler, J., Abe, K., Schöler, H.R. & Suda, T. (2003). Identification and characterization of stem cells in prepubertal spermatogenesis in mice small star, filled. *Dev Biol* 258(1): 209-25.

Ohta, H., Yomogida, K., Yamada, S., Okabe, M. & Nishimune, Y. (2000). Real-time observation of transplanted 'green germ cells': proliferation and differentiation of stem cells, *Dev Growth Differ* 42(2):105–12.

Okita, K., Ichisaka, T., Yamanaka, S. (2007). Generation of germline-competent induced pluripotent stem cells, *Nature* 448(7151): 313–17.

Orwig, K.E.& Schlatt, S. (2005). Cryopreservation and transplantation of spermatogonia and testicular tissue for preservation of male fertility, J Natl Cancer Inst Monogr 34: 51–6.

Phillips, B.T., Gassei, K. & Orwig, K.E.(2010). Spermatogonial stem cell regulation and spermatogenesis. *Philos Trans R Soc Lond B Biol Sci* 365(1546): 1663-78.

Rajpert-De Meyts, E., Jacobsen, G.K., Bartkova, J., Aubry, F., Samson, M., Bartek, J. & Skakkebaek, N.E. (2003). The immunohistochemical expression pattern of Chk2, p53, p19INK4d, MAGE-A4 and other selected antigens provides new evidence for the premeiotic origin of spermatocytic seminoma, *Histopathology* 42(3): 217-26.

Rathi, R., Honaramooz, A., Zeng, W., Turner, R. & Dobrinski, I. (2006). Germ cell development in equine testis tissue xenografted into mice, *Reproduction* 131(6): 1091–8.

Rathi, R., Zeng, W., Megee, S., Conley, A., Meyers, S. & Dobrinski, I. (2008). Maturation of testicular tissue from infant monkeys after xenografting into mice, *Endocrinology* 149(10): 5288–96.

Reding, S.C., Stepnoski, A.L., Cloninger, E.W. & Oatley, J.M. (2010). THY1 is a conserved marker of undifferentiated spermatogonia in the pre-pubertal bull testis, *Reproduction* 139(5): 893-903.

Rodriguez-Sosa, J.R., Dobson, H. & Hahnel, A. (2006). Isolation and transplantation of spermatogonia in sheep, *Theriogenology* 66(9): 2091-103.

Ryu, B.Y., Kubota, H., Avarbock, M.R. & Brinster, R.L. (2005). Conservation of spermatogonial stem cell self-renewal signalling between mouse and rat, *Proc Natl Acad Sci U S A* 102(40): 14302–07.

Saitou, M., Furuse, M., Sasaki, H., Schulzke, J. D., Fromm, M., Takano, H., Noda, T. & Tsukita, S. (2000). Complex phenotype of mice lacking occludin, a component of tight junction strands, *Mol. Biol. Cell* 11(12): 4131–42.

Schaller, J., Glander, H.J, Dethloff, J. (1993). Evidence of beta 1 integrins and fibronectin on spermatogenic cells in human testis, *Hum Reprod.* 8(11):1873-8.

Schlatt, S., Foppiani, L., Rolf, C., Weinbauer, G.F., Nieschlag, E. (2002a). Germ cell transplantation into X-irradiated monkey testes, *Hum Reprod.* 17 (1): 55–62.

Schlatt, S., Kim, S.S., Gosden, R. (2002b). Spermatogenesis and steroidogenesis in mouse, hamster and monkey testicular tissue after cryopreservation and heterotopic grafting to castrated hosts, *Reproduction* 124(3): 339-46.

Schlatt, S., Ehmcke, J., Jahnukainen, K. (2009). Testicular stem cells for fertility preservation: preclinical studies on male germ cell transplantation and testicular grafting, *Pediatr Blood Cancer* 53(2): 274–80.

Schnieders, F., Dörk, T., Arnemann, J., Vogel, T., Werner, M. &Schmidtke, J. (1996). Testis-specific protein, Y-encoded (TSPY) expression in testicular tissues, *Hum Mol Genet* 5(11): 1801-7.

Schrans-Stassen, B.H.G.J, van de Kant, H.J.G, de Rooij, D.G & van Pelt, A.M.M. (1999). Differential expression of c-kit in mouse undifferentiated and differentiating type A spermatogonia, *Endocrinology* 140(12): 5894-900.

Seandel, M., James, D., Shmelkov, S.V., Falciatori, I., Kim, J., Chavala, S., Scherr, D. S., Zhang, F., Torres, R., Gale, N. W. ancopoulos, G.D., Murphy, A., Valenzuela, D.M., Hobbs, R.M., Pandolfi, P.P. & Rafii, S. (2007). Generation of functional multipotent adult stem cells from GPR125+ germline progenitors, *Nature* 449 (7160): 346 -50.

Shinohara, T., Avarbock, M.R. & Brinster, R.L. (1999). beta1- and alpha6-integrin are surface markers on mouse spermatogonial stem cells, *Proc Natl Acad Sci USA* 96(10):5504-9.

Shinohara, T., Orwig, K.E., Avarbock, M.R, Brinster, R.L. (2003). Restoration of spermatogenesis in infertile mice by Sertoli cell transplantation, *Biol Reprod* 68(3): 1064–71.

Shinohara, T., Kato, M., Takehashi, M., Lee, J., Chuma, S., Nakatsuji,N., Kanatsu-Shinohara, M. & Hirabayashi, M. (2006). Rats produced by interspecies spermatogonial transplantation in mice and in vitro microinsemination, *Proc. Natl Acad. Sci. U S A* 103(37): 13624–8.

Stadtfeld, M., Nagaya, M., Utikal, J., Weir, G. &Hochedlinger, K. (2008). Induced pluripotent stem cells generated without viral integration, *Science* 322(5903): 945–46.

Takahashi, K., Tanabe, K., Ohnuki, M., Narita, M., Ichisaka, T., Tomoda, K., Yamanaka, S. (2007). Induction of pluripotent stem cells from adult human fibroblasts by defined factors, *Cell* 131(5): 861–72.

Takahashi, K. & Yamanaka, S. (2006). Induction of pluripotent stem cells from mouse embryonic and adult fibroblast cultures by defined factors, *Cell* 126(4): 663 -76.

Takehashi, M., Kanatsu-Shinohara, M., Miki, H., Lee, J., Kazuki, Y., Inoue, K., Ogonuki, N., Toyokuni, S., Oshimura, M., Ogura, A. & Shinohara, T. (2007). Production of knockout mice by gene targeting in multipotent germline stem cells, *Dev Biol* 312(1): 344 -52.

Tohonen,V., Ritzen, E. M., Nordqvist, K., Wedell, A. (2003). Male sex determination and prenatal differentiation of the testis, *Endocr Dev* 5: 1-23.

Tokuda, M., Kadokawa, Y., Kurahashi, H. & Marunouchi, T. (2007). CDH1 is a specific marker for undifferentiated spermatogonia in mouse testes, *Biol Reprod* 76(1): 130-41.

Tokunaga, Y., Imai, S., Torii, R. & Maeda, T. (1999). Cytoplasmic liberation of protein geneproduct 9.5 during the seasonal regulation of spermatogenesis in the monkey (Macaca fuscata), *Endocrinology* 140(4): 1875-83.

Wernig, M., Meissner, A., Foreman, R., Brambrink, T., Ku, M., Hochedlinger, K., Bernstein, B. E. & Jaenisch, R. (2007). In vitro reprogramming of fibroblasts into a pluripotent ES-cell-like state, *Nature* 448(7151): 318 -24.

Wrobel, K.H., Bickel, D., Kujat, R. & Schimmel, M. (1995). Configuration and distribution of bovine spermatogonia. *Cell Tissue Res.* 279(2): 277-89.

Ying, Y., Qi, X. & Zhao, G. Q. (2001). Induction of primordial germ cells from murine epiblasts by synergistic action of BMP4 and BMP8B signaling pathways, *Proc Natl Acad Sci USA* 98(14): 7858–62.

Yoshida, S., Sukeno, M. & Nabeshima, Y. (2007). A vasculature-associated niche for undifferentiated spermatogonia in the mouse testis, *Science* 317(5845): 1722-6.

Yoshida, S., Sukeno, M., Nakagawa, T., Ohbo, K., Nagamatsu, G., Suda, T. & Nabeshima, Y.(2006) The first round of mouse spermatogenesis is a distinctive program that lacks the self-renewing spermatogonia stage, *Development* 133(8): 1495–1505.

Yoshida, S., Takakura, A., Ohbo, K., Abe, K., Wakabayashi, J., Yamamoto, M., Suda, T. & Nabeshima, Y. (2004). Neurogenin3 delineates the earliest stages of spermatogenesis in the mouse testis, *Dev Biol* 269(2): 447-58.

Yoshinaga, K., Nishikawa, S., Ogawa, M., Hayashi, S., Kunisada, T., Fujimoto, T. & Nishikawa, S. (1991). Role of c-kit in mouse spermatogenesis: identification of spermatogonia as a specific site of c-kit expression and function, *Development* 113(2): 689-99.

11

Amniotic Fluid Stem Cells

Gianni Carraro, Orquidea H. Garcia,
Laura Perin, Roger De Filippo and David Warburton
Saban Research Institute, Children's Hospital Los Angeles
USA

1. Introduction

The amniotic fluid or liquor amnii, was first isolated and studied during the beginning of the 20th century (Brace et al., 1989). More recently, in the 1960s and 1970s there was an increased interest in characterization and culture of the cells contained in the amniotic fluid (Huisjes HJ, 1970; Marchant GS, 1971). Nevertheless, most all of these studies were directed at using amniotic fluid, and the cells contained within, for determining the health of the fetus during development, or to provide a general characterization of the amniotic fluid. Although the discovery of stem cells, in particular bone marrow stem cells, occurred in the 1960's, it was not until recently that the possibility of isolating stem cells from the amniotic fluid was investigated. Amniotic fluid stem cell isolation and characterization is therefore fairly recent, dating back to the early 1990's (Torricelli et al., 1993).

The study of amniotic fluid-derived stem cells (AFDSCs) has captured the attention of researchers and clinicians for several reasons. First, AFDSCs can be collected during amniocentesis and isolated from material that would be otherwise discarded. Therefore, their use is not subject to the ethical debate that surrounds the use of embryonic stem cells. Second, like other fetal derived stem cells, storage of AFDSCs is easy and achieved at minimal costs. AFDSC populations can be easily expanded, and have shown the capability of being stored over long periods of time with no adverse effects (Da Sacco et al., 2010). Furthermore, the "banking" of AFDSCs from developing fetuses, may guarantee a source of stem cells with a matching immune profile to that of the recipient. Most importantly, the extensive characterization of a specific subset of AFDSCs positive for the marker c-Kit+ (De Coppi et al., 2007), have displayed no tumor formation following transplant into an animal model, even after several months. These cells, known simply as amniotic fluid stem cells (AFSC) have been at the forefront of AFDSC research and will be discussed in depth later. Finally, as a source of stem cells collected before birth AFDSCs may become an invaluable source of stem cells for direct treatment of various genetic disorders treatable in utero (Turner CG et al., 2009).

The potential applications and implications of AFDSCs in regenerative medicine and therapeutic treatments are significant, however; AFDSCs research is still in its infancy and much work is required to properly characterize AFDSCs and determine their effectiveness. In this chapter, we describe the different AFDSCs that have been isolated to date, list their characteristics, and provide an overview of the different organs in which AFDSCs have been used in vitro or in vivo to develop this stem cell population into a viable therapeutic strategy.

2. The amniotic cavity

The amniotic fluid is contained in the amniotic cavity that, in humans, starts forming as early as seven days post fertilization, and is delimited by a membrane called amnion. The formation of the amniotic cavity is a result of the cavitation of the epiblast. The amnion is formed by the cells of the epiblast, by the side facing the cytotrophoblast. This is the first appearance of the amniotic ectoderm, and at this stage it is still a continuum of the portion of the epiblast that will form the embryo. The amnion formation is completed at fourteen days post fertilization and is constituted of two layers: the amniotic ectoderm (inner layer facing the amniotic fluid) and the amniotic mesoderm (outer layer). The amnion has the important function of protecting the embryo and controlling the composition and the volume of the amniotic fluid. In humans, after seventeen weeks of gestation the amnion becomes surrounded and fused with another membrane, the chorion, and is therefore incorporated into the placenta. At the beginning of the formation of the amniotic cavity, active transport of solutes from the amnion, followed by passive movement of water, comprise the amniotic fluid.

In mice the amniotic cavity starts forming at embryonic stage E0.5 as a result of apoptotic events in the epiblast. At this stage, there is still the presence of a proamniotic cavity and the amnion that will start forming during gastrulation, is not yet defined. At approximately day E7.5 the amniotic cavity is formed and one day later the embryo starts the rotation process. At the end of the rotation, the embryo will be surrounded by the amnion. Surrounding the amnion are two more membranes, the visceral yolk sac and most externally the parietal yolk sac (Kaufman MH, 1992). These membranes represent three distinct layers surrounding the mouse embryo. Differently from human, in mice, the amnion does not fuse with the chorion and is not included in the placenta.

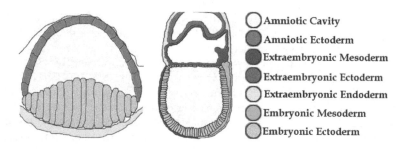

Amniotic Cavity
Amniotic Ectoderm
Extraembryonic Mesoderm
Extraembryonic Ectoderm
Extraembryonic Endoderm
Embryonic Mesoderm
Embryonic Ectoderm

Fig. 1. Amniotic cavity formation

Twelve days post fertilization the human amniotic cavity is delimitated by the amnion (that at this stage is composed by the amniotic ectoderm) and the embryonic ectoderm (left). In the 7.5-day mouse embryo (right) the amnion is formed by the amniotic mesoderm and the amniotic ectoderm.

In mammals the embryo is immersed in the amniotic fluid contained inside the amniotic cavity. In human (left) the cavity is delimited by the amniotic ectoderm and the amniotic mesoderm that constitute the amnion, and by the chorion. The amniotic ectoderm is in direct contact with the amniotic fluid. In mouse (right) the amnion is surrounded by two extra membranes, the visceral and parietal yolk sac.

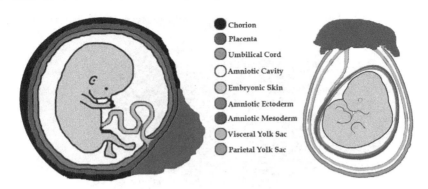

Chorion
Placenta
Umbilical Cord
Amniotic Cavity
Embryonic Skin
Amniotic Ectoderm
Amniotic Mesoderm
Visceral Yolk Sac
Parietal Yolk Sac

Fig. 2. Extra-embryonic membranes

3. The amniotic fluid

The amniotic fluid is the liquid present in the amniotic cavity and is constituted of about 98% water. This volume and composition change continuously during the different gestational stages. The volume of the amniotic fluid at the beginning of the pregnancy is multiple times the volume of the fetus, but at the end of gestation, at forty weeks, it will represent only a quarter of the volume of the fetus. Early during development, when the fetus has not yet started urination and deglutition, the plasma from the mother is surmised to play an important role in the composition of the amniotic fluid, and even though the mechanism is not completely understood, active transport of solutes is probably present between the amnion into the amniotic cavity, therefore creating a gradient for water recruitment (Bacchi Modena A and Fieni S, 2004). The exchange of fluid through the skin that occurs until keratinization is also an important contributor to the osmolarity of the amniotic fluid. After keratinization, urination, swallowing and secretion due to breathing events also contributes to the composition of the amniotic fluid. Urine start to be part of the composition of the amniotic fluid at about eight weeks and its amount will increase during gestation, reaching a flow rate of up to 900 ml/day at the end of gestation (Lotgering FK et al., 1986). Similarly, at approximately eight weeks, the fetus begins swallowing and secreting material including lung fluid and urine. Secretion of lung fluid is due to an active transport of chloride through the epithelium of the lung (Adamson TM et al., 1973). Sampling of amniotic fluid at later stages of the pregnancy is used to monitor lung development via the presence or absence of surfactant lipids and proteins secreted into the amniotic fluid.

The cells present in the amniotic fluid have both embryonic and extraembryonic origins. Approximately forty years ago, researchers attempted to characterize these cells by cytological and biochemical parameters (Morris HHB et al., 1974). Early characterization distinguished four epithelial cell types in the amniotic fluid: large eosinophilic cells, large cyanophilic cells, small round cyanophilic cells, and polygonal eosinophilic cells (Huisjes HJ, 1970). Today we know that most of the cells of the amniotic fluid are derived from the skin, digestive, urinary (Fig. 3) and pulmonary tracts of the fetus and from the surrounding amnion. We also know that the proportion and type of cells changes continuously during the different gestational stages. Some cells may also be derived from the mother, passing through the placenta into the fluid itself. The size of the cells contained in the fluid can range from 6um to 50um and the shape can vary notably from round to squamous in morphology (Siddiqui and Atala, 2004).

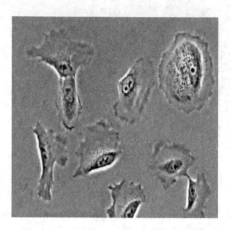

Fig. 3. Kidney amniotic fluid cells

Amniotic fluid contains cell populations derived from several different tissues. Pictured above is a population of cells isolated using kidney specific markers (40X magnification).

4. Amniotic fluid-derived stem cells

AFDSCs belong to the group of stem cells present in extra embryonic tissues; all sharing the feature of belonging to material that is discarded after birth or that can be collected during amniocentesis. Besides the amniotic fluid, the amnion, umbilical cord and placenta have shown to contain stem cells that can be isolated at birth (Bailo M et al., 2004; Banas RA et al, 2008; Brunstein CG et al., 2006; Fukuchi Y et al., 2004).

The first studies of AFDSCs, were completed using mesenchymal amniocytes isolated from sheep. These cells showed the ability to expand in vitro and to integrate into a scaffold (Kaviani A et al., 2001). In the following years, the identification of cells expressing the marker Oct4 (Prusa et al., 2003), or co-expressing Oct4, CD44 and CD105 (Tsai et al., 2004) were discovered in amniotic fluid. More recently a clonal population of AFDSCs derived from human and mouse were isolated and characterized (De Coppi P et al., 2007). These cells named AFSCs, were isolated through positive selection for the marker CD117 (or c-Kit), and represented 1% of cells derived from amniocentesis. AFSCs express the marker of "stemness", Oct4, and the embryonic stem cell (ESC) marker SSEA-4. Furthermore AFSCs express markers characteristic of mesenchymal and neural stem cells such as CD29, CD44, CD73, CD90, and CD105. Interestingly, these cells are negative for markers of hematopoietic stem cells such as CD34 and CD133.

Recently, a screen for the expression profile of cells present in the amniotic fluid was reported (Da Sacco S et al., 2010). This screening analyzed cells obtained from human amniotic fluid between gestational weeks 15 to 20 and showed that markers such as Oct4 and CD117 are stably expressed during gestation. Furthermore, while markers for ectoderm are stably expressed during gestation, markers for the early endoderm and mesoderm are more abundant during early gestation and tend to disappear after 17 to 18 weeks. During the same time, organ specific markers start to become highly expressed. A full proteome analysis (Tsangaris G et al., 2005) using bi-dimensional gel electrophoresis and mass spectrometry, has allowed the identification of specific proteins expressed in the cells present in the amniotic fluid. This analysis has confirmed that amniotic fluid contains a heterogeneous population of cells, both differentiated and with characteristics of stem cells. In the following paragraphs a detailed description of the approaches used to differentiate AFDSCs into various lineages is presented.

When considering the use of amniotic fluid stem cells for regenerative medicine and various therapeutic interventions, clinicians and researchers agree that the ease of amniotic fluid stem cell isolation and culture make them attractive candidates for further research and development. As mentioned previously, amniotic fluid stem cells are isolated from samples of amniotic fluid collected during routine amniocentesis. This routine procedure (Fig. 4.) occurs during weeks 16-20 of a pregnancy, where approximately 10-20 milliliters of amniotic fluid is collected and split into two samples (Trounson, 2007). One sample serves as the test sample to screen for genetic and gestational abnormalities, while the other sample serves as a back up. When the back-up sample is no longer needed, some diagnostic laboratories donate this "medical waste" to research laboratories for stem cell isolation and further research. Throughout this entire process, neither the mother, nor the fetus is harmed, making the collection of these cells ethically neutral.

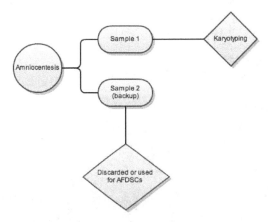

Fig. 4. Diagram for Amniotic Fluid-Derived Stem Cells isolation

The use of AFDSCs for the treatment of congenital anomalies has great potential, but in most cases is still far from clinical applications. Nerveless there is at least one case in which cells derived from amniotic fluid have been successfully used for tissue engineering. Mesenchymal cells isolated from amniotic fluid have been expanded in vitro using a chondrogenic medium and than seeded into a biodegradable scaffold and maintained in a rotating bioreactor (Kunisaki SM et al., 2006). The cells used in this report were not specifically analyzed for pluripotency or selected for specific markers, and were considered progenitor cells by the authors. Being a mixed population of cells they likely contained both committed lineages and AFDSCs, but most importantly they were able to differentiate into cartilage in vitro into a three-dimensional scaffold and maintain these characteristics for as long as fifteen weeks.

5. Amniotic fluid stem cells

Within amniotic fluid are a menagerie of cells previously described as AFDSCs, however approximately 1% of the cells contained within the fluid have been identified and designated as amniotic fluid stem cells (AFSC). AFSCs represent the most characterized clonal population of pluripotent stem cells isolated from amniotic fluid. AFSCs can be isolated by immunoselection with magnetic microsphere or FACS for the receptor for stem cell factor (c-Kit or CD117). The clonal origin of these cells was tested by integration of a single provirus (CMMP-eGFP) and analysis of subclones. Analysis of the subclones grown at limiting dilution maintained the signature integration at the same position (a 4 kilobase BamH1 fragment). The sublones were able to differentiate into lineages representative of the three embryonic germ layers. After isolation AFSCs will grow slowly for about one week (this phenomenon differs in AFSCs isolated at different gestational stages), and will then start to proliferate faster following this initial 'lag-phase' (Siddiqui MM and Atala A, 2004). AFSCs grow in absence of feeder layer when plated on Petri dishes and have a doubling time of about 36 hours (De Coppi et al, 2007).   The isolated population can then be cultured quite readily on plastic or glass.   If maintained at a sub-confluent state, AFSCs do not differentiate. Clones should be cultured in medium containing α-minimal essential medium supplemented with 20% Chang-B and 2% Chang-C solutions, 20% fetal bovine serum (FBS), 1% L-glutamine, and 1% antibiotics. Clones should be periodically monitored for the presence of a correct karyotype, and for the expression of specific markers such as Oct4, SSEA4, CD29, CD44, and the absence of markers such as CD45, CD34, and CD133 (see De Coppi et al., 2007 for a complete list of specific markers). AFSCs are pluripotent and can be differentiate in vitro into several lineages (De Coppi et al., 2007; Siddiqui MM and Atala A, 2004).   Numerous groups have reported the high renewal capacity of these cells without differentiation or loss of telomere length (Da Sacco et al., 2010).

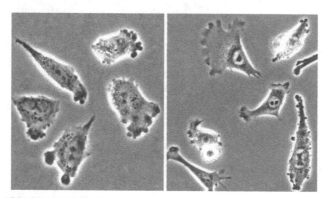

Fig. 5. Amniotic Fluid Stem Cells

Human amniotic fluid stem cells (left) and mouse amniotic fluid stem cells (right) that were isolated via selection for the surface marker CD117. Both cells have similar phenotypes (40X magnification).

5.1 Differentiation of amniotic fluid stem cells

C-kit positive amniotic fluid stem cells are pluripotent and have been successfully differentiated into all three germ layer cell types: endoderm, ectoderm and mesoderm.

From these pluripotent cells, various phenotypes have been derived in vitro. Osteogenic, endotheilial, hepatic, neurogenic, adipogenic and myogenic progenitor cell lines are a few of the lineages derived to date. Derivation of these lines has been verified by morphogenesis, phenotypic analysis and a litany of biochemical assays for characteristic of each cell type. Culture and manipulation of these cells into various progenitors has become so streamlined, that various standard protocols have been established (Delo et al., 2006). Although a significant milestone, differentiation of AFSC into various lineages in vitro is quite distinct from the in vivo potential, use and efficacy of these cells. Transplantation of these cells into a living system, or the use of these cells to create a functional organ hinge on the ability of these cells not simply to survive in vivo, however; success is dependant on the physiological functionality of these cells to perform within the anatomy. The future of regenerative medicine and cellular therapy hinges on this principle, and not surprisingly, AFSC have also shown remarkable capabilities in vivo in numerous organs.

5.1.1 Hematopoietic system

AFSC expressing CD117+ and Lin-, derived from both human and mouse, have been shown to have hematopoietic potential (Ditadi A et al., 2010). These cells were capable of differentiating into erythroid, myeloid, and lymphoid lineages in vitro as well as in vivo, in the peripheral blood of irradiated mice. Furthermore, single cells analysis was able to assess the expression of several genes important during different stages of hematopoietic differentiation.

5.1.2 Brain

A fully mature neural differentiation remains to be tested for cells derived from amniotic fluid. Neural differentiation was fist reported during the initial identification of AFSCs (De Coppi et al., 2007). Subsequently, a study for the differentiation of AFSCs into dopamine neurons (Donaldson AE et al., 2009), showed that AFSCs express specific markers of neural progenitors and immature dopamine neurons, but were unable to fully differentiate in vitro or in vivo. Analyzing other cell lines isolated from amniotic fluid (McLaughlin D et al., 2006) it was shown that phenotypic characteristics of dopaminergic neurons are present, while markers for other neurons, like cholinergic, GABAergic, and adrenergic were absent or had a weak expression.

5.1.3 Bone

AFSC cultured with an osteogenic medium, can secrete alkaline phosphatase and produce mineralized calcium, characteristic of functional osteoblasts. Furthermore, when implanted into an immunodeficient mouse, AFSC where able to produce mineralized tissue in vivo (De Coppi et al., 2007). A comparison between AFDSCs and bone morrow-derived stem cells (MSCs), has shown that while MSCs undergo a faster differentiation, AFDSCs can maintain and increase the mineralization for a longer period (Peister A et al., 2011).

5.1.4 Kidney

AFSC therapy in the kidney is progressing quickly and is arguably at the forefront of AFSC research. Research groups using AFSC in kidney have not only been able to demonstrate the ability of AFSC to populate the kidney and form renal structures, but also to protect the kidney during injury and aid in the regeneration of renal tissue. The groundbreaking studies, which follow, paved the way for much of the other organ specific experimentation, in particular, that of the lung.

In the embryonic kidney, AFSC have been shown to differentiate into tubular and glomerular structures and express characteristic kidney cell markers and genes (Perin et al., 2007). In this study, metanephric kidneys were isolated from embryonic mice, microinjected with approximately 1000 CM-dil labeled c-kit positive AFSC and placed on a membrane for cultivation in an incubator. What is remarkable is that even though the embryonic kidney was not fully formed at the beginning of the experiment, labeled AFSC were seen to integrate into developing C and S-shaped structures at day 5, and at day 6, integrated into tubular and glomerular structures. Reverse transcriptase-PCR for human kidney specific genes, not previously expressed by the AFSC, identified expression of ZO-1, claudin and glial-derived neurotrophic factor were detected. This experiment showed the ability of AFSC to survive within developing tissue, engraft into that tissue, differentiate into the appropriate cell type and aid in the population of an organ.

Furthermore, it has recently been discovered that AFSC injected into the acutely injured kidney stimulate the release of anti-inflammatory cytokines and attenuate pro-inflammatory signaling greatly reducing apoptosis and allowing for proliferation and repopulation of injured epithelia (Perin L. et al., 2011). In this study, nude mice, deprived of water for a period of 22 hours, were given an intramuscular injection of a 50% hypertonic glycerol solution in water. This type of injury induces rhabdomyolysis-related acute tubular necrosis (ATN) ultimately resulting in renal dysfunction. Following intrarenal injection of 1.2×10^6 cells, AFSC were observed, via luciferase, to persist at the site of injury most notably at 48 and 72 hours, with persistence in the kidneys for up to 6 days. Additionally, analysis of the cytokine milieu showed the markedly different expression patterns of cytokines at 14 days post transplant. Mice with ATN only, and no AFSC transplant, showed a general trend of increased pro-inflammatory cytokines and decreased anti-inflammatory cytokine expression. On the other hand, mice with ATN and intra-renal injection of AFSC demonstrated that the anti inflammatory cytokines increased over the 14 day study period, while pro-inflammatory cytokines decreased. In another study after glycerol-induced acute kidney injury (Hauser PV et al., 2010) a comparison between mesenchymal stem cells (MSCs) and AFSCs has shown that while MSCs where mainly inducing proliferation, AFSCs had an antiapoptotic effect. Thus, these data suggests that AFSCs responds in a paracrine manner in response to injury and/or stress, and modulation of immune signaling is what contributes to the alleviation of symptoms associated with the injury.

5.1.5 Lung

In utero, the developing lungs of the fetus are filled with fetal lung liquid which is actively secreted into the amniotic fluid. In the late gestational period, surfactant produced by the fetal lungs contributes to the composition of amniotic fluid and can be measured to determine the developmental stage of the surfactant system within the fetal lungs. Thus, it makes sense that when looking for regenerative therapies for lung tissue, AFSC are a logical source.

In our preliminary transplantation studies, it was found that c-kit positive AFSC can incorporate into mouse embryonic lung and express human lung epithelial cell markers (Carraro, et al., 2008). In the same study, following naphthalene injury in nude mice, and intravenous transplantation of 1×10^6 AFSC, cells were observed to preferentially remain at the site of injury when compared to uninjured controls when visualized via luciferase assay.

Additionally, following oxygen injury in the lung it was observed that AFSC appear to exhibit alveolar epithelial type II phenotypes, widely surmised to be a lung epithelial stem cell, suggesting that once in the lung these cells are stimulated to differentiate in response to injury. Furthermore, in vivo, the efficiency of AFSC diapedesis, integration and expression in upper and lower airway epithelia is increased following injury. After oxygen injury, AFSC were observed to be taken into the SP-C positive alveolar epithelial lineage, whereas after naphthalene injury AFSC are taken up into the CC10-positive Clara cell lineage. AFSC presence persisted in the lung after injury, but decreased over time. Although integration into the adult lung following injury is a relatively rare event, additional therapeutic mechanisms displayed by these cells, such as the modulation of the inflammatory milieu and their differentiation into type II lineages demonstrate great potential in the stimulation of lung repair mechanisms.

Lung researchers have also begun investigating the potential of seeding AFSC on a scaffold to regenerate tissue for transplantation. Due to the overwhelming shortage of donor lungs, and the inability of modern medicine to effectively treat or halt many progressive lung diseases such as idiopathic pulmonary fibrosis, research focus has shifted to the bioengineering of functional lung tissue. Decellularization of lungs, where all cells are removed from the extracellular matrix of an organ, has become an investigational target. In 2010 a whole lung decellularization method and tissue engineering study using neonatal lung epithelia was reported (Peterson et al., 2010). What is remarkable about this study is that while it has long been known that epithelial cells seeded on a decellularized lung matrix were capable of forming alveolar epithelia, this study demonstrated the functionality of the regenerated tissue. The decellularized, repopulated and regenerated lungs were transplanted into a rat and were able to support short-term perfusion and gas exchange. In another study, researchers were able to seed not only epithelium, but also endothelium as well on a decellularized rat lung. Following transplantation, blood gas analysis of the engineered lung demonstrated that the lung was capable of gas exchange (Ott et al., 2010). Thus decellularized lung matrix seems currently to be the most promising scaffold for whole lung regeneration and the possibility of using an autologous source of stem cells such as AFSC to repopulate the scaffold could have great potential in the future.

5.1.6 Heart

The use of AFSC as a regenerative therapy for cardiac disease and congenital disorders has shown the efficacy of transplanted cells providing both cardio protective potential, as well as the engineering of various cardiac components such as valves and tissue (Bollini et al., 2011; Schmidt et al., 2007; & Hilkfer et al., 2011).

The engineering of heart valves, obtained from normal human amniotic fluid samples, sorted via positive selection for the CD133 molecule, was elegantly demonstrated in 2007 (Schmidt et al., 2007). Both CD 133 positive and negative cell populations were cultured in media that caused differentiation towards endothelial phenotypes. CD133+ cell populations showed the ability to produce functional endothelial cells indicated by the expression of eNOS and CD141, while CD133- cells displayed a more mesenchymal phenotype. CD133- cells were then seeded on biodegradable PGA leaflets that were positioned within a mold to form a valve structure. After 14 days, CD133+ cells were seeded onto the scaffold as well. While regeneration of both extracellular matrix and endothelial layers were generated, functional testing revealed that the heart valves were sufficiently functional only under low-pressure conditions. This failure to perform at physiological levels was not due to the scaffold material, which displayed linear properties prior to being seeded with cells, but instead was a result of the incomplete formation of collagen suggesting that the method of seeding and culture upon the biodegradable scaffolding needs to be optimized further to be able to transplant these engineered valves into patients. In an acute myocardial infarction model, ischemia, produced via ligation of the left anterior descending coronary artery, was followed with intravenous transplantation of AFSC and reperfusion of the heart for 2 hours. Animals treated with 5×10^6 cells intravenously, showed a significant decrease in infarct size and number of apoptotic cardiomyocityes when compared to control animals administered saline alone (Bollini et al., 2011). Staining to determine the localization and viability of transplanted AFSC showed that two hours post transplant, cells localized to the lung, spleen and heart. AFSC within the heart co-stained for epithelia vWf and α-SMA, suggestive of the potential of these cells to commit to endothelium and smooth muscle following transplant. Long term retention and engraftment in the injured myocardial tissue did not occur however. The secretion of thymosin beta 4 in vitro, a cardio protective factor, suggests that the transplantation of AFSC in this model exert a paracrine effect.

5.2 Why use AFSC in regenerative medicine?

When selecting a stem cell population for use in a regenerative or therapeutic capacity, there are a myriad of factors that need to be considered. The pluripotentiality, the ability of the cells to differentiate into different germ layers and tissue types, is of fundamental importance if one is isolating cells to treat diseases or developmental deficiencies in which progenitor cells within the patient are compromised or overwhelmed. Additionally, the plasticity of the cells and their ability to differentiate to repopulate different populations within an organ, and repopulate them correctly is crucial. Furthermore, the behavior of the cells after injection must be carefully studied and characterized. Tumorogenicity, immunogenicity and the propensity to form teratomas and further exacerbate a disease state can rule out various cellular therapies simply due to risk. To date, amniotic fluid stem cells have demonstrated the ability to meet all of these criteria and behave remarkably well in a regenerative and therapeutic capacity. Amazingly pluripotent, less immunogenic, and not prone to teratoma formation, AFSCs have quickly risen near the top of the list of stem cell therapies to continue developing.

Furthermore, recently induced pluripotent stem (iPS) cells have been prepared from cells derived from amniotic fluid (AF-iPS), and have shown high efficiency of transformation and colony formation after just six days (Li C et al., 2009). Although not fully understood, this is probably due to the presence of an epigenetic status closer to the embryonic state (Galende E et al., 2010). Reprogramming of somatic cells using the four specific factors, Oct4, Sox2, Klf4, and c-Myc has the potential to provide pluripotent stem cells specific for patients, thus AF-iPS seem to be more easily reprogrammed to pluripotency compared to adult cells or cells from neonates.

6. Conclusion

The studies outlined in this chapter demonstrating the capability that AFSC have shown in vitro and in vivo show that AFSC are viable targets for regenerative medicine and for future therapeutic treatment strategies. Although the relatively early stage of AFSC research limits a full understanding of the behaviors, properties and characteristics of these fascinating cells, research to date demonstrates two important mechanisms of action that need to be investigated further.

First, AFSC have the potential to serve as an in vivo treatment to stimulate endogenous cell populations, repopulate injured tissue or ameliorate inflammatory or disease states. These properties are advantageous when dealing with disease or injury states in which there is enough functional tissue remaining in an organ to drive repopulation. The only caveat to endogenous cellular stimulation is that the remaining tissue (that is being stimulated) must be functional, meaning that it is free of genetic disorders or mutations. If remaining tissue within an organ meets these standards, exogenous AFSC transplantation can be used to stimulate endogenous progenitors to repopulate, protect progenitor or other cell types from further injury, or AFSC may be driven to differentiate to repopulate this tissue, as was indicated in the aforementioned embryonic studies.

Second, AFSC have the potential to engineer whole organs in vitro to be transplanted into a recipient. This strategy is advantageous in situations where, for whatever reason, enough functional tissue does not remain to repopulate with a cell transplant. Whole organ re-engineering, perhaps the holy grail of regenerative medicine, involves a symphony of factors, events and coordinated expression patterns to form intricate niche structures including endothelium, epithelium, extracellular matrix and so on. The engineering of a whole organ will in fact require a much deeper understanding of these cells as signaling cascades and response elements need to be coordinated to engineer every cell type within a specific organ. However the recent findings of Kajtsura et al (2011) support the our notiion that the genome within a single stem cell type may prove to be sufficiently plastic to simultaneously derive all of the cell lineages required for complex organ repair or engineering.

7. References

Adamson TM, Brodecky V, Lambert TF. The production and composition of lung liquid in the in-utero foetal lamb. In Comline RS, Cross KW, Dawes GS (eds): Foetal and Neonatal Physiology. Cambridge University Press, 1973.

Bacchi Modena A., Fieni S. Amniotic fluid dynamics. Acta Bio Medica Ateneo Parmense. 75: 11-13. 2004.

Bailo M., Soncini M., Vertua E., Signorini P.B., Sanzone S., Lombardi G., Arienti D., Calamani F., Zatti D., Paul P. et al. Engraftment potential of human amnion and chorion cells derived from term placenta. Transplantation 78: 1439-1448. 2004.

Banas, RA, Trumpower C., Bentlwjewsky C., Marshall V., Sing G. and Zeevi A. Immunogenicity and immunomodulatory effects of amnion-derived multipotent progenitor cells. Hum Immunol 69: 321-328. 2008

Bollini S., Cheung K.K., Riegler J., Dong X., Smart N., et al. Amniotic Fluid Stem Cells Are Cardioprotective Following Acute Myocardial Infarction. Stem Cells and Development. May 2011.

Brace RA, Wolf EJ. Normal amniotic fluid volume changes throughout pregnancy. Am J Obstet Gynecol. 1989 Aug; 161:382-8.

Brunstein CG, Wagner JE. Cord blood transplantation for adults. Vox Sang. 91(3):195-205. 2006

Carraro G, Perin L, Sedrakyan S, Giuliani S, Tiozzo C, Lee J, Turcatel G, De Langhe SP, Driscoll B, Bellusci S, Minoo P, Atala A, De Filippo RE, Warburton D. Human amniotic fluid stem cells can integrate and differentiate into epithelial lung lineages. *Stem Cells* 2008; 26: 2902-2911.

De Coppi P., Bartsch Jr. G., Siddiqui M.M., Xu T., Santos C.C., et al. Isolation of amniotic stem cell lines with potential for therapy. Nture Biotechnology 25 (1): 100-106(2007).

Da Sacco S., De Filippo R.E., & Perin L. Amniotic fluid as a source of pluripotent and multipotent stem cells for organ regeneration. Curr Opin Organ Transplant. 2010.

Delo DM., De Coppi P, Bartsch Jr G., & Atala A. Amniotic Fluid and Placental Stem Cells. Methods in Enzymology 419: 426-436. 2006.

Ditadi A, de Coppi P, Picone O, Gautreau L, Smati R, Six E, Bonhomme D, Ezine S, Frydman R, Cavazzana-Calvo M, Andrea-Schmutz I. Human and murine amniotic fluid c-Kit+Lin- cells display hematopoietic activity. Blood. 113(17):3953-60. 2009.

Donaldson AE, Cai J, Yang M, Iacovitti L. Human amniotic fluid stem cells do not differentiate into dopamine neurons in vitro or after transplantation in vivo. Stem Cells Dev. 18(7):1003-12. 2009.

Fukuchi Y, Nakajima H, Sugiyama D, Hirose I, Kitamura T, Tsuji K. Human placenta-derived cells have mesenchymal stem/progenitor cell potential. Stem Cells. 22(5):649-58. 2004.

Galende E, Karakikes I, Edelmann L, Desnick RJ, Kerenyi T, Khoueiry G, Lafferty J, McGinn JT, Brodman M, Fuster V, Hajjar RJ, Polgar K. Amniotic fluid cells are more efficiently reprogrammed to pluripotency than adult cells. Cell Reprogram. 12:2. 117-125. 2010.

Hauser PV, De Fazio R, Bruno S, Sdei S, C Grange C, Bussolati B, Benedetto C, Camussi G. Stem Cells Derived from Human Amniotic Fluid Contribute to Acute Kidney Injury Recovery. The American Journal of Pathology. 177:4. 2011-2021. 2010.

Hilkfer A., Kasper C., Hass R., & Haverich A. Mesenchymal stem cells and proenitor cells in connective tissue engineering and regenerative medicine : is there a future for transplantation? Langenbeck's Archives of Surgery, 396: 4, 489-497. 2011.

Huisjes HJ. Origin of the cells in the liquor amnii. Americ. J. Obstet. Gynec. 106: 1222-1228. 1970.

Kajstura J, Rota M, Hall SR, Hosoda T, D'Amario D, Sanada F, Zheng H, Ogórek B, Rondon-Clavo C, Ferreira-Martins J, Matsuda A, Arranto C, Goichberg P, Giordano G, Haley KJ, Bardelli S, Rayatzadeh H, Liu X, Quaini F, Liao R, Leri A, Perrella MA, Loscalzo J, Anversa P. Evidence for human lung stem cells. N Engl J Med. 2011 12;364(19):1795-806.

Kaufman, MH. The Atlas of Mouse Development. Academic Press, CA. 1992.

Kaviani A, Perry TE, Dzakovic A, Jennings RW, Ziegler MM, Fauza DO. The amniotic fluid as a source of cells for fetal tissue engineering. J Pediatr Surg. 36(11):1662-5. 2001.

Kunisaki SM, Jennings RW, Fauza DO. Fetal cartilage engineering from amniotic mesenchymal progenitor cells. Stem Cells Dev. 15(2):245-53. 2006.

Li C, Zhou J, Shi G, Ma Y, Yang Y, Gu J, Yu H, Jin S, Wei Z, Chen F, Jin Y. Pluripotency can be rapidly and efficiently induced in human amniotic fluid-derived cells. Hum Mol Genet. 18(22):4340-9. 2009.

Lotgering FK, Wallenburg HCS. Mechanisms of production and clearance of amniotic fluid. *Semin Perinatol* ;10: 94. 1986.

Marchant GS. Evaluation of Methods of Amniotic Fluid Cell Culture. American Journal of Medical Technology. 37: 391-396. 1971.

McLaughlin D, Tsirimonaki E, Vallianatos G, Sakellaridis N, Chatzistamatiou T, Stavropoulos-Gioka C, Tsezou A, Messinis I, Mangoura D. Stable expression of a neuronal dopaminergic progenitor phenotype in cell lines derived from human amniotic fluid cells. J Neurosci Res. 83(7):1190-200. 2006.

Morris HHB and Bennett MJ. The classification and origin of amniotic fluid cells. Acta Cytologica. 18: 2. 149-154. 1974.

Ott HC, Clippinger B, Conrad C, Schuetz C, Pomerantseva I, Ikonomou L, Kotton D, Vacanti JP. Regeneration and orthotopic transplantation of a bioartificial lung. Nature Medicine: Vol. 16, No. 8. 2010.

Peister A, Woodruff MA, Prince JJ, Gray DP, Hutmacher DW, Guldberg RE. Cell sourcing for bone tissue engineering: Amniotic fluid stem cells have a delayed, robust differentiation compared to mesenchymal stem cells. Stem Cell Res. 2011.

Peterson T.H., Calle E.A., Zhao L., Lee E.J., Gui L., et al. Tissue-Engineered Lungs for in Vivo Implantation. Science, 2010.

Perin L, Sedrakyan S, Giuliani S, Da Sacco S, Carraro G, Shiri L, Lemley KV, Rosol M, Wu S, Atala A, Warburton D, De Filippo R. Protectice Effect of Human Amniotic Fluid Stem Cells in an Immunodeficient Mouse Model of Acute Tubular Necrosis. PLoS ONE 5(2): e9357.

Perin L, Giuliani S, Jin D, Sedrakyan S, Carraro G, Habibian R, Warburton D, Atala A, De Filippo RE. Renal differentiation of amniotic fluid stem cells. *Cell Prolif*. 40:9. 2007.

Prusa AR, Marton E, Rosner M, Bernaschek G, Hengstschl√ §ger M. Oct-4-expressing cells in human amniotic fluid: a new source for stem cell research? Hum Reprod. Jul;18(7):1489-93. 2003.

Schmidit D., Achermann J., Odermatt B., Breymann C., Mol A., et al. Prenatally Fabricated Autologous Human Living Heart Valves Based on Amniotic Fluid-Derived Progenitor Cells as Single Cell Source. Circulation, 116: 164-170. 2007.

Siddiqui MM and Atala A. Amniotic fluid-derived pluripotent cells. Handbook of stem cells. 2:16. 175-179. 2004.

Torricelli F, Brizzi L, Bernabei PA, Gheri G, Di Lollo S, Nutini L, Lisi E, Di Tommaso M, Cariati E. Identification of hematopoietic progenitor cells in human amniotic fluid before the 12th week of gestation. Ital J Anat Embryol. Apr-Jun;98(2):119-26. 1993.

Trounson, A. A fluid means of stem cell generation. Nature Biotechnology 25 (1): 62-63 (2007).

Tsai MS, Lee JL, Chang YJ, Hwang SM. Isolation of human multipotent mesenchymal stem cells from second-trimester amniotic fluid using a novel two-stage culture protocol. Hum Reprod. 19(6):1450-6. 2004.

Tsangaris G, Weitzdrfer R, Pollak D, Lubec G, Fountoulakis M. The amniotic fluid cell proteome. Electrophoresis. 26(6):1168-73. 2005.

Turner CG, Fauza DO. Fetal tissue engineering. Clin Perinatol. 36(2):473-88. 2009.

12

Very Small Embryonic/Epiblast-Like Stem Cells (VSELs) Residing in Adult Tissues and Their Role in Tissue Rejuvenation and Regeneration

Dong-Myung Shin[1], Janina Ratajczak[1],
Magda Kucia[1] and Mariusz Z. Ratajczak[1]
[1]Stem Cell Institute at the James Graham Brown Cancer Center,
University of Louisville, KY,
USA

1. Introduction

Embryonic development and later rejuvenation of adult tissues are regulated by a population of stem cells (SCs) that, by undergoing self-renewal, maintain their own pool and, by giving rise to differentiated progenitors, replace cells used up during life (Ratajczak et al., 2007). Thus, SCs are guardians of tissue/organ integrity and regulate the life span of an adult organism. The most important SCs, from a regenerative potential point of view, are pluripotent stem cells (PSCs). According to their definition, such cells must meet certain *in vitro* and *in vivo* criteria. PSCs must: i) give rise to cells from all three germ layers; ii) complete blastocyst development; and iii) form teratomas after inoculation into experimental animals.

The SC compartment shows a high degree of hierarchy (Hayashi & Surani, 2009). In embryonic development, the most primitive stem cells are the fertilized oocyte (zygote) and the first blastomers in the morula. These cells are called totipotent, possessing the ability to give rise to both embryo and placenta. The developing morula gives rise to the blastocyst, where PSCs are found in the inner cell mass (ICM). These cells may give rise to all three germ layers of the developing embryo; however, they have lost the ability to differentiate into placenta. The PSCs at this stage can be expanded *ex vivo* as immortalized embryonic stem cell (ESC) lines (Evans & Kaufman, 1981).

After implantation of the blastocyst, PSCs from the blastocyst ICM give rise to pluripotent epiblast stem cells (EpiSCs) that will form the entire embryo proper (Brons et al., 2007; Tesar et al., 2007). During the gastrulation process, cell lineage determination programs are initiated and EpiSCs respond to the signals from surrounding extra-embryonic tissues, which leads to their differentiation into several types of tissue-committed stem cells (TCSCs) (Ratajczak et al., 2007). TCSCs are monopotent (unipotent), which means they are restricted in their differentiation potential to cells for one tissue only (e.g., epidermis, intestinal epithelium, liver, skeletal muscles, or lympho-hematopoietic). TCSCs terminate expression of pluripotent genes and, at the same time, turn on lineage-specific molecular programs.

The first population of SCs, which at around embryonic day 7.25 (E7.25) become specified in the proximal epiblast, are primordial germ cells (PGCs), and alkaline phosphatase (AP)-

positive PGCs grow into extra-embryonic mesoderm at the base of the allantois as an appendage arising from around the posterior primitive streak (Surani et al., 2007). These cells transcribe pluripotency-related genes, such as *Oct-4, Nanog,* and *Sox2,* and are the only population of SCs that maintains expression of these genes during gastrulation. When PGCs are cultured over murine embryonic fibroblasts and exposed *ex vivo* to three growth factors (kit ligand, leukemia inhibitory factor, and basic fibroblast growth factor), they continue to proliferate and form large colonies of embryonic germ cells (EGCs), which, like ESCs, can be expanded indefinitely (Matsui et al., 1992). At around E12.5, PGCs arrive at the genital ridges, lose their markers of pluripotency, and initiate their commitment to becoming gametes (oocytes and sperm).

As mentioned above, SCs show a developmental hierarchy (Hayashi & Surani, 2009), and PSCs that emerge during embryogenesis give rise to more differentiated SC populations with the ability to self renew, but with a more limited ability for multilineage differentiation (Surani et al., 2007). Evidence is accumulating that differentiation potential is regulated by epigenetic reprogramming (Surani et al., 2007). PSCs from the ICM show global DNA demethylation, which results in i) activation of the X chromosome, ii) expression of germ-line, lineage-characteristic genes (e.g *Stella, Mvh, Dazl,* and *Sycp3*), and iii) expression of repetitive sequence families (e.g. *LINE1, SINE,* and *IAP*). After implantation of the blastocyst in the uterus, ICM-derived PSCs give rise to EpiSCs and again methylate i) the X chromosome, ii) promoters for genes characteristic of PSCs in the ICM (*Rex-1* and *Stella*), and iii) repetitive sequences (Hayashi et al., 2008). Whereas most EpiSCs undergo further differentiation into TCSCs by stable repression of promoters for pluripotent-specific genes, some EpiSCs in the proximal epiblast (precursors of PGCs) revert to a state that resembles ICM PSCs by undergoing genome-wide DNA demethylation (Hayashi & Surani, 2009). This leads to re-activation of the X chromosome and promoters for germline-lineage genes and repetitive sequences.

Unlike differentiated somatic cells, PSCs commonly express the pluripotency core transcription factors (TFs) such as Oct-4, Nanog, and Sox2 (Kim et al., 2008). These TFs form the pluripotency core circuitry by reinforcing the expression of genes involved in keeping PSCs in an undifferentiated state and, at the same time, repressing their differentiation. The biological significance of these core TFs has been experimentally proven by the generation of inducible pluripotent stem cells (iPSCs), in which fully differentiated somatic cells can be reprogrammed into ESC-like stem cells after transduction by so-called Yamanaka factors (*Oct-4, Sox2, Klf4,* and *cMyc*) (Takahashi & Yamanaka, 2006; Wernig et al., 2007).

Another hallmark of pluripotency is the presence of transcriptionally active chromatin structures at the promoters of core TFs due to methylation and histone modifications of promoter DNA (Cedar & Bergman, 2009). Thus, promoters for core TFs in PSCs are de-methylated and highly enriched for histone codes associated with active transcription, such as acetylated histones and trimethylation on lysine 4 of histone 3 (H3K4me3). In addition to the expression of pluripotency core TFs, undifferentiated PSCs also exhibit specific epigenetic marks called bivalent domains (BDs) (Azuara et al., 2006; Boyer et al., 2006; Lee et al., 2006; Stock et al., 2007). In BDs, the transcriptionally active H3K4me3 code coexists with repressive histone codes, such as trimethylated lysine 27 in histone 3 (H3K27me3). The BDs are mainly detected in the promoter regions of homeodomain-containing developmental master TFs, such as *Dlx-, Irx-, Lhx-, Pou-, Pax-,* and *Six*-family proteins. Due to the overwhelming effect of the transcription-repressive activity of H3K27me3, the transcription of BD-controlled   genes is transiently repressed to prevent premature differentiation.

Very Small Embryonic/Epiblast-Like Stem Cells (VSELs) Residing in Adult Tissues and Their Role in
Tissue Rejuvenation and Regeneration

227

However, in response to developmental stimuli, BDs in promoters of these genes are switched into the monovalent type that promotes transcription. Therefore, both positive (expression of Oct-4-Nanog-Sox2) and negative (repression of differentiation-inducing TFs by bivalent domains) mechanisms are indispensable for controlling the pluripotent state of PSCs.

As mentioned before, PSCs are detected only during very early embryonic development and they disappear after differentiation into TCSCs and germline cells (Niwa, 2007). However, recent evidence has accumulated demonstrating that PSCs may reside in adult tissues and are able to differentiate into TCSCs (Ratajczak et al., 2007). These cells have been variously described in the literature as i) multipotent adult progenitor cells (MAPCs), ii) marrow-isolated adult multilineage-inducible (MIAMI) cells, iii) multipotent adult (MA) SCs, or iv) OmniCytes (Beltrami et al., 2007; D'Ippolito et al., 2004; Jiang et al., 2002; Pochampally et al., 2004). Thus, the physical presence of PSCs in adult tissues may better explain stem cell plasticity, according to which TCSCs are purportedly plastic and can trans-dedifferentiate into SCs for other tissues.

However, several questions remain to be addressed regarding these rare PSCs. First, the developmental origin of these cells is unresolved. As shown in **Figure 1,** PSCs during embryogenesis/gastrulation may become eliminated after giving rise to TCSCs, or conversely, they may survive among TCSCs and serve as a back-up/reserve source for these cells. Thus, it is important to elucidate whether PSCs found in adult tissue cells are functional under steady-state conditions or are merely remnants from developmental embryogenesis that reside in a dormant state in adult tissues. Second, is the question of

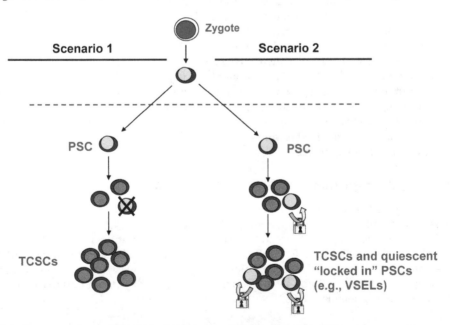

Fig. 1. **Developmental specification of PSCs into TCSCs. Scenario I:** During embryogenesis/gastrulation, PSCs are eliminated after giving rise to TCSCs and PGCs. **Scenario II:** PSCs survive and serve as a back-up/reserve source of TCSCs.

whether the dormant state of these cells is regulated by cell-intrinsic epigenetic reprogramming similar to other PSCsduring embryogenesis. Finally, there is the question of whether their dormant state is influenced by microenvironmental cues, such as their (i) location in non-physiological niches, (ii) exposure to inhibitors, or (iii) deprivation of appropriate stimulatory signals. The answer to these questions could be key to successful application of these adult-tissue-derived PSCs in the clinical setting. In this chapter, we will discuss these issues in more detail.

2. Very small embryonic-like stem cells (VSELs) residing in adult tissues

Recently, our group purified a population of very small embryonic-like stem cells (VSELs) from BM by employing a multiparameter fluorescence-activated cell sorter (FACS) (Kucia et al., 2006b). These rare Sca-1+Lin-CD45- cells reside in several adult murine organs (*e.g.,* brain, liver, skeletal muscles, heart, and kidney) (Zuba-Surma et al., 2008) and recently were detected also in human umbilical cord-blood and mobilized peripheral-blood (Kucia et al., 2006a; Paczkowska et al., 2009; Wojakowski et al., 2009). VSELs are very small in size (~3-6 μm) and express pluripotent markers, such as Oct-4, Nanog, Rex-1, and SSEA-1 (Kucia et al., 2006b). They are morphologically, similarly to ESCs, possessing large nuclei containing unorganized chromatin (euchromatin) and exhibiting a significantly higher nuclear/cytoplasm (N/C) ratio and a lower cytoplasmic area than hematopoietic stem cells (HSCs). The true expression of *Oct-4* and *Nanog* in BM-derived murine VSELs was recently confirmed by demonstrating transcriptionally active chromatin structures for both *Oct-4* and *Nanog* promoters (Shin et al., 2009). If cultured under a C2C12 myoblast feeder layer, freshly isolated VSELS form spheres corresponding to embryoid bodies (EBs). These VSEL-derived spheres (VSEL-DSs) contain primitive SCs that, after replating into tissue-specific differentiation media, are induced to differentiate into cells from all three germ layers (Kucia et al., 2008a). From experiments with mouse models, it has been proposed that VSELs are mobilized into peripheral blood in response to injury and circulate to the organ of injury in an attempt to enrich and regenerate damaged tissues (e.g., following heart infarct or stroke) (Kucia et al., 2008b; Paczkowska et al., 2009; Wojakowski et al., 2009). This physiological mechanism probably plays a significant role in the regeneration of some small tissue and organ injuries; however, further studies are needed to demonstrate that these cells do in fact home to the damaged organs.

3. Molecular signature of VSELs residing in BM

To investigate the relationship between VSELs and embryonic PSCs (e.g. embryonic stem cells [ESCs], epiblast stem cells [EpiSCs], primordial germ cells [PGCs], and embryonic germ cells [EGs]), we employed several molecular strategies to evaluate VSEL molecular signatures (**Figure 2**). Highly purified Sca-1+Lin-CD45- VSELs from murine BM were evaluated for i) expression of pluripotent genes, epiblast/germ line markers, and developmentally crucial imprinted genes; ii) the presence of BDs; and iii) reactivation of the X chromosome in female VSELs.

3.1 VSELs express PSC genes

PSCs express the essential pluripotency TF *Oct-4*. The importance of this TF is well-established by the fact that transduction with *Oct-4* is obligatory in several protocols for

Very Small Embryonic/Epiblast-Like Stem Cells (VSELs) Residing in Adult Tissues and Their Role in
Tissue Rejuvenation and Regeneration

229

generating iPSCs. We found that VSELs express Oct-4 at both the mRNA and protein level (Kucia et al., 2006a). However, recently some doubts have been raised about whether cells isolated from adult tissues express these embryonic genes, and it has been suggested that positive PCR data showing *Oct-4* expression may be due to amplification of *Oct-4* pseudogenes (Lengner et al., 2007; Liedtke et al., 2007). Thus, to prove true expression of the *Oct-4* gene in VSELs, we investigated the epigenetic state of the *Oct-4* promoter. Our DNA methylation studies of the *Oct-4* promoter using bisulfite sequencing revealed that it is hypomethylated in highly purified Sca-1$^+$Lin$^-$CD45$^-$ VSELs, similarly to cells isolated from ESC-derived EBs (28% and 13.2%, respectively) (Shin et al., 2009). Next, to evaluate the state of histone codes for the *Oct-4* promoter, we performed the chromatin-immunoprecipitation (ChIP) assay to verify its association with acetylated histone 3 (H3Ac) and dimethylated lysine 9 of histone 3 (H3K9me2), the molecular marks for open- and closed-type chromatin, respectively. By employing the carrier-ChIP assay (using the human hematopoietic cell-line THP-1 as carrier) we found that *Oct-4* promoter chromatin is associated with H3Ac and its association with H3K9me2 is relatively low (Shin et al., 2009). We also evaluated the epigenetic state of another core TF, *Nanog,* and observed that its promoter has a higher level of methylation in VSELs (~50%). However, in quantitative ChIP experiments performed in parallel, it was confirmed that the H3Ac/H3K9me2 ratio favors transcription and supports its active state (Shin et al., 2009). Based on these results, we conclude that VSELs truly express *Oct-4* and *Nanog*. Of note, we also reported that VSELs express several other markers of PSCs, such as SSEA-1 antigen, as well as *Sox2* and *Klf4* TFs (Shin et al., 2010b).

3.2 Expression of epiblast markers

As a result of the epigenetic reprogramming that occurs during implantation of the blastocyst, EpiSCs exhibit transcription profiles different from ESCs. For example, the expression of *Nanog, Sox2,* and *Stella* is reduced in EpiSCs through DNA methylation of their promoters (Surani et al., 2007). In functional assays, EpiSCs, unlike ESCs, show a highly restricted capacity to complement blastocyst development (Brons et al., 2007; Tesar et al., 2007). However, pluripotent EpiSCs may differentiate *in vivo* into TCSCs, which during embryogenesis orchestrate organogenesis and later in adult life are involved in rejuvenation of tissues and organs. Like EpiSCs, highly purified BM-derived Oct-4$^+$ VSELs do not complement blastocyst development and therefore cannot enable *in vitro* differentiation into cells from all three germ layers. Therefore, we have hypothesized that VSELs may be epiblast-derived precursors of TCSCs (Ratajczak et al., 2010). To investigate the similarity between VSELs and EpiSCs, we examined the expression of genes that are characteristic of EpiSCs (*Gbx2, Fgf5,* and *Nodal*) and ESCs from the blastocyst ICM (*Rex-1*) in adult BM-derived VSELs. It is known that *Gbx2, Fgf5,* and *Nodal* are upregulated in EpiSCs, but are expressed at lower levels in ESCs isolated from the ICM (Hayashi et al., 2008). In contrast, the level of *Rex-1* transcripts is highly expressed in ICM cells. We found that VSELs highly express *Gbx2, Fgf5,* and *Nodal,* but express the *Rex-1* transcript at a low level compared to the established murine ESC cell line, ESC-D3. This suggests that VSELs are more differentiated than ICM-derived ESCs and share several markers with more differentiated EpiSCs (Shin et al., 2010b).

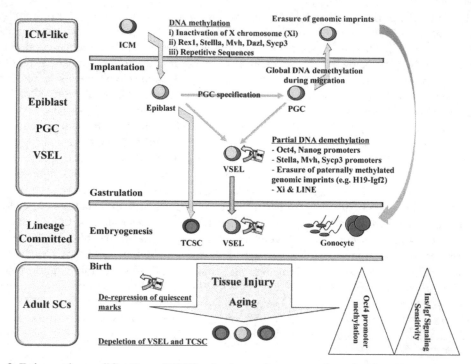

Fig. 2. **Epigenetic modification of VSELs during embryogenesis and aging.** Epigenetic modifications control the differentiation potential of SCs during embryogenesis and aging. The DNA methylation processes during development of ICM-derived epiblast SCs specify them to TCSCs. However, at the beginning of gastrulation, the proximal epiblast-specified PGCs can reset their epigenetic profile to one that characterizes ICM-derived PSCs. Subsequently, during PGC migration to the genital ridges, global DNA demethylation leads to the erasure of genomic imprints. Consistent with the hypothesis that VSELs originate from an epiblast-derived PGC population, they show a PGC-like epigenetic profile, including partial DNA demethylation of several pluripotency, germ-line, and genomic imprints. These epigenetic profiles of developing VSELs are retained after their deposition into adult tissues. This parent-specific reprogramming of the genomic imprinting of VSELs deposited in adult tissues (e.g., BM) functions as i) a "lock-in mechanism" to prevent their inappropriate proliferation and ii) a mechanism to restrict their sensitivity to Ins/Igf signaling. During the aging process, while residing in adult tissues, VSELs exposed to oxidative stress or chronic Ins/Igf signaling de-repress locked-in genomic imprints and progressively methylate DNA in the Oct-4 promoter (Ratajczak et al 2011a). As a result of these epigenetic changes, the total number and pluripotency of VSELs decreases with age (Ratajczak et al. 2008), which leads to impaired tissue regeneration and rejuvenation.

3.3 Expression of germline markers

During gastrulation, EpiSCs lose expression of core pluripotency TFs. On the other hand, during specification of proximal epiblast EpiSCs into PGCs, the expression of these early embryonic genes is re-activated by resetting epigenetic programs in these cells (Hayashi &

Very Small Embryonic/Epiblast-Like Stem Cells (VSELs) Residing in Adult Tissues and Their Role in
Tissue Rejuvenation and Regeneration

231

Surani, 2009). Thus, PGCs reset epigenetic marks to an ICM-like state, which results in re-activation of pluripotency and germline-related genes (Hayashi & Surani, 2009). The specification of PGCs is initiated at E7.25 by expression of germline master regulators, such as *Fragilis, Blimp1,* and *Stella,* in response to signals from extra-embryonic tissues (Surani et al., 2007). At this time, around 40 proximal epiblast-derived PGCs are detected. At E8.5, PGCs enter back into the embryo proper through the primitive streak and start migration through the hindgut endoderm and mesentry to the aorta-gonads-mesonephros (AGM) region, and at around E11.5 they reach the genital ridge in which PGCs differentiate into monopotent gametes (sperm and egg). Our data indicate some relationship between VSELs and PGCs (Shin et al., 2010b). Accordingly, VSELs are reported to highly express genes that are involved in germ-line specification of the epiblast (e.g., *Stella, Prdm14, Fragilis, Blimp1, Nanos3,* and *Dnd1*). The expression of Stella, Blimp1, and Mvh has been confirmed at the protein level by immunostaining. Furthermore, the *Stella* promoter in VSELs is partially demethylated and displays transcriptionally active histone modifications (H3Ac and H3K4me3) and is less enriched for transcriptionally repressive histone marks (H3K9me2 and H3K27me3) (Shin et al., 2010b). It can be concluded that VSELs express several germline-specific genes and display a *Stella* promoter chromatin structure that is characteristics of germline specification. VSELs also highly express *Dppa2, Dppa4,* and *Mvh,* which characterize late migratory PGCs; however, they do not express *Sycp3, Dazl,* and *LINE1* genes that are expressed in post-migratory PGCs (Maatouk et al., 2006; Maldonado-Saldivia et al., 2007). Thus, our results *in toto* support the conclusion that VSELs deposited into murine BM show some similarities in gene expression and epigenetic signatures to epiblast-derived migratory PGCs (at ~E10.5–E11.5).

3.4 VSELs are marked by BDs

As mentioned above, in undifferentiated ESCs, most of the homeodomain-containing developmental TFs are repressed by BDs (Bernstein et al., 2006), which are chromatin structures in which transcriptionally opposite histone codes physically co-exist in the same promoter. In undifferentiated ESCs, BD epigenetic codes at the promoters of these TFs are temporarily repressed, preventing their premature differentiation. During differentiation, the transient repressive epigenetic marks in these TFs become monovalent and thereafter activate or repress expression of the appropriate TFs. Our preliminary data indicate that murine VSELs display BDs in the promoters of several homeodomain-containing developmental TFs (*Sox21, Nkx2.2, Dlx1, Lbx1h, Hlxb9, Pax5,* and *HoxA3*). The presence of transcriptionally active histone codes, such as H3K4me3, physically coexisting with repressive histone codes, such as H3K27me3, was confirmed by employing the carrier-ChIP assay (submitted for publication).

3.5 VSELs from female mice partially activate an X chromosome

The process of X-chromosome inactivation is mediated by expression of the large noncoding RNA *Xist,* which is transcribed on the inactivated X chromosome. Coating of the X chromosome to be inactivated by spreading of Xist RNA induces the silenced chromatin structure (Payer & Lee, 2008). As already mentioned above, it is well known that female PSCs (*e.g.,* murine and human ESCs isolated from the blastocyst ICM, as well as PGCs) reactivate the X chromosome that was inactivated after fertilization, and, as a result, female PSCs display two equivalently activated X chromosomes (Surani et al., 2007). Our initial studies in murine female VSELs show that these cells partially reactivate the inactivated X chromosome. As mentioned above, female murine VSELs partially hypermethylate the *Xist* promoter (~80%), unlike somatic cells which show 50% DNA methylation. This result strongly suggests that murine VSELs, like ESCs and PGCs, can undergo the process of X chromosome reactivation (submitted for publication).

4. Developmental origin of VSELs

Taking into consideration all the molecular signatures characteristic of VSELs, we propose that VSELs are epiblast-derived PSCs deposited early during embryogenesis in developing organs as a potential reserve pool of precursors for TCSCs. Thus, VSELs have an important role in tissue rejuvenation and regeneration (Shin et al., 2010a). Because of the gene expression profile and epigenetic state of the core TFs, expression of epiblast and germline genes suggests that VSELs deposited in adult BM originate from migratory PGCs that have gone astray from the "orthodox" migration route.

From the second trimester on, VSELs are easily found as a Sca-1+Lin−CD45− population in murine fetal liver, which is the main embryonic hematopoietic tissue. VSELs that emerge in fetal liver (FL-VSELs) follow the developmental route of hematopoietic stem cells (HSCs) and subsequently colonize BM together with HSCs (Zuba-Surma et al., 2009). FL-VSELs and their BM-derived counterparts express a similar pattern of pluripotent and epiblast/germline genes at the mRNA and protein levels. Accordingly, the promoters for *Oct-4*, *Nanog*, and *Stella* show significant DNA demethylation and enriched histone modifications for an open, transcriptionally active structure in these promoters (Shin et al., 2010a).

Mounting evidence also indicates that PGCs could be related to HSCs, another population of highly migratory SCs (De Miguel et al., 2009). In support of this notion, the first primitive HSCs appear in the extra-embryonic tissues in yolk sac blood islands at the time when proximal epiblast-specified PGCs enter the extra-embryonic mesoderm (Mikkola & Orkin, 2006). In addition, the appearance of definitive HSCs in the AGM region of the embryo proper coincides with migration of PGCs to the genital ridges through the AGM (De Miguel et al., 2009). Furthermore, PGCs isolated from murine embryos have been proven to be able to grow HSC colonies while, on the other hand, robust hematopoietic differentiation has been observed in some classical germline tumors (Kritzenberger & Wrobel, 2004; Ohtaka et al., 1999; Rich, 1995; Saito et al., 1998; Woodruff et al., 1995). All this suggests developmental overlap between PGCs and HSCs.

On the other hand, VSELs share several characteristics with both PGCs and HSCs. In particular, VSELS i) share several BM- and FL-derived markers characteristic of the epiblast/germ line (Shin et al., 2010b), ii) follow the developmental route of HSCs (Zuba-Surma et al., 2009), and iii), in appropriate culture conditions, can also be differentiated toward the hematopoietic lineage. All of this suggests that VSELs are the most primitive murine BM-residing population of SCs and function as precursors for long-term repopulating HSCs (Ratajczak et al., 2011b).

Thus, PGCs, HSCs , and VSELs together form a unique highly migratory population of interrelated SCs that may be envisioned as a kind of 4th (highly migratory) germ layer. Due to this unique developmental origin, VSELs show characteristic epigenetic reprogramming and gene expression in stemness, germline, and imprinted genes (as described below) that maintain their pluripotency, but also prevent inappropriate proliferation and teratoma formation (Shin et al., 2009).

Very Small Embryonic/Epiblast-Like Stem Cells (VSELs) Residing in Adult Tissues and Their Role in
Tissue Rejuvenation and Regeneration

233

5. Epigenetic changes of imprinted genes that regulate VSEL pluripotency

Unlike ESCs, highly purified BM-derived Oct-4+ VSELs do not proliferate *in vitro* if cultured alone and do not grow teratomas *in vivo*. On the other hand, cells from VSEL-DSs have restored their proliferation potential, demonstrating that their quiescent state can be modulated. This suggests that VSELs are a quiescent cell population and that some mechanisms must exist to prevent their unleashing of proliferation and teratoma formation. Like VSELs, PGCs in cultures freshly isolated from embryos proliferate only for a few days before disappearing, either because they differentiate or die (De Felici & McLaren, 1983). They also neither grow teratomas nor complement blastocyst development (Surani et al., 2007). However, when PGCs are cultured over a feeder layer supplemented by a specific combination of growth factors, they continue to proliferate and can be reprogrammed into EGCs (Shamblott et al., 1998; Turnpenny et al., 2003). Therefore, it is possible that these two SC populations employ a similar molecular mechanism to regulate their pluripotency and to prevent cell proliferation.

The hallmark of epigenetic reprogramming during PGC development is erasure of genomic imprinting (Surani et al., 2007), which is an epigenetic process ensuring paternal-specific, mono-allelic expression of imprinted genes (Reik & Walter, 2001). Around 80 imprinted genes (expressed from maternal or paternal chromosomes only) have been reported in the mouse genome and their proper mono-allelic expression regulates totipotency and pluripotency of the zygote and developmentally early SCs, respectively. Furthermore, most imprinted genes, such as insulin-like growth factor 2 (*Igf2*), H19, Igf2 receptor (*Igf2R*), and *p57KIP2* (also known as *Cdkn1c*) are directly involved in embryo development. Since the majority of imprinted genes exist as gene clusters enriched for CpG islands, their expression is coordinately regulated by the DNA methylation state of CpG-rich cis-elements known as differentially methylated regions (DMRs) (Delaval & Feil, 2004). The differential methylation state of DMRs is mediated by DNA methyltransferases (*Dnmts*), depending on the parental allele of origin. Depending on the developmental period of methylation, there are two types of DMRs: "primary DMRs" are differentially methylated during gametogenesis and "secondary DMRs" acquire allele-specific methylation after fertilization. So far, 15 primary DMRs have been identified in the mouse genome. Interestingly, most DMRs are methylated at the maternal allele and only three DMRs (at *Igf2-H19, Rasgrf1*, and *Meg3* loci) are paternally methylated (Kobayashi et al., 2006). In addition to DNA methylation of DMRs, histone modifications also contribute to monoallelic expression of imprinted genes (Fournier et al., 2002; Mager et al., 2003).

Shortly after PGC specification at E7.25, PGCs initiate epigenetic reprogramming programs, resulting in global DNA demethylation and changes in histone modifications (Seki et al., 2007). As a result, epigenetic marks for genomic imprinting in both parental chromosomes are erased during migration into the genital ridge and new genomic imprints are established during differentiation into gametes in a sex-dependent manner. The erasure of genomic imprints could be a mechanism to protect the Oct-4-expressing germline SCs from uncontrolled expansion and teratoma formation. For example, while the nuclei of early migrating PGCs at E8.5–9.5 can be successfully used as donors for nuclear transfer, nuclei from post-migratory PGCs after E11.5 are incompetent to support full-term development (Yamazaki et al., 2003).

Since VSELs, as discussed above, share similar molecular signatures as PGCs, we have proposed that VSELs, like PGCs, modify methylation of imprinted genes, which prevents them from unleashing proliferation and may explain their quiescent state in adult tissues. Indeed, as shown in **Figure 3** and **Table 1**, VSELs freshly isolated from murine BM erase the paternally methylated imprints (e.g., *Igf2-H19* and *Rasgrf1* loci), while they hypermethylate the maternally methylated ones (e.g., *Igf2* receptor (*Igf2R*), *Kcnq1-p57KIP2*, and *Peg1* loci). Because paternally expressed imprinted genes (*Igf2* and *Rasgrf1*) enhance embryo growth and maternally expressed genes (*H19*, *p57KIP2*, and *Igf2R*) inhibit cell proliferation (Reik & Walter, 2001), the unique genomic imprinting pattern observed in VSELs demonstrates growth-repressive imprinting in these cells. As coordinated with genomic imprinting reprogramming programs, VSELs highly express growth-repressive imprinted gene transcripts (*H19*, *p57KIP2*, and *Igf2R*) and downregulate growth-promoting ones (*Igf2* and *Rasgrf1*), which explains the quiescent state of VSELs (Shin et al., 2009). Importantly, all the growth-repressive patterns of genomic imprinting are progressively recovered during the formation of VSEL-DSs, in which SCs proliferate and differentiate. These results suggest that epigenetic reprogramming of genomic imprinting should maintain the quiescence of Oct-4+ VSELs deposited in the adult body and protect them from premature aging and tumor formation. Therefore, the modulation of mechanisms controlling genomic imprinting in VSELs is crucial for developing more powerful strategies to unleash the regenerative potential of these cells for efficient employment in the clinical setting.

6. VSELs and ageing

Tissue regeneration depends on the proper function of SCs, and we envision that aging can be partially explained by a decline in the regenerative potential of VSELs (Ratajczak et al., 2008). In support of this notion, the number of VSELs in murine BM gradually declines with age, ranging from 0.052 ± 0.018% at 2 months to 0.003 ± 0.002% at 3 years of age (Kucia et al., 2008a). Furthermore, the frequency of VSEL-DS formation decreases with age, thus little VSEL-DS formation was observed in cells isolated from older mice (>2 years). Accordingly, VSELs from older mice (2 years) also show lower expression of pluripotency master regulators, such as *Oct-4, Nanog, Sox2, Klf4,* and *cMyc,* while the *Oct-4* promoter in VSELs becomes hypermethylated with age and shows a closed chromatin structure (Ratajczak et al., 2011a). The age-dependent decrease of the pool size and function of VSELs in BM may explain the decline of regeneration potential during aging. This hypothesis has been further corroborated by looking for differences in the content of these cells among BM mononuclear cells (BMMNCs) in long- and short-lived mouse strains. The concentration of VSELs was much higher in the BM of long-lived (e.g., C57B6) compared to short-lived (DBA/2J) mice (Kucia et al., 2006b).

We have also reported that while long-lived Laron dwarf mice, with low levels of circulating Igf1, have a higher number of VSELs in BM compared to normal littermates (Ratajczak et al. 2011a), short-lived bovine-growth-hormone-expressing transgenic mice, with high circulating Igf1 levels, prematurely deplete this population of PSCs (submitted for publication). These observations suggest interesting links between high caloric uptake, increases in chronic insulin/insulin growth factor signaling, and premature depletion of VSELs.

In support of this linkage, it is well known that changes in insulin/insulin-like growth factors (Ins/Igf) signaling molecules play a crucial role in aging. In particular, insulin-like growth factor 1 (*Igf1*) signaling negatively regulates the life span of animals, from worms

Very Small Embryonic/Epiblast-Like Stem Cells (VSELs) Residing in Adult Tissues and Their Role in
Tissue Rejuvenation and Regeneration

235

and flies to mammals (Russell & Kahn, 2007), whileIgf1 and insulin level in blood is regulated positively by caloric uptake (Piper & Bartke, 2008). Overall, the genomic imprinting reprogramming in VSELs leads to impaired Ins/Ingf signaling due to i) downregulation of expression of *Igf2*, ii) upregulation of expression of *Igf2R*, which serves as a molecular sink for Igf2, and iii) a decrease in expression of *Rasgrf1*, which is a small GTP exchange factor (GEF) for Ins/Igf signal transduction. This suggests that the epigenetic mechanism governing the VSEL quiescent state regulates the sensitivity to Ins/Igf signaling and could, if overactivated, lead to premature depletion of primitive VSELs in tissues (Ratajczak et al., 2011a).

Thus, high chronic calorie uptake, followed by high plasma insulin and Igf-1 levels may, over time, prematurely deplete VSELs from adult organs and thus accelerate aging.

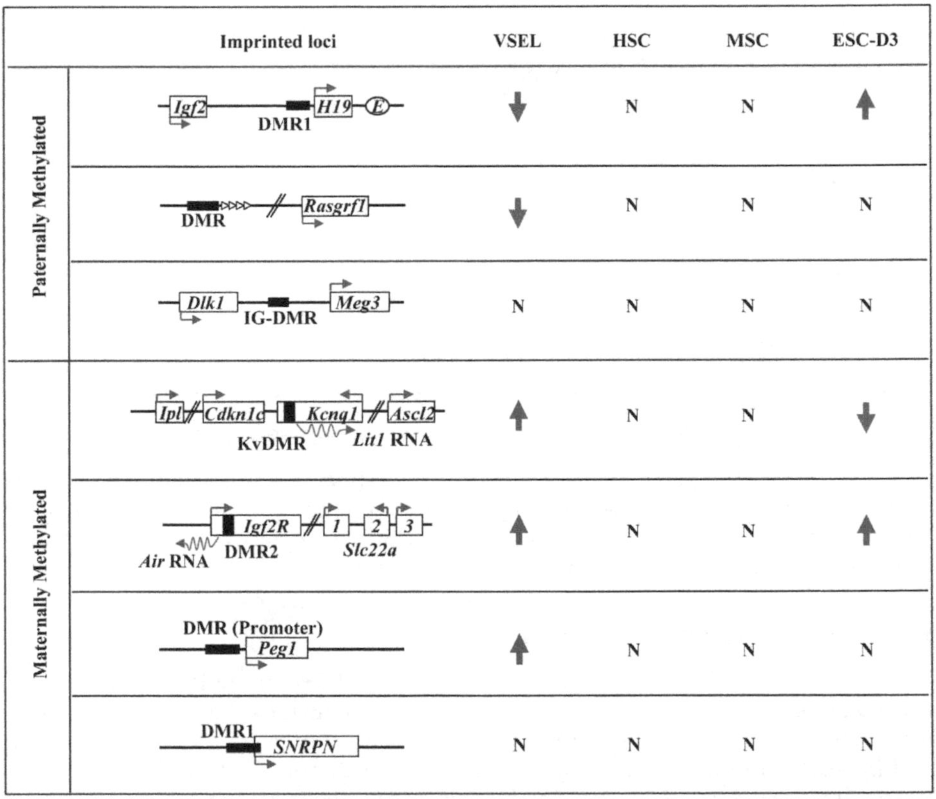

Fig. 3. **The unique DNA methylation pattern and expression of imprinted genes in VSELs.** Arrows in the schematic diagram of paternally (Igf2-H19 and Rasgrf1) or maternally (Igf2R and Kcnq1) methylated loci indicate the transcriptional activity of the indicated gene. Red (up) and blue (down) arrows indicate upregulated and downregulated gene expression, respectively. M = maternal chromosome, P = paternal chromosome. DMR1, IG-DMR, KvDMR, DMR2 = DMRs for Igf2-H19, Rasgrf1, Kcnq1, and Igf2R loci, respectively.

Imprinted gene	Expression	Proliferation	VSEL
Igf2	Pat	+	↓
Rasgrf1	Pat	+	↓
Dlk1	Pat	+	N
Air	Pat	+	↓
Lit1	Pat	+	↓
H19	Mat	−	↑
Meg3	Mat	−	N
Igf2R	Mat	−	↑
p57^{KIP2}/Cdkn1c	Mat	−	↑
SNRPN	Mat	−	N

Table 1 . Expression profiles of crucial imprinted genes in murine VSELs.

The expression level of paternally (pat) or maternally (mat) expressed imprinted genes in murine BM-derived VSELs is indicated by red-up (up-regulated) and blue-down (down-regulated) arrows. The effect of the indicated imprinted genes on cell proliferation is marked as '+' (proliferation promoting) or '−' (repressing).

7. Regeneration potential of VSELs *in vivo*

To address the most important question of whether these primitive VSELs could be efficiently employed in the clinic, we have tested their potential role in several *in vivo* tissue-regeneration animal models. First, VSELs can be specified *in vivo* into mesenchymal stem cells (MSCs). Accordingly, in the first study by Taichman *et al*, VSELs isolated from GFP+ mice were implanted into SCID mice, and 4 weeks later the formation of bone-like tissues was observed (Taichman *et al.*, 2010). Second, freshly isolated BM-derived VSELs from GFP+ mice were injected into the hearts of mice that had undergone ischemia/reperfusion injury. After 35 days of follow-up, VSEL-treated mice exhibited improved global and regional left ventricular (LV) systolic function (as determined by echocardiography) and attenuated myocyte hypertrophy in surviving tissue (as determined by histology and echocardiography) when compared with vehicle-treated controls (Zuba-Surma et al., 2010). Finally, we observed that VSELs, if plated over the supportive OP9 cell line, give rise to

Very Small Embryonic/Epiblast-Like Stem Cells (VSELs) Residing in Adult Tissues and Their Role in
Tissue Rejuvenation and Regeneration

237

colonies of CD45+CD41+Gr-1-Ter119- cells that, when transplanted into wild-type animals, protected them from lethal irradiation and differentiated *in vivo* into all   major hematopoietic lineages (e.g., Gr-1+, B220+ and CD3+ cells) (Ratajczak et al., 2011b). Thus, we propose that VSELs are a population of BM-residing PSCs that give rise to long-term-engrafting hematopoietic SCs.

8. Conclusion

In the past few years, several attempts have been made to purify a population of PSCs from adult tissues. We propose that the VSELs described by our team play a physiological role in rejuvenation of the pool of TCSCs under steady-state conditions. VSELs developmentally originate from epiblast-derived migrating PGCs and they could be deposited in adult organs early in development as a reserve pool of primitive SCs for tissue repair and regeneration. Therefore, VSELs share several molecular signatures with epiblast and migrating PGCs with respect to gene expression and epigenetic programs. Based on the developmental origin of VSELs, their proliferation, like PGCs, is controlled by the DNA methylation state of some of the developmentally crucial imprinted genes (e.g. *H19, Igf2,* and *Rasgrf1*). During the ageing process, proliferation-repressive epigenetic marks progressively disappear, resulting in the increased sensitivity to Ins/Igf signaling and, concomitantly, to depletion of the primitive VSEL population. The decrease in the number and pluripotency of these cells will affect pools of TCSCs and have an impact on tissue rejuvenation and life span. Furthermore, VSELs can be specified into several tissue-residing TCSCs (e.g. MSCs, HSCs, and cardiac SCs) in response to tissue/organ injury. Therefore, VSELs isolated from adult tissues are an alternative and ethically uncontroversial source of SCs for regenerative medicine. However, to successfully employ VSELs for this purpose, it is very important to establish experimental protocols for reprogramming of the growth-repressive genomic imprinted state of VSELs into the regular somatic pattern to unleash their regenerative potential.

9. Acknowledgment

This work was supported by NIH R01 CA106281-01, NIH R01 DK074720, and the Henry M. and Stella M. Hoenig Endowment to MZR and NIH P20RR018733 from the National Center for Research Resources to MK.

10. Conflicts of interest statement

The authors declare that they have no competing financial interests.

11. References

Azuara, V., Perry, P., Sauer, S., Spivakov, M., Jorgensen, H.F., John, R.M., Gouti, M., Casanova, M., Warnes, G., Merkenschlager, M., *et al.* (2006). Chromatin signatures of pluripotent cell lines. *Nat Cell Biol* 8: 532–538.

Beltrami, A.P., Cesselli, D., Bergamin, N., Marcon, P., Rigo, S., Puppato, E., D'Aurizio, F., Verardo, R., Piazza, S., Pignatelli, A., *et al.* (2007). Multipotent cells can be generated in vitro from several adult human organs (heart, liver, and bone marrow). *Blood* 110: 3438-3446.

Bernstein, B.E., Mikkelsen, T.S., Xie, X., Kamal, M., Huebert, D.J., Cuff, J., Fry, B., Meissner, A., Wernig, M., Plath, K., *et al.* (2006). A Bivalent Chromatin Structure Marks Key Developmental Genes in Embryonic Stem Cells. *Cell* 125: 315-326.

Boyer, L.A., Plath, K., Zeitlinger, J., Brambrink, T., Medeiros, L.A., Lee, T.I., Levine, S.S., Wernig, M., Tajonar, A., Ray, M.K., *et al.* (2006). Polycomb complexes repress developmental regulators in murine embryonic stem cells. *Nature* 441: 349-353.

Brons, I.G.M., Smithers, L.E., Trotter, M.W.B., Rugg-Gunn, P., Sun, B., Chuva de Sousa Lopes, S.M., Howlett, S.K., Clarkson, A., Ahrlund-Richter, L., Pedersen, R.A., *et al.* (2007). Derivation of pluripotent epiblast stem cells from mammalian embryos. *Nature* 448: 191-195.

Cedar, H. & Bergman, Y. (2009). Linking DNA methylation and histone modification: patterns and paradigms. *Nat Rev Genet* 10: 295-304.

D'Ippolito, G., Diabira, S., Howard, G.A., Menei, P., Roos, B.A. & Schiller, P.C. (2004). Marrow-isolated adult multilineage inducible (MIAMI) cells, a unique population of postnatal young and old human cells with extensive expansion and differentiation potential. *J Cell Sci* 117: 2971-2981.

De Felici, M. & McLaren, A. (1983). In vitro culture of mouse primordial germ cells. *Exp Cell Res* 144: 417-427.

De Miguel, M.P., Arnalich Montiel, F., Lopez Iglesias, P., Blazquez Martinez, A. & Nistal, M. (2009). Epiblast-derived stem cells in embryonic and adult tissues. *Int J Dev Biol* 53: 1529-1540.

Delaval, K. & Feil, R. (2004). Epigenetic regulation of mammalian genomic imprinting. *Current Opinion in Genetics & Development* 14: 188-195.

Evans, M.J. & Kaufman, M.H. (1981). Establishment in culture of pluripotential cells from mouse embryos. *Nature* 292: 154-156.

Fournier, C., Goto, Y., Ballestar, E., Delaval, K., Hever, A.M., Esteller, M. & Feil, R. (2002). Allele-specific histone lysine methylation marks regulatory regions at imprinted mouse genes. *EMBO J* 21: 6560-6570.

Hayashi, K., Lopes, S.M.C.d.S., Tang, F. & Surani, M.A. (2008). Dynamic Equilibrium and Heterogeneity of Mouse Pluripotent Stem Cells with Distinct Functional and Epigenetic States. *Cell Stem Cell* 3: 391-401.

Hayashi, K. & Surani, M.A. (2009). Resetting the Epigenome beyond Pluripotency in the Germline. *Cell Stem Cell* 4: 493-498.

Jiang, Y., Jahagirdar, B.N., Reinhardt, R.L., Schwartz, R.E., Keene, C.D., Ortiz-Gonzalez, X.R., Reyes, M., Lenvik, T., Lund, T., Blackstad, M., *et al.* (2002). Pluripotency of mesenchymal stem cells derived from adult marrow. *Nature* 418: 41-49.

Kim, J., Chu, J., Shen, X., Wang, J. & Orkin, S.H. (2008). An Extended Transcriptional Network for Pluripotency of Embryonic Stem Cells. *Cell* 132: 1049-1061.

Kobayashi, H., Suda, C., Abe, T., Kohara, Y., Ikemura, T. & Sasaki, H. (2006). Bisulfite sequencing and dinucleotide content analysis of 15 imprinted mouse differentially methylated regions (DMRs): paternally methylated DMRs contain less CpGs than maternally methylated DMRs. *Cytogenetic and Genome Research* 113: 130-137.

Kritzenberger, M. & Wrobel, K.-H. (2004). Histochemical in situ identification of bovine embryonic blood cells reveals differences to the adult haematopoietic system and

Very Small Embryonic/Epiblast-Like Stem Cells (VSELs) Residing in Adult Tissues and Their Role in
Tissue Rejuvenation and Regeneration

239

suggests a close relationship between haematopoietic stem cells and primordial germ cells. *Histochemistry and Cell Biology* 121: 273–289.

Kucia, M., Halasa, M., Wysoczynski, M., Baskiewicz-Masiuk, M., Moldenhawer, S., Zuba-Surma, E., Czajka, R., Wojakowski, W., Machalinski, B. & Ratajczak, M.Z. (2006a). Morphological and molecular characterization of novel population of CXCR4+ SSEA-4+ Oct-4+ very small embryonic-like cells purified from human cord blood - preliminary report. *Leukemia* 21: 297–303.

Kucia, M., Reca, R., Campbell, F.R., Zuba-Surma, E., Majka, M., Ratajczak, J. & Ratajczak, M.Z. (2006b). A population of very small embryonic-like (VSEL) CXCR4+SSEA-1+Oct-4+ stem cells identified in adult bone marrow. *Leukemia* 20: 857–869.

Kucia, M., Wysoczynski, M., Ratajczak, J. & Ratajczak, M. (2008a). Identification of very small embryonic like (VSEL) stem cells in bone marrow. *Cell and Tissue Research* 331: 125–134.

Kucia, M.J., Wysoczynski, M., Wu, W., Zuba-Surma, E.K., Ratajczak, J. & Ratajczak, M.Z. (2008b). Evidence That Very Small Embryonic-Like Stem Cells Are Mobilized into Peripheral Blood. *Stem Cells* 26: 2083–2092.

Lee, T.I., Jenner, R.G., Boyer, L.A., Guenther, M.G., Levine, S.S., Kumar, R.M., Chevalier, B., Johnstone, S.E., Cole, M.F., Isono, K.-i., *et al.* (2006). Control of Developmental Regulators by Polycomb in Human Embryonic Stem Cells. *Cell* 125: 301–313.

Lengner, C.J., Camargo, F.D., Hochedlinger, K., Welstead, G.G., Zaidi, S., Gokhale, S., Scholer, H.R., Tomilin, A. & Jaenisch, R. (2007). Oct4 Expression Is Not Required for Mouse Somatic Stem Cell Self-Renewal. *Cell Stem Cell* 1: 403–415.

Liedtke, S., Enczmann, J.g., Waclawczyk, S., Wernet, P. & K?ler, G. (2007). Oct4 and Its Pseudogenes Confuse Stem Cell Research. *Cell Stem Cell* 1: 364–366.

Maatouk, D.M., Kellam, L.D., Mann, M.R.W., Lei, H., Li, E., Bartolomei, M.S. & Resnick, J.L. (2006). DNA methylation is a primary mechanism for silencing postmigratory primordial germ cell genes in both germ cell and somatic cell lineages. *Development* 133: 3411–3418.

Mager, J., Montgomery, N.D., de Villena, F.P.-M. & Magnuson, T. (2003). Genome imprinting regulated by the mouse Polycomb group protein Eed. *Nat Genet* 33: 502–507.

Maldonado-Saldivia, J., van den Bergen, J., Krouskos, M., Gilchrist, M., Lee, C., Li, R., Sinclair, A.H., Surani, M.A. & Western, P.S. (2007). Dppa2 and Dppa4 Are Closely Linked SAP Motif Genes Restricted to Pluripotent Cells and the Germ Line. *Stem Cells* 25: 19–28.

Matsui, Y., Zsebo, K. & Hogan, B.L.M. (1992). Derivation of pluripotential embryonic stem cells from murine primordial germ cells in culture. *Cell* 70: 841–847.

Mikkola, H.K.A. & Orkin, S.H. (2006). The journey of developing hematopoietic stem cells. *Development* 133: 3733–3744.

Niwa, H. (2007). How is pluripotency determined and maintained? *Development* 134: 635–646.

Ohtaka, T., Matsui, Y. & Obinata, M. (1999). Hematopoietic Development of Primordial Germ Cell-Derived Mouse Embryonic Germ Cells in Culture. *Biochemical and Biophysical Research Communications* 260: 475–482.

Paczkowska, E., Kucia, M., Koziarska, D., Halasa, M., Safranow, K., Masiuk, M., Karbicka, A., Nowik, M., Nowacki, P., Ratajczak, M.Z., *et al.* (2009). Clinical Evidence That

Very Small Embryonic-Like Stem Cells Are Mobilized Into Peripheral Blood in Patients After Stroke. *Stroke* 40: 1237–1244.

Payer, B. & Lee, J.T. (2008). X Chromosome Dosage Compensation: How Mammals Keep the Balance. *Annual Review of Genetics* 42: 733–772.

Piper, M.D.W. & Bartke, A. (2008). Diet and Aging. *Cell Metabolism* 8: 99–104.

Pochampally, R.R., Smith, J.R., Ylostalo, J. & Prockop, D.J. (2004). Serum deprivation of human marrow stromal cells (hMSCs) selects for a subpopulation of early progenitor cells with enhanced expression of OCT-4 and other embryonic genes. *Blood* 103: 1647–1652.

Ratajczak, J., Shin, D.M., Wan, W., Liu, R., Masternak, M.M., Piotrowska, K., Wiszniewska, B., Kucia, M., Bartke, A. & Ratajczak, M.Z. (2011a). Higher number of stem cells in the bone marrow of circulating low Igf-1 level Laron dwarf mice - novel view on Igf-1, stem cells and aging. *Leukemia* 25: 729–733.

Ratajczak, J., Wysoczynski, M., Zuba-Surma, E., Wan, W., Kucia, M., Yoder, M.C. & Ratajczak, M.Z. (2011b). Adult murine bone marrow-derived very small embryonic-like stem cells differentiate into the hematopoietic lineage after coculture over OP9 stromal cells. *Experimental Hematology* 39: 225–237.

Ratajczak, M., Shin, D.-M., Liu, R., Marlicz, W., Tarnowski, M., Ratajczak, J. & Kucia, M. (2010). Epiblast/Germ Line Hypothesis of Cancer Development Revisited: Lesson from the Presence of Oct-4<sup>+</sup> Cells in Adult Tissues. *Stem Cell Reviews and Reports* 6: 307–316.

Ratajczak, M.Z., Machalinski, B., Wojakowski, W., Ratajczak, J. & Kucia, M. (2007). A hypothesis for an embryonic origin of pluripotent Oct-4+ stem cells in adult bone marrow and other tissues. *Leukemia* 21: 860–867.

Ratajczak, M.Z., Zuba-Surma, E.K., Shin, D.-M., Ratajczak, J. & Kucia, M. (2008). Very small embryonic-like (VSEL) stem cells in adult organs and their potential role in rejuvenation of tissues and longevity. *Experimental Gerontology* 43: 1009–1017.

Reik, W. & Walter, J. (2001). Genomic imprinting: parental influence on the genome. *Nat Rev Genet* 2: 21–32.

Rich, I.N. (1995). Primordial germ cells are capable of producing cells of the hematopoietic system in vitro. *Blood* 86: 463–472.

Russell, S.J. & Kahn, C.R. (2007). Endocrine regulation of ageing. *Nat Rev Mol Cell Biol* 8: 681–691.

Saito, A., Watanabe, K., Kusakabe, T., Abe, M. & Suzuki, T. (1998). Mediastinal mature teratoma with coexistence of angiosarcoma, granulocytic sarcoma and a hematopoietic region in the tumor: a rare case of association between hematological malignancy and mediastinal germ cell tumor. *Pathol Int* 48: 749–753.

Seki, Y., Yamaji, M., Yabuta, Y., Sano, M., Shigeta, M., Matsui, Y., Saga, Y., Tachibana, M., Shinkai, Y. & Saitou, M. (2007). Cellular dynamics associated with the genome-wide epigenetic reprogramming in migrating primordial germ cells in mice. *Development* 134: 2627–2638.

Shamblott, M.J., Axelman, J., Wang, S., Bugg, E.M., Littlefield, J.W., Donovan, P.J., Blumenthal, P.D., Huggins, G.R. & Gearhart, J.D. (1998). Derivation of pluripotent stem cells from cultured human primordial germ cells. *Proc Natl Acad Sci U S A* 95: 13726–13731.

Shin, D.-M., Liu, R., Klich, I., Ratajczak, J., Kucia, M. & Ratajczak, M. (2010a). Molecular characterization of isolated from murine adult tissues very small embryonic/epiblast like stem cells (VSELs). *Molecules and Cells* 29: 533–538.

Shin, D.M., Liu, R., Klich, I., Wu, W., Ratajczak, J., Kucia, M. & Ratajczak, M.Z. (2010b). Molecular signature of adult bone marrow-purified very small embryonic-like stem cells supports their developmental epiblast/germ line origin. *Leukemia* 24: 1450–1461.

Shin, D.M., Zuba-Surma, E.K., Wu, W., Ratajczak, J., Wysoczynski, M., Ratajczak, M.Z. & Kucia, M. (2009). Novel epigenetic mechanisms that control pluripotency and quiescence of adult bone marrow-derived Oct4+ very small embryonic-like stem cells. *Leukemia* 23: 2042–2051.

Stock, J.K., Giadrossi, S., Casanova, M., Brookes, E., Vidal, M., Koseki, H., Brockdorff, N., Fisher, A.G. & Pombo, A. (2007). Ring1-mediated ubiquitination of H2A restrains poised RNA polymerase II at bivalent genes in mouse ES cells. *Nat Cell Biol* 9: 1428–1435.

Surani, M.A., Hayashi, K. & Hajkova, P. (2007). Genetic and Epigenetic Regulators of Pluripotency. *Cell* 128: 747–762.

Taichman, R.S., Wang, Z., Shiozawa, Y., Jung, Y., Song, J., Balduino, A., Wang, J., Patel, L.R., Havens, A.M., Kucia, M., *et al.* (2010). Prospective Identification and Skeletal Localization of Cells Capable of Multilineage Differentiation In Vivo. *Stem Cells and Development* 19: 1557–1570.

Takahashi, K. & Yamanaka, S. (2006). Induction of Pluripotent Stem Cells from Mouse Embryonic and Adult Fibroblast Cultures by Defined Factors. *Cell* 126: 663–676.

Tesar, P.J., Chenoweth, J.G., Brook, F.A., Davies, T.J., Evans, E.P., Mack, D.L., Gardner, R.L. & McKay, R.D.G. (2007). New cell lines from mouse epiblast share defining features with human embryonic stem cells. *Nature* 448: 196–199.

Turnpenny, L., Brickwood, S., Spalluto, C.M., Piper, K., Cameron, I.T., Wilson, D.I. & Hanley, N.A. (2003). Derivation of Human Embryonic Germ Cells: An Alternative Source of Pluripotent Stem Cells. *STEM CELLS* 21: 598–609.

Wernig, M., Meissner, A., Foreman, R., Brambrink, T., Ku, M., Hochedlinger, K., Bernstein, B.E. & Jaenisch, R. (2007). In vitro reprogramming of fibroblasts into a pluripotent ES-cell-like state. *Nature* 448: 318–324.

Wojakowski, W., Tendera, M., Kucia, M., Zuba-Surma, E., Paczkowska, E., Ciosek, J., Halasa, M., Kr, M., Kazmierski, M., Buszman, P., *et al.* (2009). Mobilization of Bone Marrow-Derived Oct-4+ SSEA-4+ Very Small Embryonic-Like Stem Cells in Patients With Acute Myocardial Infarction. *Journal of the American College of Cardiology* 53: 1–9.

Woodruff, K., Wang, N., May, W., Adrone, E., Denny, C. & Feig, S.A. (1995). The clonal nature of mediastinal germ cell tumors and acute myelogenous leukemia : A case report and review of the literature. *Cancer Genetics and Cytogenetics* 79: 25–31.

Yamazaki, Y., Mann, M.R., Lee, S.S., Marh, J., McCarrey, J.R., Yanagimachi, R. & Bartolomei, M.S. (2003). Reprogramming of primordial germ cells begins before migration into the genital ridge, making these cells inadequate donors for reproductive cloning. *Proc Natl Acad Sci U S A* 100: 12207–12212.

Zuba-Surma, E.K., Guo, Y., Taher, H., Sanganalmath, S.K., Hunt, G., Vincent, R.J., Kucia, M., Abdel-Latif, A., Tang, X.L., Ratajczak, M.Z., *et al.* (2010). Transplantation of expanded bone marrow-derived very small embryonic-like stem cells (VSEL-SCs) improves left ventricular function and remodeling after myocardial infarction. *Journal of Cellular and Molecular Medicine*: no-no.

Zuba-Surma, E.K., Kucia, M., Rui, L., Shin, D.-M., Wojakowski, W., Ratajczak, J. & Ratajczak, M.Z. (2009). Fetal Liver Very Small Embryonic/Epiblast Like Stem Cells Follow Developmental Migratory Pathway of Hematopoietic Stem Cells. *Annals of the New York Academy of Sciences* 1176: 205–218.

Zuba-Surma, E.K., Kucia, M., Wu, W., Klich, I., Jr., J.W.L., Ratajczak, J. & Ratajczak, M.Z. (2008). Very small embryonic-like stem cells are present in adult murine organs: ImageStream-based morphological analysis and distribution studies. *Cytometry Part A* 73A: 1116–1127.

13

Multipotent Dental Stem Cells: An Alternative Adult Derived Stem Cell Source for Regenerative Medicine

Tammy Laberge[1,2] and Herman S. Cheung[1,2]
[1]Department of Biomedical Engineering, College of Engineering, University of Miami
[2]Geriatrics Research, Education and Clinical Center, Miami VA Healthcare System
USA

1. Introduction

The pluripotent nature of embryonic stem cells (ESCs) makes them amenable for regenerative therapies because they can differentiate into cells that form all tissue types within the body (Zandstra and Nagy, 2001). The potential drawbacks to the use of ESCs for cellular therapies include the obvious ethical dilemmas of obtaining ESCs, the potential of cancer or tumor formation and the risk of immunogenic rejection (Wobus and Boheler, 2005). Therefore adult stem cell sources with multipotent and pluripotent potential have been sought as an alternative for ESCs including mesenchymal stem cell (MSCs) and tissue-derived specific stem cells.

Interestingly, the isolation of a population of dental stem cells derived ectodermally from the neural crest (NC) have been shown to be multipotent and give rise to multifarious cell types that result in the development of many of the body's organs or tissues (Huang et al., 2009a; Huang et al., 2009b). Stem cells extracted from dental tissues including dental pulp, periodontal ligament, apical papilla and dental follicle precursor cells have an expansive differentiation potential with respect to mesodermal and ectodermal lineages. Currently there are six types of dental stem cells that are well characterized and described both in vitro and in vivo (Gronthos et al., 2000; Huang et al., 2009a; Karaöz et al., 2010; Miura et al., 2003; Morsczeck et al., 2005; Seo et al., 2004; Sonoyama et al., 2006).

Some dental stem cells lines have been shown to express ESC markers Oct4, Nanog, Sox2 and Klf4 and NC markers p75, Sox10, Slug and Nestin suggesting that dental stem cells may be able to become many of the same tissues as ESCs (Huang et al., 2009a). Further, dental stem cells have been shown to differentiate into neurogenic, adipogenic, cardiomyogenic, chondrogenic, myogenic and osteogenic lineages (Huang et al., 2009a; Karaöz et al., 2010; Miura et al., 2003; Seo et al., 2004; Sonoyama et al., 2006; Zhang et al., 2006). Since dental stem cells have been shown to differentiate into a multitude of cell types, their potential for use in tissue regeneration may be boundless.

We are currently using dental stem cells to investigate the mechanisms of mechanotransduction elicited during dynamic cyclic compression for chondrogenesis. Our long term goal is to develop technology and protocols utilizing dental stem cells and biomechanical force for reparative medicine and tissue regeneration of cartilage. This review will discuss the most current findings in tissue engineering with respect to dental stem cells both for whole tooth regeneration and potential use in future stem cell therapies.

2. Characteristics and sources of stem cells

2.1 What is a stem cell?

The general properties that define a stem cells are: 1. Stem cells are cells that are clonogenic and have the ability for self-renewal; 2. Stem cells are unspecialized cells that when correctly stimulated have the ability to differentiate into specialized cell types (Blau et al., 2001; Bongso and Fong, 2009).

There are two broader categories of stem cells: embryonic stem cells (ESCs) and adult stem cells. Embryonic stem cells are derived from the blastocyst stage of a developing embryo (Fortier, 2005; Thomson et al., 1998) and are capable of forming all three germ layers (ectoderm, endoderm, and mesoderm)(Bongso and Fong, 2009). Harvesting ESCs requires the destruction of the embryo (Lanzendorf et al., 2001) which leads to ethical dilemmas when obtaining these cells. The use of adult stem cells avoids these ethical issues. Adult stem cells have been obtained from multiple tissues including bone marrow (Pittenger et al., 1999), adipose tissue (Zuk et al., 2001), muscle (Deasy et al., 2001), umbilical cord tissue (Schugar et al., 2009), intestine (Wong, 2004), and skin (Blanpain et al., 2004). While most of this book focuses on the embryonically derived stem cells, this chapter focuses on the adult or postnatal stem cells with special emphasis on those derived from dental tissues.

2.2 Stem cell potency

Stem cell potency refers to the ability of the cell to differentiate into specific tissue type(s). Totipotent is defined as the ability to differentiate into any of the cell types of the entire organism, both embryonic and adult cell types (Dannan, 2009; Mummery et al., 2011; Smith, 2006). An example of a totipotent cell is a fertilized egg cell because it is able to differentiate into embryonic, extra-embryonic (ie. placenta) and adult tissues of the entire organism (Alison et al., 2002; Dannan, 2009; Mummery et al., 2011). Pluripotent stem cells have the potential to differentiate into all cell lineages including the three germ layers: ectoderm, mesoderm, or endoderm but not the extra-embryonic tissues (Alison et al., 2002; Dannan, 2009; Fortier, 2005; Mummery et al., 2011; Smith, 2006). ESCs are considered the gold standard of stem cells because of their pluripotency and their ability to be maintained indefinitely in culture (Thomson et al., 1998). Pluripotency has also been demonstrated in adult stem cells including bone marrow mesenchymal stem cells (BMMSCs) (Jiang et al., 2002). Multipotent stem cells have the ability to differentiate into multiple cell lineages that can form more than one tissue type (Alison et al., 2002; Mummery et al., 2011; Smith, 2006). Mesenchymal stem cells (MSCs) derived from adipose tissue are an example of a multipotent stem cell and are able to differentiate into multiple tissues of the mesodermal lineage including bone, fat and cartilage (Zuk et al., 2002).

2.3 Bone marrow mesenchymal stem cells

Stem cells obtained from bone marrow are a major source of adult MSCs and are widely studied. Bone marrow stromal cells can be harvested from bone marrow by mechanical disruption, but the cell suspension will contain both hematopoietic stem cells and BMMSCs (Bianco et al., 2001). BMMSCs are isolated as colony forming unit-fibroblasts (CFU-Fs) from the bone marrow cell suspension. In order to separate the two types of stem cells, the cell suspension is cultured in vitro at low density. A small number of BMMSCs will adhere to the plate and begin to form colonies while the non-adherent hematopoietic cells are then removed by repeat washings (Bianco et al., 2001; Chamberlain et al., 2007). BMMSCs isolated in this manner are capable of 20–25 passages in vitro without significant changes to the cell phenotype (Bianco et al., 2001; Conget and Minguell, 1999). Gronthos et al. (2003) further showed that BMMSCs could be isolated from bone marrow aspirates by determining which CFU-F colonies were highly reactive to the antibody STRO-1 (STRO-1[Bright]) and also reactive to the antibody VCAM-1 (VCAM-1[+]). These new studies isolated BMMSCs in bone marrow aspirates based on STRO-1[Bright]/ VCAM-1[+] cell surface markers by florescence activated cell sorting (FACS) and were capable of proliferating up to 40 population doublings (Gronthos et al., 2003).

BMMSCs show a great level of plasticity and have shown the potential to differentiate into multiple tissue types in vitro including muscle, adipose, cartilage, bone, connective tissue, neurons and endothelial cells (Gronthos et al., 2003; Pittenger et al., 1999; Woodbury et al., 2000; Young and Black, 2004). Interestingly, when transplanted into immunodeficient mice, BMMSCs undergo osteogenic differentiation in vivo and form bone (Kuznetsov et al., 1997). In 2006, the minimum criteria to define human multipotent mesenchymal stromal cells was established as: Cells that are plastic adherent in standard culture; Cells that have the ability to differentiate in vitro into osteoblasts, adipocytes and chondroblasts; Cells that express the cell surface markers CD73, CD90 and CD105 in 95% of the cell population as determined by flow cytometry and lack the expression (≤ 2% positive) of CD14, CD34, CD45 or CD11b, CD79a or CD19 and HLA class II (Dominici et al., 2006).

2.4 Dental stem cells

Dental stem cells are an alternative source of adult stem cells that are easily accessible by tooth extraction with a local anesthetic or when a primary tooth is replaced. This section discusses where dental stem cells arise during tooth formation and the types of tissue they form. We also characterize the many types of the dental stem cells utilized in research today and compare the utility of dental stem cells versus BMMSCs.

There are six types of human dental stem cells that have been well described in the literature: 1. Dental pulp stem cells (DPSCs) (Gronthos et al., 2000); 2. Stem cells isolated from human exfoliated deciduous teeth (SHEDs) (Miura et al., 2003); 3. Stem cells derived from human natal dental pulp (hNDPs) (Karaöz et al., 2010); 4. Periodontal ligament stem cells (PDLSCs) (Seo et al., 2004); 5. Stem cells isolated from the apical papilla (SCAPs) (Sonoyama et al., 2008); 6. Stem cells isolated from dental follicle precursor cells (DFPCs) (Morsczeck et al., 2005).

Within the body, MSCs have been localized to perivascular niches (Crisan et al., 2009; Kolf et al., 2007) and recent studies have also shown that dental stem cells are also localized to perivascular niches within the tooth structure (Chen et al., 2006; Shi and Gronthos, 2003). Dental stem cells arise from dental mesenchyme which has early interaction with the neural crest during normal tooth development (Huang et al., 2009b). Therefore, dental stem cells may display characteristics of both mesoderm and ectoderm due to their ectomesenchymal origins (Huang et al., 2009b).

2.4.1 Mammalian tooth formation

A mature tooth is comprised externally of hard structures of enamel, dentin and cementum and internally possesses a soft dental pulp (Figure 1). Tooth formation or odontogenesis is a complex process involving multiple tooth-associated cell types. Odontogenesis occurs as a tooth bud is formed from an aggregation of embryonic cells. These cells have ectodermal and ectomesodermal origins from the first branchial arch and the neural crest respectively (Ten Cate, 1998; Tucker and Sharpe, 2004). Tooth development has three stages. 1. The bud stage, where epithelial cells begin to proliferate into ectomesenchyme and condense in the jaw forming the tooth bud. 2. The cap stage, where ectomesenchmyal cells aggregate and begin to surround and enclose the epithelial cells which invaginate further into the mesenchyme and form the dental follicle, the enamel organ or cap and the dental papilla (Slatter, 2002; Ten Cate, 1998; Tucker and Sharpe, 2004). The dental follicle is of ectomesodermal origins and forms a sac surrounding the developing tooth that supports the tooth prior to eruption. The enamel organ is of ectodermal origins and eventually forms the enamel, whereas the dental papilla is of mesodermal origins and eventually forms the primary dentin and the pulp. 3. The bell stage, where the tooth undergoes extensive differentiation with the epithelial cells differentiating into ameloblasts and mesenchymal cells differentiating into odontoblasts. After the bell stage, the hard structures are formed with ameloblasts forming enamel while odontoblasts form dentin (Figure 1). Secondary dentin aids in root formation. Later in tooth development further differentiation of the dental follicle occurs with the formation of cementoblasts, fibroblasts and osteoblasts to form the cementum, the periodontal ligament and bone respectively (Figure 1).

2.4.2 Sources of dental stem cells

2.4.2.1 Dental Pulp Tissue

The soft dental pulp is located in the middle of the tooth surrounded by the harder structures of the tooth including dentin, cementum and enamel (Figure 1). The dental pulp contains a mix of cell types including fibroblasts which form the extracellular matrix and collagen and odontoblasts that form reparative dentin (Gronthos et al., 2002; Liu et al., 2006). The dental pulp region also contains nerve fibers and blood vessels and is accessible to external stimuli through the apical foramen (Figure1). Three types of stem cells have been identified from dental pulp tissue: DPSCs, SHEDs and hNDPs. DPSCs are present in the pulp of the adult tooth, whereas SHEDs are only present in the pulp of primary teeth or "baby teeth." Lastly, hNDPs are a unique type of dental pulp stem cells isolated only from the pulp of newborn teeth. Very few newborns are born with teeth, approximately one in every two to three thousand births (Leung and Robson, 2006), so hNDPs are very rare.

2.4.2.1.1 Dental Pulp Stem Cells

DPSCs are a heterogeneous population of cells that were first isolated by Gronthos et al. (2000) and exhibited some characteristics of BMMSCs, including the production of fibroblast-like cells that were clonogenic and had a high proliferation rate. Interestingly, DPSCs had a higher proliferation rate than BMMSCs (Gronthos et al., 2000) . DPSCs also had a similar protein expression pattern to BMMSCs in vitro including vascular adhesion molecule 1, alkaline phosphatase, collagen I, collagen III, osteonectin, osteopontin, osteocalcin, bone sialoprotein, α-smooth muscle actin, fibroblast growth factor 2 and the cell surface marker CD 146 (Gronthos et al., 2000). Immunohistochemistry staining further showed that like BMMSCs, primary cultures of DPSCs did not stain for the cell surface markers CD14, CD34, and CD45 or other markers including MyoD, neurofilament, collagen II , and peroxisome-proliferator activated receptor γ-2 (Gronthos et al., 2000).

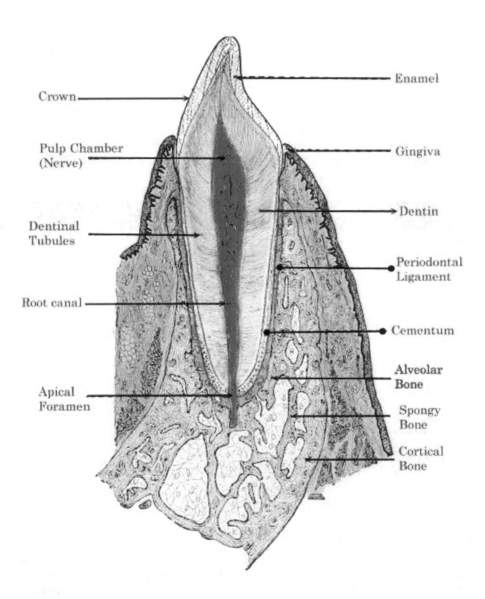

Fig. 1. Mature tooth anatomy. Image copied with permission from Dr. Martin S. Spiller, D.M.D. from DoctorSpiller.com.

Recently FACS has been used to sort DPSCs based on cell surface markers which found that in addition to the markers identified above, DPSCs expressed the following: CD9, CD10, CD13, CD29, CD44, CD49d, CD59, CD73, CD90, CD105, CD106, CD166 and STRO-1(Lindroos et al., 2008; Nam and Lee, 2009). Further, DPSC did not express CD14, CD 31, CD 45 (Nam and Lee, 2009) (Summarized in Table 1).

When cultured under osteogenic conditions DPSCs were capable of forming calcified deposits sparsely throughout the culture; these results were unlike BMMSCs which formed sheets of calcium deposits (Gronthos et al., 2000). In vivo transplantation of DPSCs into immunocompromised mice resulted in the production of a dentin-pulp-like complex with a collagen matrix containing blood vessels and lined with odontoblasts (Gronthos et al., 2000) suggesting that DPSCs are multipotent. Further studies also found DPSCs to be multipotent, capable of differentiating into myoblasts, osteoblasts, odontoblast-like cells, chondrocytes, adipocytes and neural cells (Gronthos et al., 2002; Liu et al., 2006; Pierdomenico et al., 2005; Zhang et al., 2006).

Letter name	BMMSCs	DPSCs	SHEDs	hNDPs	PDLSCs	SCAPs	DFPCs
CD9	+	+			+		+
CD 10		+		-	+		+
CD 13	+	+	+	+	+	+	+
CD 14	-	-	-		-	-	
CD 18							-
CD 19		-					
CD 24		-			-	+	
CD 29		+	+		+	+	+
CD 34	-	-	-	-	-	-	-
CD 44	+	+	+	+	+	+	+
CD 45	-	-	-	-	-	-	-
CD 53							+
CD 59		+			+		+
CD73	+	+	+	+	+	+	+
CD 90	+	+	+	+	+	+	+
CD 105	+	+	+		+	+	+
CD 106	+	+	+		+	+	+
CD 146	+	+	+	+	+	+	+
CD 150						-	
CD 166		+	+	+	+		+
STRO-1	+	+	+		+	+	+

Table 1. Cell surface markers expressed in dental stem cells compared to bone marrow mesenchymal stem cells as determined by flow cytometry. Table adapted from Karaöz et al. 2011, Rodriguez-Lozano et al. 2011, Huang, G.T. et al. 2009, Nam and Lee 2009, Lindroos et al. 2008 and Shi et al. 2005. BMMSCs, bone marrow mesenchymal stem cells; DPSCs, dental pulp stem cells; SHEDs, stem cells from human exfoliated deciduous teeth; SCAPs, stem cells from apical papilla; DFPCs, dental follicle precursor cells; hNDPs, stem cells derived from human natal dental pulp; + = marker present; - = marker absent.

2.4.2.1.2 Stem Cells from Human Exfoliated Deciduous Teeth

SHEDs are found in the pulp of the naturally exfoliated deciduous teeth or "baby teeth." When the permanent tooth erupts from the gums the deciduous tooth in displaced. SHED cells were first isolated by Miura et al. (2003) from the remnant pulp in the crown of human deciduous incisors of children 7-8 years old.

Similar to DPSCs, SHEDs met the criteria to be defined as a stem cell population as they were highly proliferative, capable of self-renewal and had the ability to differentiate into multiple cell types (Miura et al., 2003). SHEDs also had a fibroblast-like morphology similar to DPSCs. However, SHEDs were capable of a greater number of population doublings and had a higher proliferation rate than both BMMSCs and DPSCs (Miura et al., 2003). SHEDs have also been isolated and identified as immature dental pulp stem cells (IDPSCs) (Kerkis et al., 2006) and found to express embryonic stem cell markers Oct-4 (POU transcription factor), Nanog, stage specific embryonic antigens (SSEA-3, SSEA-4), and tumorigenic recognition antigens (TRA-1-60, TRA-1-81). SHEDs have also been shown to express neural stem cell markers SRY (sex determining region Y)-box 2 (Sox-2), nestin, and ATP-binding cassette, subfamily G, member 2 (ABCg2)(Morsczeck et al., 2010).

SHEDs were further characterized using FACS as having the following cell surface markers: CD13, CD29, CD31, CD44, CD73, CD90, CD105, CD146, CD166, and STRO-1 and similar to BMMSCs and DPSCs, SHEDs did not express CD14, CD34 or CD45 (Kerkis et al., 2006; Morsczeck et al., 2010; Pivoriuunas et al., 2010; Shi et al., 2005; Wang et al., 2010) (Summarized in Table 1).

A distinguishing feature of SHEDs not demonstrated for DPSCs is SHEDs formed sphere-like clusters when cultured in neuronal differentiation media (Miura et al., 2003). While Miura et al. (2003) demonstrated that SHEDs could differentiate into neural cells, adipocytes and odontoblasts, Kerkis et al. (2006) showed that SHEDs also had chondrogenic and myogenic potential. SHEDs were shown to express chondrogenic markers Sox-9, type II collagen and type X collagen when cultured for 14 days with bone morphogenic protein 2 (BMP2), a chondrogenic signaling protein in the TGFβ family (Koyama et al., 2009). Interestingly, Koyama et al. (2009) did not find any expression of the chondrogenic markers in their untreated populations of SHED cultures.

When SHED were transplanted into immunocompromised mice they exhibited an osteoinductive capacity in vivo but were not able to regenerate the dentin-pulp-like complex that DPSCs cells were able to form (Miura et al., 2003). Kerkis et al. (2006) also showed that when SHEDs were transplanted into immunocompromised mice via intraperitoneal injection they engrafted into the lungs, liver, spleen, brain and kidney and the tissue formed by the SHEDs was indistinguishable from the host tissue for liver, spleen, brain and kidney (Kerkis et al., 2006).

2.4.2.1.3 Stem Cells Derived from Human Natal Dental Pulp

Natal teeth are deciduous teeth that arise in newborns that are smaller than primary teeth and have little or no root development (Leung and Robson, 2006). Karaöz et al. (2010) isolated and characterized hNDPs from the remnant pulp of natal teeth. A small number of hNDPs adhered to plastic in culture and displayed a fibroblast-like spindle shaped morphology that eventually became flattened in later passages (Karaöz et al., 2010). Similar to DPSCs, hNDPs had a higher proliferation rate the BMMSCs, were clonogenic, and had the ability to differentiate into multiple cell types, satisfying the criteria to be classified as a stem cell population.

Using flow-cytometry Karaöz et al. (2010) showed that like BMMSCs, hNDPs expressed CD13, CD44, CD73, CD90, CD146, and CD166 but did not express CD14, CD31 or CD45 (Summarized in Table 1). Stem cells derived from human natal dental pulp expressed many of the same cell surface markers seen in DPSCs and SHEDs (Table 1).

Cultures of NDPs with chondrogenic, osteogenic, adipogenic, myogenic and neurogenic media expressed the appropriate differentiation markers associated with their culture media. Further, the multipotent nature of hNDPs was demonstrated by their differentiation in vitro into chondroblasts, osteoblasts, adipocytes, myoblasts and neuro-glial-like cells respectively (Karaöz et al., 2010). Interestingly, hNDPs expressed detectable levels of the embryonic stem cell markers Rex-1, Oct4 and Nanog as well as the transcription factors Sox-2 and FoxD3 suggesting that these cells display some of the characteristics for pluripotency (Karaöz et al., 2010).

2.4.2.2 Periodontal Ligament Stem Cells

The periodontal ligament is the part of the tooth derived from the neural crest and made of soft connective tissue that resides between the cementum and the alveolar bone of the jaw (Figure 1). It is responsible for anchoring and supporting the tooth within the tooth socket. The periodontal ligament is composed of a heterogeneous population of cells containing fibroblasts, osteoblasts and cementoblasts (Bartold et al., 2000; Gay et al., 2007; Lekic et al., 2001; Seo et al., 2004; Shimono et al., 2003). Early studies have suggested that the PDL tissue had regenerative or repair abilities when an injury was incurred by the periodontal tissue (Reviewed in Bartold et al. (2005) and Shimono et al. (2003)).

Periodontal ligament stem cells were first isolated by Seo et al. (2004) from impacted third molar adult teeth. Immunohistochemical staining of PDLSCs stained positive for early mesenchymal stem cell markers STRO-1 and CD146 suggesting that these cells has similar stem cell characteristics to BMMSCs (Seo et al., 2004). PDLSCs demonstrated other characteristics of BMMSCs and DPSCs including fibroblastic-like cell morphology that adhered to plastic and formed clonogenic cell clusters with the ability to differentiate into multiple cell types (Seo et al., 2004). PDLSCs had a higher proliferation rate than BMMSCs, but similar rate to DPSCs after 24 hours in culture (Seo et al., 2004).

Multipotent human PDLSCs cells have been characterized using FACS sorting and were shown to express the following cell surface markers: CD9, CD10, CD13, CD29, CD44, CD59, CD73, CD90, CD105, CD106, CD146, CD166 and STRO-1 (Feng et al., 2010; Lindroos et al., 2008; Shi et al., 2005; Wada et al., 2009). Like BMMSCs, DPSCs and SHEDs, PDLSCs do not express CD14, CD31 or CD45 (Shi et al., 2005)(Summarized in Table 1). PDLSCs have also been shown to express the embryonic stem cell markers Oct4, Sox-2, Nanog and Klf-4 and neural crest markers Nestin, Slug, p75 and Sox-10 (Huang et al., 2009a).

Like BMMSCs and DPSCs, PDLSC's formed calcium deposits when cultured in osteogenic media, however, unlike BMMSCs and DPSCs these deposits were sparsely distributed though out the culture (Gay et al., 2007; Seo et al., 2004). Increased protein expression of osteoblastic/cementoblastic markers alkaline phosphatase, bone sialoprotein, matrix extracellular protein, osteocalcin and TGFβ receptor 1 was observed after osteogenic induction (Seo et al., 2004). PDLSCs were also capable of differentiation into adipocytes as demonstrated by the formation of oil red O positive droplets and the upregulation of adipocyte specific transcripts after 21-25 days of culture in adipogenic inducing media (Gay et al., 2007; Seo et al., 2004). Gay et al. (2007) showed that PDLSCs could undergo chondrogenic differentiation in vitro after 21 days culture.

When transplanted into immunocompromised mice PDLSCs formed a cementum/PDL-like structure with attached collagen fibers (Seo et al., 2004). However, despite the expression of osteogenic / cementoblastic markers in vitro (Gay et al., 2007; Seo et al., 2004), PDLSCs were unable to form dentin or bone in vivo (Seo et al., 2004). By implanting PDLSCs into immunocompromised rats with periodontal defects, Seo et al. (2004) were able to show that PDLSCs were capable of periodontal tissue repair.

2.4.2.3 Stem Cells from the Apical Papilla

SCAPs were first isolated by Sonoyama et al. (2006) from impacted wisdom teeth of adults aged 18-20. The apical papilla is a part of the soft tissue found at the apices of the immature permanent tooth that eventually becomes the pulp tissue in the mature tooth (Huang et al., 2009b; Sonoyama et al., 2006; Sonoyama et al., 2008). Histological characterization of the apical papilla by Sonoyama et al. (2008) showed that the apical papilla is separate from the pulp canal and apical cell rich zone of the immature tooth.

SCAPs expressed the early mesenchymal stem cell markers STRO-1 and CD146 suggesting that these cells were a stem cell population. Further characterization of this cell population showed that SCAPs formed adherent fibroblastic cell cultures that were clonogenic and capable of over 70 population doublings with the ability to transform into odontoblastic/ osteoblastic, adipogenic, chondrogenic and neural cell types (Abe et al., 2007; Sonoyama et al., 2006; Sonoyama et al., 2008). Sonoyama et al. (2006) also showed that SCAPs had a greater proliferation rate and population doubling than DPSCs isolated from the same tooth. SCAPs were also distinct from DPSCs with respect to expression levels of survivin, telomerase and the cell surface marker CD24, all which are thought to be associated with cell proliferation (Sonoyama et al., 2006).

Analysis of cell surface markers by flow cytometry showed that SCAPs expressed CD13, CD24, CD29, CD73, CD90, CD105, CD106, CD146, CD166 and STRO-1 but did not express CD14, CD18, CD34, CD45, or CD150 (Abe et al., 2007; Sonoyama et al., 2006) (Summarized in Table1).

In vitro culture of SCAPs, DPSCs and BMMSCs showed that SCAPs and DPSCs had similar osteo/dentinogenic potential to BMMSCs, but had a weaker response to adipogenic differentiation than BMMSCs (Sonoyama et al., 2008). After neural induction, immunostaining showed that SCAPs expressed the following neuronal markers: βIII tubulin, glial fibrillary acid protein, glutamic acid decarboxylase, nestin, neuronal nuclear antigen, neuronal filament M, neuron-specific enolase and 2', 3'-cyclic nucleotide 3'-phosphodiesterase (Abe et al., 2007; Sonoyama et al., 2008). When transplanted into immunocompromised mice SCAPs underwent in vivo differentiation into odontoblasts which regenerated the dentin-pulp-like structure and connective tissue (Sonoyama et al., 2006).

2.4.2.4 Dental Follicle Progenitor Cells

As described above, the dental follicle is the ectomesodermal tissue surrounding the developing tooth that leads to the formation of cementoblasts, periodontal ligament and osteoblasts. Morszceck et al. (2005) isolated human DFPCs from the dental follicle area of impacted wisdom teeth and noted that a small number had stem cell characteristics. DFPCs formed clonogenic, fibroblastic-like colonies in culture that adhered to plastic (Morszceck et al., 2005). Like SHEDs, DFPCs expressed neural stem cell associated markers Sox-2, nestin, and ABCg2 (Morszceck et al., 2010).

Interestingly, multipotent DFPCs have been reported in mice and rats that are capable of undergoing osteogenic, adipogenic, chondrogenic and neurogenic differentiation (Luan et al., 2006; Yao et al., 2008). However, only osteogenic differentiation has been demonstrated consistently for human DFPCs in vitro (Honda et al.; Kémoun et al., 2007; Lindroos et al., 2008; Morsczeck et al., 2005). For human DFPCs neural induction has also been demonstrated by Morsczeck et al. (2010) but conflicting results for adipogenic and chondrogenic differentiation have been observed (Honda et al.; Kémoun et al., 2007; Lindroos et al., 2008).

Immunohistochemistry and FACS sorting have shown that DFPCs express the following cell surface markers: CD9, CD10, CD13, CD29, CD44, CD53, CD59, CD73, CD90, CD105, CD106, CD146, CD166 and STRO-1 but do not express CD34 or CD45 (Lindroos et al., 2008; Morsczeck et al., 2010; Yagyuu et al., 2010).

When Morsczeck et al. (2005) transplanted human DFPCs into severe combined immunodeficiency (SCID) mice they saw an increase in bone sialoprotein, osteocalcin and collagen I expression in vivo but did not see any evidence of cementum or bone formation. However, transplantation of mouse DFPCs into SCID mice demonstrated that DFPCs were capable of regenerating the PDL in vivo (Yokoi et al., 2007). Recently, when cryopreserved DFPCs were transplanted into immunocompromised rats, a mineralized tissue structure was formed in vivo containing cementocyte/osteocyte cells, but the exact identity of the tissue type could not be determined as dentin, cementum or bone (Yagyuu et al., 2010).

3. Tissue engineering

3.1 Dental stem cells in tissue engineering and regenerative medicine

When tissues become damaged or non-functional tissue engineering is used to replace, repair or restore damaged tissue in the body (Levenberg and Langer, 2004). Tissue engineering and regenerative medicine requires an abundant cell source capable of differentiation into the required tissue. Therefore, stem cells with their ability to self-renew, proliferate and differentiate make an ideal cell source for this type of tissue repair and replacement (Barrilleaux et al., 2006).

Whole tooth regeneration is the goal of many researchers and much of tissue engineering involving dental stem cells is used to reconstruct or repair damaged and diseased dental tissue (Dannan, 2009; Huang et al., 2009b; Shi et al., 2005; Sonoyama et al., 2006; Yen and Sharpe, 2008; Yokoi et al., 2007). When a patient's dental pulp cavity becomes infected or diseased, often the entire pulp is removed and replaced with a filling. Due to the ability of DPSCs to form the dentine-pulp-like complex in vivo, it has been suggested that this may soon be an option for regenerative therapy of teeth (Caton et al., 2010). SHEDs also have shown potential for regenerating the dental-pulp-like tissue in vivo when transplanted into immunocompromised mice (Cordeiro et al., 2008) and therefore may be useful for future regenerative endodontic procedures. Further, Seo et al. (2004) showed that PDLs participated in periodontal tissue repair and formed a PDL/cementum-like complex when transplanted into immunocompromised mice suggesting that we will soon be able to regenerate tissues surrounding the teeth. Unfortunately one of the challenges remaining for whole tooth regeneration is that we are currently unable to regenerate human enamel (Mitsiadis and Papagerakis, 2011).

Two significant advancements in the area of whole tooth engineering are the ability to generate dental tissue structures in vitro and the ability to deliver these dental stem cells in vivo (Cordeiro et al., 2008; Yen and Sharpe, 2008). An important development in tissue engineering is the use of hydroxyapatite/ tricalcium phosphate (HA/TCP) particles and other carrier particles that allow dental stem cells cultured in vitro and delivered in vivo (Caton et al., 2010; Sharma et al., 2010). Also important to for dental tissue engineering is developing appropriate biodegradable scaffolds that can be seeded with stem cells for use in transplants and that provide the correct 3D space for differentiation (Caton et al., 2010; Dannan, 2009; Huang, 2009; Sharma et al., 2010; Yen and Sharpe, 2008). Scaffolds are made from both synthetic polymers like polylactic acid (PLA), polyglycolic acid (PGA), polylacticco-glycolic acid (PLGA), and polycaprolactone (PCL)) or natural polymers like collagen, fibrin, polysaccharides and alginates (Sharma et al., 2010). PGA fibers have been shown to be useful for engineering dental pulp-like tissue (Bohl et al., 1998).

Dental stem cells are also used to repair or supplement other types of tissues including bone, heart and neuronal tissue (d'Aquino et al., 2009; Gandia et al., 2008; Huang et al., 2009b; Wang et al., 2010). The potential of stem cells to regenerate bone tissue was demonstrated in a study by d'Aquino et al. (2007). These researchers showed that in vivo transplantation of human DPSCs in woven bone chips or polymer scaffolds into immunocompromised rats resulted in adult bone formation complete with de novo synthesis of blood vessels (d'Aquino et al., 2007). Potential treatment with DPSCs has also been tested using cardiac tissue in rats that have been subjected to a myocardial infarction. After transplanting DPSCs into the site of infarction via injection, there was a decrease in the size of the infarct and increased vessel formation near the infarct (Gandia et al., 2008). Interestingly, SHED cells have been used by researchers to produce dopaminergic neuron cells (Wang et al., 2010) to alleviate the effects of Parkinson's disease in rats. Wang et al. (2010) used a two-step induction protocol to stimulate SHED cells to form neurospheres which were then treated with a neurogenic cocktail to stimulate their differentiation into dopaminergic neurons. The formation of neurons by SHED cells suggests that dental cells may become an invaluable resource for neurodegenerative disease therapies. Another suggested application of stem cell therapy for SHEDs is for the treatment of wound healing (Nishino et al., 2011). Using a mouse model, SHEDs were transplanted into an excisional wound and were found to accelerate healing after 5 days when compared to control (Nishino et al., 2011). The potential use of dental stem cells has become even more viable for tissue regeneration and other therapies with the recent advances in cryopreservation. These advances allow proliferation and long term storage of these cells for future cell therapy treatments while maintaining their differentiation potential (Ding et al., 2010; Papaccio et al., 2006; Seo et al., 2005; Woods et al., 2009; Zhang et al., 2006).

3.2 Dental stem cells and dynamic compression

Our lab is exploring the area of cellular based tissue engineering and in particular the effects of dynamic cyclic compression on chondrogenesis in two types of human dental stem cells, PDLSCs and SHEDs.

Earlier work in our lab on biomechanical force has shown that short intervals of cyclic compression cause rabbit BMMSCs to up-regulate TGFβ (Huang et al., 2005). TGFβ3 has been shown to induce chondrogenic differentiation of BMMSCs in vitro (Barry et al., 2001) and the extracellular signal-related kinase (ERK) 1/2 signal transduction pathway of mitogen activated protein kinases (MAPKs) has been implicated in this process (Lee et al., 2004). The application of dynamic mechanical compression has been shown to induce chondrogenic differentiation of stem cells via an autocrine signaling pathway (Huang et al., 2005). Interestingly, just two hours of cyclic compression applied to BMMSCs stimulated TGFβ gene expression and the expression of both of its receptors (Huang et al., 2005). This stimulation in turn resulted in an up-regulation of the early response genes c-Fos and c-Jun as well as chondrogenic specific genes Sox-9, aggrecan and collagen type II (Huang et al., 2005).

Our lab has developed a line of adult dental stem cells derived from the PDL that are multipotent and express some ESC markers (Huang et al., 2009a). Using in vitro cultures in chondrogenic media we were able to show that after two weeks in culture with TGFβ3, PDLSCs increased expression of the chondrogenic markers collagen II and aggrecan (Huang et al., 2009a). Further, we see that PDLSCs express chondrogenic markers when subject to dynamic cyclic compression in a custom built bioreactor. After applying 15% strain at 1 Hertz for four hours we see a two to three fold increase in PDLSCs chondrogenic gene expression of Sox-9 and aggrecan as well as a 50% increase in ERK1/2 activity (Fritz, 2009). These results suggest that human PDLSCs, like BMMSCs, subject to dynamic cyclic compression require the ERK1/2 signaling pathway for chondrogenic expression (Fritz, 2009).

Recently we examined the effects of shorter durations of dynamic cyclic compression on SHEDs. As in previous experiments (Fritz, 2009; Pelaez et al., 2009), fibrin gel constructs were cast into 1.5-mm deep and 8-mm diameter Teflon molds set on top of a clean microscope slide. We loaded 1×10^7 SHEDs into 85 μL fibrin gel mixture containing 5 U/mL thrombin in PBS and 40 mg/mL fibrinogen in high-glucose DMEM. The fibrin gel constructs were allowed to solidify for one hour before removing from the Teflon mold and then placed in fibrin gel media containing high-glucose DMEM, 1% penicillin/streptomycin and 1× ITS supplement (BD Biosciences, San Jose, CA) and 0.0875 IU/mL aprotinin from bovine lung (Sigma-Aldrich, St. Louis, MO) for 24 hours in a water-jacketed incubator at 37°C and 5% CO_2. The compression chambers were loaded with the fibrin gel constructs and 650 μL of fibrin gel media. Fibrin gel constructs were then subjected them to 1Hertz dynamic cyclic compression with 15% strain in a custom built bioreactor placed in a water-jacketed incubator at 37°C and 5% CO_2. Twelve samples for each treatment were subjected to 0 minutes, 15 minutes, 30 minutes, 60 minutes and 240 minutes of compression. Fibrin gel constructs were removed from the bioreactor and flash frozen in liquid nitrogen.

Messenger RNA expression was determined using methods similar to Fritz (2009) and Pelaez et al. (2009). Briefely, fibrin gel constructs were homogenized using a IKA Ultra Turrax® T8 Homogenizer in 1 mL TRIzol (Invitrogen, Carlsbad, CA) and RNA was extracted according to manufacturers recommended protocol. Purified RNA concentration was quantified on a NanoDrop ND-1000 spectrophotometer. Reverse transcription of mRNA was performed using MultiScribe™ Reverse Transcriptase (Applied Biosciences, Foster City, CA) according to the manufacturer's suggested protocol. Quantitative real-time PCR was performed in a MxPro 3005P machine (Stratagene) using SYBR® Green PCR Master Mix (Applied Biosciences, Foster City, CA) according to manufacturer's suggested protocols. All samples were run in triplicate. GADPH was used as a reference gene. Fold changes of the chondrogenic genes (Sox-9, c-fos, and TGFβ3) were calculated from the log-transformed C_T values and expressed relative to the No Compression treatment group using a modification of the delta-delta C_T method (Livak and Schmittgen, 2001; Vandesompele et al., 2002).

Protein was extracted from the fibrin gel scaffolds and levels of p-ERK assessed using the methods described in Fritz (2009). Briefly, fibrin gel constructs were homogenized in 1 mL of RIPA cell lysis buffer 2 (Enzo Life Sciences Int'l, Inc., Plymouth Meeting, PA) plus 0.5 µL/mL protease inhibitor cocktail (Sigma-Aldrich, St. Louis, MO) and 1 mM phenymethanesulfonyl fluoride (Sigma-Aldrich, St. Louis, MO). The homogenate was kept on ice for 40 minutes and vortexed every 10 minutes. The homogenate centrifuged and the remaining supernatant was saved for protein analyses. The level of p-ERK 1/2 in each sample was determined using [pThr^{202}/Tyr^{204}]Erk1/2 EIA kit (Enzo Life Sciences Int'l, Inc., Plymouth Meeting, PA). Manufacturer suggested protocols were performed for the EIA assays and all samples were analyzed in duplicates.

All data are reported as mean ± S.E.M. (N=number of samples). 0 minutes, 15 minutes, 30 minutes, 60 minutes and 240 minutes of compression were compared level of p-ERK 1/2 and for mRNA expression of Sox-9, c-fos, and TGFβ3. Significant differences were determined by using a One-way ANOVA in Sigma Stat 3.00 (SPSS Inc.).

The effects of dynamic compression on chondrogenesis and ERK 1/2 signal transduction was observed (Figure 2). As expected, we saw an increase in the levels of the early response gene c-fos after 60 minutes of dynamic compression (Figure 2). Surprisingly, we did not see any change in the other early response gene c-jun (Data not shown) as seen in BMMSCs described above. We also saw an increase in the gene expression of both TGFβ3 and Sox-9 after 30 minutes of dynamic compression which lasted for at least 60 minutes of compression (Figure 2). Unlike the PDLSCs response to dynamic compression, SHEDs did not express Sox-9 after four hours. Further, we noticed and increase in the phosphorylation of ERK 1/2 as early as 15 minutes which was sustained for at least 60 minutes, but was no longer elevated after 4 hours (Figure 2).

SHEDs clearly have a different response to dynamic compression than PDLSCs. Like PDLSCs we see an early rise in the phosphorylation of ERK 1/2 suggesting that this signal transduction pathway is responding to compressive forces in SHEDS. The rise in TGFβ3 likely triggers the chondrogenic differentiation. Similar to PDLSCs, we see an increase in Sox-9, a transcription factor for chondrocyte differentiation, suggesting that SHEDs are indeed beginning to undergo chondrogenic differentiation. However, unlike PDLSCs, we did not see any aggrecan expression in our experiment which arises later in chondrogenic differentiation. Therefore we can suggest that SHEDs, like PDLSCs, respond to compressive force by undergoing chondrogenic differentiation and this is likely mediated though the ERK 1/2 signal transduction pathway. However, although chondrogenic differentiation is triggered within 30 minutes by dynamic compression, it is not completed during these short time intervals. This may be due to the decrease in TGFβ3 gene expression after 4 hours, which may be required to maintain chondrogenic differentiation in the dynamically compressed constructs as there was no supplementation of TGFβ3 in the media. Interestingly, the control samples did not show any gene expression for aggrecan but these samples were maintained in media without any supplemental TGFβ3. Koyama et al. (2009) did not show any chondrogenic gene expression in control cultures of SHEDs, but felt it may be due to the fact that some of their cultures were infected. We would suggest repeating that experiment to determine if SHEDs cultures express any of the chondrogenic markers without TGFβ3 supplementation.

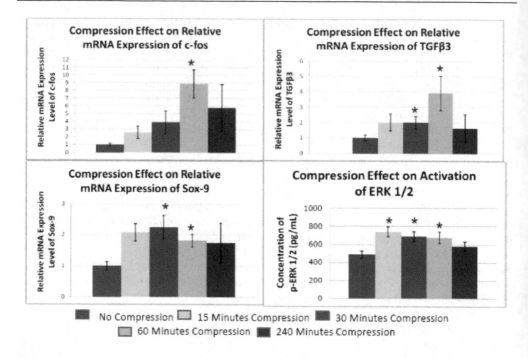

No Compression **☐ 15 Minutes Compression** **■ 30 Minutes Compression**
☐ 60 Minutes Compression **■ 240 Minutes Compression**

Fig. 2. The effects of different durations of dynamic cyclic compression (15% strain) on relative messenger RNA expression of c-fos, TGFβ3 and Sox-9 and on the phosphorylation level of ERK 1/2. All treatments N=6. Values are means ± S.E.M.; *$P < 0.05$, significantly different from No Compression treatment.

4. Dental stem cells versus embryonic stem cells

There are advantages and disadvantages for using dental stem cells compared to the using embryonic stem cells for tissue engineering and regenerative medicine. One advantage of using dental stem cells compared to ESCs is in the ease of obtaining these cells as they can be obtained from tissue during a standard tooth extraction or through loss of primary teeth (Huang et al., 2009b). ESCs are obtained from the inner cell mass of the embryoblast (Biswas and Hutchins, 2007) which requires access to the early embryo. An advantage of using embryonic stem cells is their pluripotent potential and their ability to differentiate into all three germ layers (Alison et al., 2002; Mummery et al., 2011; Thomson et al., 1998). Studies on dental stem cells have only shown them to only be multipotent (Gronthos et al., 2000; Karaöz et al., 2010; Miura et al., 2003; Morsczeck et al., 2005; Seo et al., 2004; Sonoyama et al., 2006). Interestingly, one PDL cell line has shown a broad differentiation potential and expresses some of the pluripotent markers expressed by ESCs (Huang et al., 2009a). A previous disadvantage of culturing ESCs is that they require a mouse embryonic feeder layer but recent studies have shown that ESCs can be cultured using human serum and human feeder cells and these cultures can be maintained for an extensive period of time (Ellerström et al., 2006). Dental stem cells do not require a feeder layer but only have a limited number of passages (See above).

Many of the problems encountered with stem cells delivery and scaffold choice are the same for both dental stem cells and ESCs. The use of dental stem cells or ESCs for tissue engineering or regenerative repair often produce similar results and many of the same types of problems arise. Currently whole tooth regeneration is not possible using ESCs or dental stem cells. Similar to dental stem cells, human ESCs have been used to form osteoblasts both in vitro and in vivo and had the capacity to form mineralized tissue (Bielby et al., 2004). Like DPSCs, ESCs have been used to repair cardiac function in infarcted myocardium. Human ESCs were injected into an infarcted mouse myocardium and were shown to improve cardiac function after four weeks but this improvement was not maintained after three months (van Laake et al., 2008). ESCs have also been used to explore neuronal regeneration for patients affected with Parkinson disease. Using the monkey as a primate model, ESCs have been used to generate dopaminergic neurons to aid in the relief of Parkinson disease (Takagi et al., 2005).

5. Concluding remarks

This review shows that dental stem cells are a viable alternative to embryonic stem cells for regenerative medicine. Dental stem cells are easily obtainable from the dental pulp of teeth and from other dental tissues which are often discarded as waste. Further, dental stem cells, like BMMSCs, form clonogenic, highly proliferative, multipotent cell populations in vitro and maintain their differentiation potential in vivo. Dental stem cells also show potential for cell therapy with respect to whole tooth regeneration. More work needs to be done to optimize the use of dental stem cells for use in cell therapies of other tissue types in the future including bone and cartilage formation. The potential of dental stem cells as an alternative choice to embryonic stem cells seems realistic for future stem cell therapies and regenerative medicine.

6. References

Abe, S., S. Yamaguchi, and T. Amagasa. 2007. Multilineage Cells from Apical Pulp of Human Tooth with Immature Apex. *Oral Science International*. 4:45-58.

Alison, M.R., R. Poulsom, S. Forbes, and N.A. Wright. 2002. An introduction to stem cells. *J Pathol*. 197:419-423.

Barrilleaux, B., D.G. Phinney, D.J. Prockop, and K.C. O'Connor. 2006. Review: ex vivo engineering of living tissues with adult stem cells. *Tissue Eng*. 12:3007-3019.

Barry, F., R.E. Boynton, B. Liu, and J.M. Murphy. 2001. Chondrogenic Differentiation of Mesenchymal Stem Cells from Bone Marrow: Differentiation-Dependent Gene Expression of Matrix Components. *Experimental Cell Research*. 268:189-200.

Bartold, P.M., C.A.G. McCulloch, A.S. Narayanan, and S. Pitaru. 2000. Tissue engineering: a new paradigm for periodontal regeneration based on molecular and cell biology. *Periodontology 2000*. 24:253-269.

Bianco, P., M. Riminucci, S. Gronthos, and P.G. Robey. 2001. Bone marrow stromal stem cells: nature, biology, and potential applications. *Stem Cells*. 19:180-192.

Bielby, R.C., A.R. Boccaccini, J.M. Polak, and L.D. Buttery. 2004. In vitro differentiation and in vivo mineralization of osteogenic cells derived from human embryonic stem cells. *Tissue Eng.* 10:1518-1525.

Biswas, A., and R. Hutchins. 2007. Embryonic stem cells. *Stem Cells Dev.* 16:213-222.

Blanpain, C., W.E. Lowry, A. Geoghegan, L. Polak, and E. Fuchs. 2004. Self-Renewal, Multipotency, and the Existence of Two Cell Populations within an Epithelial Stem Cell Niche. *Cell.* 118:635-648.

Blau, H.M., T.R. Brazelton, and J.M. Weimann. 2001. The Evolving Concept of a Stem Cell: Entity or Function? *Cell.* 105:829-841.

Bohl, K.S., J. Shon, B. Rutherford, and D.J. Mooney. 1998. Role of synthetic extracellular matrix in development of engineered dental pulp. *Journal of Biomaterials Science, Polymer Edition.* 9:749-764.

Bongso, A., and C.-Y. Fong. 2009. Human Embryonic Stem Cells: Their Nature, Properties, and Uses. *In* Trends in Stem Cell Biology and Technology. H. Baharvand, editor. Humana Press. 1-17.

Caton, J., N. Bostanci, E. Remboutsika, C. De Bari, and T.A. Mitsiadis. 2010. Future dentistry: cell therapy meets tooth and periodontal repair and regeneration. *J Cell Mol Med.*

Chamberlain, G., J. Fox, B. Ashton, and J. Middleton. 2007. Concise Review: Mesenchymal Stem Cells: Their Phenotype, Differentiation Capacity, Immunological Features, and Potential for Homing. *Stem Cells.* 25:2739-2749.

Chen, S.C., V. Marino, S. Gronthos, and P.M. Bartold. 2006. Location of putative stem cells in human periodontal ligament. *Journal of Periodontal Research.* 41:547-553.

Conget, P.A., and J.J. Minguell. 1999. Phenotypical and functional properties of human bone marrow mesenchymal progenitor cells. *J Cell Physiol.* 181:67-73.

Cordeiro, M.M., Z. Dong, T. Kaneko, Z. Zhang, M. Miyazawa, S. Shi, A.J. Smith, and J.E. Nör. 2008. Dental Pulp Tissue Engineering with Stem Cells from Exfoliated Deciduous Teeth. *Journal of Endodontics.* 34:962-969.

Crisan, M., C.-W. Chen, M. Corselli, G. Andriolo, L. Lazzari, and B. Péault. 2009. Perivascular Multipotent Progenitor Cells in Human Organs. *Annals of the New York Academy of Sciences.* 1176:118-123.

d'Aquino, R., A. De Rosa, G. Laino, F. Caruso, L. Guida, R. Rullo, V. Checchi, L. Laino, V. Tirino, and G. Papaccio. 2009. Human dental pulp stem cells: from biology to clinical applications. *J Exp Zool B Mol Dev Evol.* 312B:408-415.

d'Aquino, R., A. Graziano, M. Sampaolesi, G. Laino, G. Pirozzi, A. De Rosa, and G. Papaccio. 2007. Human postnatal dental pulp cells co-differentiate into osteoblasts and endotheliocytes: a pivotal synergy leading to adult bone tissue formation. *Cell Death Differ.* 14:1162-1171.

Dannan, A. 2009. Dental-derived stem cells and whole tooth regeneration: an overview. *Journal of Clinical Medicine and Research.* 1:63-71.

Deasy, B.M., R.J. Jankowski, and J. Huard. 2001. Muscle-derived stem cells: characterization and potential for cell-mediated therapy. *Blood Cells Mol Dis.* 27:924-933.

Ding, G., W. Wang, Y. Liu, Y. An, C. Zhang, S. Shi, and S. Wang. 2010. Effect of cryopreservation on biological and immunological properties of stem cells from apical papilla. *J Cell Physiol.* 223:415-422.

Dominici, M., K. Le Blanc, I. Mueller, I. Slaper-Cortenbach, F. Marini, D. Krause, R. Deans, A. Keating, D. Prockop, and E. Horwitz. 2006. Minimal criteria for defining multipotent mesenchymal stromal cells. The International Society for Cellular Therapy position statement. *Cytotherapy*. 8:315-317.

Ellerström, C., R. Strehl, K. Moya, K. Andersson, C. Bergh, K. Lundin, J. Hyllner, and H. Semb. 2006. Derivation of a Xeno-Free Human Embryonic Stem Cell Line. *Stem Cells*. 24:2170-2176.

Feng, F., K. Akiyama, Y. Liu, T. Yamaza, T.M. Wang, J.H. Chen, B.B. Wang, G.T.J. Huang, S. Wang, and S. Shi. 2010. Utility of PDL progenitors for in vivo tissue regeneration: a report of 3 cases. *Oral Diseases*. 16:20-28.

Fortier, L.A. 2005. Stem cells: classifications, controversies, and clinical applications. *Vet Surg*. 34:415-423.

Fritz, J.R. 2009. The Chondrogenesis of PDLs by Dynamic Unconfined Compression is Dependent on p42/44 and not p38 or JNK. *In* Biomedical Engineering. Vol. Masters of Science. University of Miami, Coral Gables, Fl. 47.

Gandia, C., A. Armiñan, J.M. García-Verdugo, E. Lledó, A. Ruiz, M.D. Miñana, J. Sanchez-Torrijos, R. Payá, V. Mirabet, F. Carbonell-Uberos, M. Llop, J.A. Montero, and P. Sepúlveda. 2008. Human Dental Pulp Stem Cells Improve Left Ventricular Function, Induce Angiogenesis, and Reduce Infarct Size in Rats with Acute Myocardial Infarction. *Stem Cells*. 26:638-645.

Gay, I.C., S. Chen, and M. MacDougall. 2007. Isolation and characterization of multipotent human periodontal ligament stem cells. *Orthod Craniofac Res*. 10:149-160.

Gronthos, S., J. Brahim, W. Li, L.W. Fisher, N. Cherman, A. Boyde, P. DenBesten, P.G. Robey, and S. Shi. 2002. Stem cell properties of human dental pulp stem cells. *J Dent Res*. 81:531-535.

Gronthos, S., M. Mankani, J. Brahim, P.G. Robey, and S. Shi. 2000. Postnatal human dental pulp stem cells (DPSCs) in vitro and in vivo. *Proc Natl Acad Sci U S A*. 97:13625-13630.

Gronthos, S., A.C. Zannettino, S.J. Hay, S. Shi, S.E. Graves, A. Kortesidis, and P.J. Simmons. 2003. Molecular and cellular characterisation of highly purified stromal stem cells derived from human bone marrow. *J Cell Sci*. 116:1827-1835.

Honda, M.J., M. Imaizumi, H. Suzuki, S. Ohshima, S. Tsuchiya, and K. Satomura. Stem cells isolated from human dental follicles have osteogenic potential. *Oral Surgery, Oral Medicine, Oral Pathology, Oral Radiology, and Endodontology*. In Press, Corrected Proof.

Huang, C.Y., D. Pelaez, J. Dominguez-Bendala, F. Garcia-Godoy, and H.S. Cheung. 2009a. Plasticity of stem cells derived from adult periodontal ligament. *Regen Med*. 4:809-821.

Huang, C.Y., P.M. Reuben, and H.S. Cheung. 2005. Temporal expression patterns and corresponding protein inductions of early responsive genes in rabbit bone marrow-derived mesenchymal stem cells under cyclic compressive loading. *Stem Cells*. 23:1113-1121.

Huang, G.T. 2009. Pulp and dentin tissue engineering and regeneration: current progress. *Regen Med*. 4:697-707.

Huang, G.T., S. Gronthos, and S. Shi. 2009b. Mesenchymal stem cells derived from dental tissues vs. those from other sources: their biology and role in regenerative medicine. *J Dent Res*. 88:792-806.

Jiang, Y., B.N. Jahagirdar, R.L. Reinhardt, R.E. Schwartz, C.D. Keene, X.R. Ortiz-Gonzalez, M. Reyes, T. Lenvik, T. Lund, M. Blackstad, J. Du, S. Aldrich, A. Lisberg, W.C. Low, D.A. Largaespada, and C.M. Verfaillie. 2002. Pluripotency of mesenchymal stem cells derived from adult marrow. *Nature*. 418:41-49.

Karaöz, E., B. Doğan, A. Aksoy, G. Gacar, S. Akyüz, S. Ayhan, Z. Genç, S. Yürüker, G. Duruksu, P. Demircan, and A. Sarıboyacı. 2010. Isolation and in vitro characterisation of dental pulp stem cells from natal teeth. *Histochemistry and Cell Biology*. 133:95-112.

Kémoun, P., S. Laurencin-Dalicieux, J. Rue, J.-C. Farges, I. Gennero, F. Conte-Auriol, F. Briand-Mesange, M. Gadelorge, H. Arzate, A. Narayanan, G. Brunel, and J.-P. Salles. 2007. Human dental follicle cells acquire cementoblast features under stimulation by BMP-2/-7 and enamel matrix derivatives (EMD) in vitro. *Cell and Tissue Research*. 329:283-294.

Kerkis, I., A. Kerkis, D. Dozortsev, G.C. Stukart-Parsons, S.M. Gomes Massironi, L.V. Pereira, A.I. Caplan, and H.F. Cerruti. 2006. Isolation and characterization of a population of immature dental pulp stem cells expressing OCT-4 and other embryonic stem cell markers. *Cells Tissues Organs*. 184:105-116.

Kolf, C.M., E. Cho, and R.S. Tuan. 2007. Mesenchymal stromal cells. Biology of adult mesenchymal stem cells: regulation of niche, self-renewal and differentiation. *Arthritis Res Ther*. 9:204.

Koyama, N., Y. Okubo, K. Nakao, and K. Bessho. 2009. Evaluation of pluripotency in human dental pulp cells. *J Oral Maxillofac Surg*. 67:501-506.

Kuznetsov, S.A., P.H. Krebsbach, K. Satomura, J. Kerr, M. Riminucci, D. Benayahu, and P.G. Robey. 1997. Single-colony derived strains of human marrow stromal fibroblasts form bone after transplantation in vivo. *J Bone Miner Res*. 12:1335-1347.

Lanzendorf, S.E., C.A. Boyd, D.L. Wright, S. Muasher, S. Oehninger, and G.D. Hodgen. 2001. Use of human gametes obtained from anonymous donors for the production of human embryonic stem cell lines. *Fertil Steril*. 76:132-137.

Lee, J.W., Y.H. Kim, S.H. Kim, S.H. Han, and S.B. Hahn. 2004. Chondrogenic differentiation of mesenchymal stem cells and its clinical applications. *Yonsei Med J*. 45 Suppl:41-47.

Lekic, P., J. Rojas, C. Birek, H. Tenenbaum, and C.A.G. McCulloch. 2001. Phenotypic comparison of periodontal ligament cells in vivo and in vitro. *Journal of Periodontal Research*. 36:71-79.

Leung, A.K., and W.L. Robson. 2006. Natal teeth: a review. *J Natl Med Assoc*. 98:226-228.

Levenberg, S., and R. Langer. 2004. Advances in Tissue Engineering. *In* Current Topics in Developmental Biology. Vol. Volume 61. P.S. Gerald, editor. Academic Press. 113-134.

Lindroos, B., K. Maenpaa, T. Ylikomi, H. Oja, R. Suuronen, and S. Miettinen. 2008. Characterisation of human dental stem cells and buccal mucosa fibroblasts. *Biochem Biophys Res Commun*. 368:329-335.

Liu, H., S. Gronthos, and S. Shi. 2006. Dental pulp stem cells. *Methods Enzymol.* 419:99-113.

Livak, K.J., and T.D. Schmittgen. 2001. Analysis of Relative Gene Expression Data Using Real-Time Quantitative PCR and the 2−ΔΔCT Method. *Methods.* 25:402-408.

Luan, X., Y. Ito, S. Dangaria, and T.G. Diekwisch. 2006. Dental follicle progenitor cell heterogeneity in the developing mouse periodontium. *Stem Cells Dev.* 15:595-608.

Mitsiadis, T.A., and P. Papagerakis. 2011. Regenerated teeth: the future of tooth replacement? *Regenerative Medicine.* 6:135-139.

Miura, M., S. Gronthos, M. Zhao, B. Lu, L.W. Fisher, P.G. Robey, and S. Shi. 2003. SHED: stem cells from human exfoliated deciduous teeth. *Proc Natl Acad Sci U S A.* 100:5807-5812.

Morsczeck, C., W. Gotz, J. Schierholz, F. Zeilhofer, U. Kuhn, C. Mohl, C. Sippel, and K.H. Hoffmann. 2005. Isolation of precursor cells (PCs) from human dental follicle of wisdom teeth. *Matrix Biol.* 24:155-165.

Morsczeck, C., F. Völlner, M. Saugspier, C. Brandl, T. Reichert, O. Driemel, and G. Schmalz. 2010. Comparison of human dental follicle cells (DFCs) and stem cells from human exfoliated deciduous teeth (SHED) after neural differentiation in vitro. *Clinical Oral Investigations.* 14:433-440.

Mummery, C., I. Wilmut, A. van de Stolpe, and B.A.J. Roelen. 2011. Stem Cells: Scientific Facts and Fiction. Academic Press, London, England. 324 pp.

Nam, H., and G. Lee. 2009. Identification of novel epithelial stem cell-like cells in human deciduous dental pulp. *Biochem Biophys Res Commun.* 386:135-139.

Nishino, Y., Y. Yamada, K. Ebisawa, S. Nakamura, K. Okabe, E. Umemura, K. Hara, and M. Ueda. 2011. Stem cells from human exfoliated deciduous teeth (SHED) enhance wound healing and the possibility of novel cell therapy. *Cytotherapy.* 13:598-605.

Papaccio, G., A. Graziano, R. d'Aquino, M.F. Graziano, G. Pirozzi, D. Menditti, A. De Rosa, F. Carinci, and G. Laino. 2006. Long-term cryopreservation of dental pulp stem cells (SBP-DPSCs) and their differentiated osteoblasts: a cell source for tissue repair. *J Cell Physiol.* 208:319-325.

Pelaez, D., C.Y. Huang, and H.S. Cheung. 2009. Cyclic compression maintains viability and induces chondrogenesis of human mesenchymal stem cells in fibrin gel scaffolds. *Stem Cells Dev.* 18:93-102.

Pierdomenico, L., L. Bonsi, M. Calvitti, D. Rondelli, M. Arpinati, G. Chirumbolo, E. Becchetti, C. Marchionni, F. Alviano, V. Fossati, N. Staffolani, M. Franchina, A. Grossi, and G.P. Bagnara. 2005. Multipotent mesenchymal stem cells with immunosuppressive activity can be easily isolated from dental pulp. *Transplantation.* 80:836-842.

Pittenger, M.F., A.M. Mackay, S.C. Beck, R.K. Jaiswal, R. Douglas, J.D. Mosca, M.A. Moorman, D.W. Simonetti, S. Craig, and D.R. Marshak. 1999. Multilineage potential of adult human mesenchymal stem cells. *Science.* 284:143-147.

Pivoriuunas, A., A. Surovas, V. Borutinskaite, D. Matuzeviccius, G. Treigyte, J. Savickiene, V. Tunaitis, R. Aldonyte, A. Jarmalavicciuute, K. Suriakaite, E. Liutkeviccius, A. Venalis, D. Navakauskas, R. Navakauskiene, and K.E. Magnusson. 2010. Proteomic analysis of stromal cells derived from the dental pulp of human exfoliated deciduous teeth. *Stem Cells Dev.* 19:1081-1093.

Rodriguez-Lozano, F.J., C. Bueno, C.L. Insausti, L. Meseguer, M.C. Ramirez, M. Blanquer, N. Marin, S. Martinez, and J.M. Moraleda. 2011. Mesenchymal stem cells derived from dental tissues. *Int Endod J.*

Schugar, R.C., S.M. Chirieleison, K.E. Wescoe, B.T. Schmidt, Y. Askew, J.J. Nance, J.M. Evron, B. Peault, and B.M. Deasy. 2009. High harvest yield, high expansion, and phenotype stability of CD146 mesenchymal stromal cells from whole primitive human umbilical cord tissue. *J Biomed Biotechnol.* 2009:789526.

Seo, B.M., M. Miura, S. Gronthos, P.M. Bartold, S. Batouli, J. Brahim, M. Young, P.G. Robey, C.Y. Wang, and S. Shi. 2004. Investigation of multipotent postnatal stem cells from human periodontal ligament. *Lancet.* 364:149-155.

Seo, B.M., M. Miura, W. Sonoyama, C. Coppe, R. Stanyon, and S. Shi. 2005. Recovery of stem cells from cryopreserved periodontal ligament. *J Dent Res.* 84:907-912.

Sharma, S., V. Sikri, N. Sharma, and V. Sharma. 2010. Regeneration of tooth pulp and dentin : trends and advances. *Annals of Neurosciences.* 17:31-43.

Shi, S., P.M. Bartold, M. Miura, B.M. Seo, P.G. Robey, and S. Gronthos. 2005. The efficacy of mesenchymal stem cells to regenerate and repair dental structures. *Orthod Craniofac Res.* 8:191-199.

Shi, S., and S. Gronthos. 2003. Perivascular niche of postnatal mesenchymal stem cells in human bone marrow and dental pulp. *J Bone Miner Res.* 18:696-704.

Shimono, M., T. Ishikawa, H. Ishikawa, H. Matsuzaki, S. Hashimoto, T. Muramatsu, K. Shima, K.-I. Matsuzaka, and T. Inoue. 2003. Regulatory mechanisms of periodontal regeneration. *Microscopy Research and Technique.* 60:491-502.

Slatter, D.H. 2002. Textbook of small animal surgery. Vol. 2. Saunders, Philadelphia, P.A. 3070.

Smith, A. 2006. A glossary for stem-cell biology. *Nature.* 441:1060-1060.

Sonoyama, W., Y. Liu, D. Fang, T. Yamaza, B.M. Seo, C. Zhang, H. Liu, S. Gronthos, C.Y. Wang, S. Wang, and S. Shi. 2006. Mesenchymal stem cell-mediated functional tooth regeneration in swine. *PLoS One.* 1:e79.

Sonoyama, W., Y. Liu, T. Yamaza, R.S. Tuan, S. Wang, S. Shi, and G.T. Huang. 2008. Characterization of the apical papilla and its residing stem cells from human immature permanent teeth: a pilot study. *J Endod.* 34:166-171.

Takagi, Y., J. Takahashi, H. Saiki, A. Morizane, T. Hayashi, Y. Kishi, H. Fukuda, Y. Okamoto, M. Koyanagi, M. Ideguchi, H. Hayashi, T. Imazato, H. Kawasaki, H. Suemori, S. Omachi, H. Iida, N. Itoh, N. Nakatsuji, Y. Sasai, and N. Hashimoto. 2005. Dopaminergic neurons generated from monkey embryonic stem cells function in a Parkinson primate model. *J Clin Invest.* 115:102-109.

Ten Cate, A.R. 1998. Oral histology: development, structure, and function. Mosby, St. Louis. 528 pp.

Thomson, J.A., J. Itskovitz-Eldor, S.S. Shapiro, M.A. Waknitz, J.J. Swiergiel, V.S. Marshall, and J.M. Jones. 1998. Embryonic stem cell lines derived from human blastocysts. *Science.* 282:1145-1147.

Tucker, A., and P. Sharpe. 2004. The cutting-edge of mammalian development; how the embryo makes teeth. *Nat Rev Genet.* 5:499-508.

van Laake, L.W., R. Passier, P.A. Doevendans, and C.L. Mummery. 2008. Human Embryonic Stem Cell–Derived Cardiomyocytes and Cardiac Repair in Rodents. *Circulation Research.* 102:1008-1010.

Vandesompele, J., K. De Preter, F. Pattyn, B. Poppe, N. Van Roy, A. De Paepe, and F. Speleman. 2002. Accurate normalization of real-time quantitative RT-PCR data by geometric averaging of multiple internal control genes. *Genome biology.* 3:RESEARCH0034.

Wada, N., D. Menicanin, S. Shi, P.M. Bartold, and S. Gronthos. 2009. Immunomodulatory properties of human periodontal ligament stem cells. *J Cell Physiol.* 219:667-676.

Wang, J., X. Wang, Z. Sun, H. Yang, S. Shi, and S. Wang. 2010. Stem cells from human-exfoliated deciduous teeth can differentiate into dopaminergic neuron-like cells. *Stem Cells Dev.* 19:1375-1383.

Wobus, A.M., and K.R. Boheler. 2005. Embryonic Stem Cells: Prospects for Developmental Biology and Cell Therapy. *Physiological Reviews.* 85:635-678.

Wong, M.H. 2004. Regulation of Intestinal Stem Cells. *J Investig Dermatol Symp Proc.* 9:224-228.

Woodbury, D., E.J. Schwarz, D.J. Prockop, and I.B. Black. 2000. Adult rat and human bone marrow stromal cells differentiate into neurons. *Journal of Neuroscience Research.* 61:364-370.

Woods, E.J., B.C. Perry, J.J. Hockema, L. Larson, D. Zhou, and W.S. Goebel. 2009. Optimized cryopreservation method for human dental pulp-derived stem cells and their tissues of origin for banking and clinical use. *Cryobiology.* 59:150-157.

Yagyuu, T., E. Ikeda, H. Ohgushi, M. Tadokoro, M. Hirose, M. Maeda, K. Inagake, and T. Kirita. 2010. Hard tissue-forming potential of stem/progenitor cells in human dental follicle and dental papilla. *Arch Oral Biol.* 55:68-76.

Yao, S., F. Pan, V. Prpic, and G.E. Wise. 2008. Differentiation of stem cells in the dental follicle. *J Dent Res.* 87:767-771.

Yen, A.H., and P.T. Sharpe. 2008. Stem cells and tooth tissue engineering. *Cell Tissue Res.* 331:359-372.

Yokoi, T., M. Saito, T. Kiyono, S. Iseki, K. Kosaka, E. Nishida, T. Tsubakimoto, H. Harada, K. Eto, T. Noguchi, and T. Teranaka. 2007. Establishment of immortalized dental follicle cells for generating periodontal ligament in vivo. *Cell and Tissue Research.* 327:301-311.

Young, H.E., and A.C. Black, Jr. 2004. Adult stem cells. *Anat Rec A Discov Mol Cell Evol Biol.* 276:75-102.

Zandstra, P.W., and A. Nagy. 2001. Stem cell bioengineering. *Annu Rev Biomed Eng.* 3:275-305.

Zhang, W., X.F. Walboomers, S. Shi, M. Fan, and J.A. Jansen. 2006. Multilineage differentiation potential of stem cells derived from human dental pulp after cryopreservation. *Tissue Eng.* 12:2813-2823.

Zuk, P.A., M. Zhu, P. Ashjian, D.A. De Ugarte, J.I. Huang, H. Mizuno, Z.C. Alfonso, J.K. Fraser, P. Benhaim, and M.H. Hedrick. 2002. Human adipose tissue is a source of multipotent stem cells. *Mol Biol Cell.* 13:4279-4295.

Zuk, P.A., M. Zhu, H. Mizuno, J. Huang, J.W. Futrell, A.J. Katz, P. Benhaim, H.P. Lorenz, and M.H. Hedrick. 2001. Multilineage cells from human adipose tissue: implications for cell-based therapies. *Tissue Eng.* 7:211-228.

Permissions

The contributors of this book come from diverse backgrounds, making this book a truly international effort. This book will bring forth new frontiers with its revolutionizing research information and detailed analysis of the nascent developments around the world.

We would like to thank Michael S. Kallos, for lending his expertise to make the book truly unique. He has played a crucial role in the development of this book. Without his invaluable contribution this book wouldn't have been possible. He has made vital efforts to compile up to date information on the varied aspects of this subject to make this book a valuable addition to the collection of many professionals and students.

This book was conceptualized with the vision of imparting up-to-date information and advanced data in this field. To ensure the same, a matchless editorial board was set up. Every individual on the board went through rigorous rounds of assessment to prove their worth. After which they invested a large part of their time researching and compiling the most relevant data for our readers. Conferences and sessions were held from time to time between the editorial board and the contributing authors to present the data in the most comprehensible form. The editorial team has worked tirelessly to provide valuable and valid information to help people across the globe.

Every chapter published in this book has been scrutinized by our experts. Their significance has been extensively debated. The topics covered herein carry significant findings which will fuel the growth of the discipline. They may even be implemented as practical applications or may be referred to as a beginning point for another development. Chapters in this book were first published by InTech; hereby published with permission under the Creative Commons Attribution License or equivalent.

The editorial board has been involved in producing this book since its inception. They have spent rigorous hours researching and exploring the diverse topics which have resulted in the successful publishing of this book. They have passed on their knowledge of decades through this book. To expedite this challenging task, the publisher supported the team at every step. A small team of assistant editors was also appointed to further simplify the editing procedure and attain best results for the readers.

Our editorial team has been hand-picked from every corner of the world. Their multi-ethnicity adds dynamic inputs to the discussions which result in innovative outcomes. These outcomes are then further discussed with the researchers and contributors who give their valuable feedback and opinion regarding the same. The feedback is then collaborated with the researches and they are edited in a comprehensive manner to aid the understanding of the subject.

Apart from the editorial board, the designing team has also invested a significant amount of their time in understanding the subject and creating the most relevant covers. They scrutinized every image to scout for the most suitable representation of the subject and create an appropriate cover for the book.

The publishing team has been involved in this book since its early stages. They were actively engaged in every process, be it collecting the data, connecting with the contributors or procuring relevant information. The team has been an ardent support to the editorial, designing and production team. Their endless efforts to recruit the best for this project, has resulted in the accomplishment of this book. They are a veteran in the field of academics and their pool of knowledge is as vast as their experience in printing. Their expertise and guidance has proved useful at every step. Their uncompromising quality standards have made this book an exceptional effort. Their encouragement from time to time has been an inspiration for everyone.

The publisher and the editorial board hope that this book will prove to be a valuable piece of knowledge for researchers, students, practitioners and scholars across the globe.

List of Contributors

Peter Oettgen
Division of Cardiology, Division of Molecular and Vascular Medicine, Department of Medicine, and the Center for Vascular Biology Research, Beth Israel Deaconess Medical Center, Harvard Medical School, Boston, MA, USA

Kyoko Kawasaki
Helen Diller Family Comprehensive Cancer Center, University of California-San Francisco, USA

Keiji Miyazawa
Department of Biochemistry, Interdisciplinary Graduate School of Medicine and Engineering, University of Yamanashi, Japan

Toshio Miki
Eli and Edythe Broad Center for Regenerative Medicine and Stem Cell Research at USC, Department of Biochemistry and Molecular Biology, Keck School of Medicine, University of Southern California, Los Angeles, USA

N.I. Nativ, M.A. Ghodbane, T.J. Maguire, F. Berthiaume, and M.L. Yarmush
Department of Biomedical Engineering, Rutgers University, Piscataway, NJ, USA

M.L. Yarmush
Center for Engineering in Medicine, Massachusetts General Hospital, USA

Kevin C. Keller and Nicole I. zur Nieden
Department of Cell Biology & Neuroscience and Stem Cell Center, College of Natural and Agricultural Sciences, University of California Riverside, United States of America

Raymond C.B. Wong, Ellen L. Smith and Peter J. Donovan
Department of Biological Chemistry, USA
Sue and Bill Gross Stem Cell Research Center, University of California at Irvine, Irvine, USA

Peter J. Donovan
Department of Developmental and Cell Biology, USA

Koji Tanabe and Kazutoshi Takahashi
Center for iPS Cell Research and Application, Japan

Naoki Nishishita and Shin Kawamata
Foundation for Biomedical Research and Innovation, TRI308, 1-5-4 Minatojima-Minamimachi, Chuo-ku, Japan
Riken Center for Developmental Biology, 2-2-3, Minatojima-Minamimachi, Chuo-ku, Japan

Noemi Fusaki
DNAVEC Corporation 6, Okubo, Tsukuba, Japan
Japan Science and Technology Agency (JST), PRESTO, 4-1-8 Honcho, Kawaguchi, Saitama, Japan

Oz Pomp, Chen Sok Lam, Hui Theng Gan, Srinivas Ramasamy and Sohail Ahmed
Institute of Medical Biology, Agency for Science Technology& Research, Singapore

Sandeep Goel
Laboratory for the Conservation of Endangered Species, Centre for Cellular and Molecular Biology, Hyderabad, India

Hiroshi Imai
Graduate School of Agriculture, Kyoto University, Kyoto, Japan

Gianni Carraro, Orquidea H. Garcia, Laura Perin, Roger De Filippo and David Warburton
Saban Research Institute, Children's Hospital Los Angeles, USA

Dong-Myung Shin, Janina Ratajczak, Magda Kucia and Mariusz Z. Ratajczak
Stem Cell Institute at the James Graham Brown Cancer Center, University of Louisville, KY, USA

Tammy Laberge and Herman S. Cheung
Department of Biomedical Engineering, College of Engineering, University of Miami, USA
Geriatrics Research, Education and Clinical Center, Miami VA Healthcare System, USA

Printed in the USA
CPSIA information can be obtained
at www.ICGtesting.com
JSHW011448221024
72173JS00004B/985